Advances in Oncology Nursing

Editor

MARGARET BARTON-BURKE

NURSING CLINICS
OF NORTH AMERICA

www.nursing.theclinics.com

Consulting Editor
STEPHEN D. KRAU

March 2017 • Volume 52 • Number 1

ELSEVIER

1600 John F. Kennedy Boulevard • Suite 1800 • Philadelphia, Pennsylvania, 19103-2899

http://www.theclinics.com

NURSING CLINICS OF NORTH AMERICA Volume 52, Number 1
March 2017 ISSN 0029-6465, ISBN-13: 978-0-323-53017-0

Editor: Kerry Holland
Developmental Editor: Casey Potter

Nursing Clinics of North America (ISSN 0029-6465) is published quarterly by Elsevier Inc., 360 Park Avenue South, New York, NY 10010-1710. Months of issue are March, June, September, and December. Periodicals postage paid at New York, NY and additional mailing offices. Subscription price per year is, $155.00 (US individuals), $465.00 (US institutions), $275.00 (international individuals), $567.00 (international institutions), $220.00 (Canadian individuals), $567.00 (Canadian institutions), $100.00 (US students), and $135.00 (international students). To receive student/resident rate, orders must be accompanied by name of affiliated institution, date of term, and the signature of program/residency coordinator on institution letterhead. Orders will be billed at individual rate until proof of status is received. Foreign air speed delivery is included in all *Clinics* subscription prices. All prices are subject to change without notice. **POSTMASTER:** Send address changes to *Nursing Clinics*, Elsevier Health Sciences Division, Subscription Customer Service, 3251 Riverport Lane, Maryland Heights, MO 63043. **Customer Service: Telephone: 1-800-654-2452** (U.S. and Canada); **1-314-447-8871 (outside U.S. and Canada). Fax: 1-314-447-8029. E-mail: journalscustomerservice-usa@elsevier.com** (for print support) and **journalsonlinesupport-usa@elsevier.com** (for online support).

Nursing Clinics of North America is covered in *EMBASE/Excerpta Medica, MEDLINE/PubMed (Index Medicus), Social Sciences Citation Index, Current Contents, ASCA, Cumulative Index to Nursing, RNdex Top 100,* and Allied Health Literature and International Nursing Index (INI).

Contributors

CONSULTING EDITOR

STEPHEN D. KRAU, PhD, RN, CNE
Associate Professor, Vanderbilt University School of Nursing, Nashville, Tennessee

EDITOR

MARGARET BARTON-BURKE, PhD, RN, FAAN
Immediate Past President, Oncology Nursing Society 2014-2016; Director, Department of Nursing Research, Memorial Sloan Kettering Cancer Center, New York, New York

AUTHORS

MARGARET BARTON-BURKE, PhD, RN, FAAN
Immediate Past President, Oncology Nursing Society 2014-2016; Director, Department of Nursing Research, Memorial Sloan Kettering Cancer Center, New York, New York

STELLA AGUINAGA BIALOUS, MSN, RN, DrPH, FAAN
Associate Professor In Residence, School of Nursing, University of California San Francisco, San Francisco, California

ALISON BOWERS, RN, BN (Child), MClin Res
Research Ethics and Governance Officer, West Moreton Hospital and Health Service; PhD Candidate, School of Nursing, Queensland University of Technology, Brisbane, Queensland, Australia

SEAN BURKE, BS
Research Assistant, Department of Nursing Research, Memorial Sloan Kettering Cancer Center, New York, New York

RAYMOND JAVAN CHAN, RN, BN, MAppSc (Research), PhD, FACN
Associate Professor, Cancer Nursing Professorial Precinct, Royal Brisbane and Women's Hospital, Queensland University of Technology, Brisbane, Queensland, Australia

KATHRYN CICCOLINI, RN, BSN, OCN, DNC
Department of Dermatology, Memorial Sloan Kettering Cancer Center, New York, New York

JULIE EGGERT, PhD, GNP-BC, AGN-BC, AOCN, FAAN
Mary Cox Professor, Healthcare Genetics Doctoral Program Coordinator, School of Nursing, College of Behavioral, Social and Health Sciences, Clemson University, Clemson, South Carolina; Advanced Genetics Nurse, Inherited Cancer Clinic, Bon Secours St. Francis Cancer Center, Greenville, South Carolina

LORRAINE EVANGELISTA, PhD, RN, FAAN
Professor & Associate Director of the Doctoral Program, Nursing Science, School of Nursing, University of California, Los Angeles, Los Angeles, California

LAURA A. FENNIMORE, DNP, RN, NEA-BC
Professor, Acute and Tertiary Care Department, University of Pittsburgh School of Nursing, Pittsburgh, Pennsylvania

ERICA FISCHER-CARTLIDGE, MSN, CNS, CBCN, AOCNS
Clinical Nurse Specialist, Memorial Sloan Kettering Cancer Center, New York, New York

PAMELA K. GINEX, EdD, RN, OCN
Nurse Scientist, Department of Nursing, Memorial Sloan Kettering Cancer Center, New York, New York

JEANINE GORDON, MSN, RN, OCN, NE-BC
Nurse Leader, Memorial Sloan Kettering Cancer Center, New York, New York

SANTOSH KESARI, MD, PhD, FANA, FAAN
Professor of Translational Neurosciences and Neurotherapeutics, John Wayne Cancer Institute, Providence Saint John's Health Center, Santa Monica, California

SALLY MALISKI, PhD, RN, FAAN
Professor Emeriti, University of California, Los Angeles, School of Nursing, Los Angeles, California; Dean and Professor, University of Kansas Medical Center, University of Kansas School of Nursing, Kansas City, Kansas

MARIA MEKAS, BSN, RN
Department of Dermatology, Memorial Sloan Kettering Cancer Center, New York, New York

ELIZABETH A. NESS, MS, BSN, RN
Director, Office of Education and Compliance, Center for Cancer Research, National Cancer Institute, Bethesda, Maryland

ADELINE NYAMATHI, PhD, ANP, FAAN
Distinguished Professor; Associate Dean for Research and International Scholarship, University of California, Los Angeles, School of Nursing, Los Angeles, California

LINDA R. PHILLIPS, PhD, RN, FAAN
Professor Emerita, University of California, Los Angeles, School of Nursing, Los Angeles, California

LORRIE L. POWEL, PhD, RN
Associate Professor and Tenet Health System/Jo Ellen Smith, RN, Endowed Chair of Nursing, Louisiana State University Health Science Center School of Nursing, New Orleans, Louisiana

CHERYL ROYCE, MS, RN, CRNP
Director, Office of Research Nursing, Center for Cancer Research, National Cancer Institute, Bethesda, Maryland

MARLON GARZO SARIA, PhD, RN, AOCNS, FAAN
Assistant Professor of Translational Neurosciences and Neurotherapeutics, Advanced Practice Registered Nurse, John Wayne Cancer Institute, Providence Saint John's Health Center, Santa Monica, California; University of California, Los Angeles, School of Nursing, Los Angeles, California

LINDA SARNA, PhD, RN, FAAN
Professor and Dean; Lulu Wolf-Hassenplug Endowed Chair in Nursing, University of California, Los Angeles, School of Nursing, Los Angeles, California

STEPHEN M. SEIBERT, BS
Doctorate of Medicine Program, Albert Einstein College of Medicine, Bronx, New York

ANNETTE L. STANTON, PhD
Professor of Psychology and Psychiatry/Biobehavioral Sciences, Department of Psychology, University of California, Los Angeles, Los Angeles, California

JOSEPH D. TARIMAN, PhD, RN, ANP-BC, FAAN
Assistant Professor, School of Nursing, DePaul University, Chicago, Illinois

TRACY TRUANT, RN, MSN, PhD(c)
Doctoral Candidate, School of Nursing, University of British Columbia, Vancouver, British Columbia, Canada

PATSY YATES, PhD, RN, FACN, FAAN
School of Nursing, Queensland University of Technology, Kelvin Grove, Queensland, Australia

Contents

In addition to the need for basic education about genetics/genomics, other approaches are suggested to include awareness campaigns, continuing education courses, policy review, and onsite clinical development. These alternative learning strategies encourage oncology nurses across the continuum of care, from the bedside/seatside to oncology nurse research, to integrate genomics into all levels of practice and research in the specialty of oncology nursing. All nurses are warriors in the fight against cancer. The goal of this article is to identify genomic information that oncology nurses, at all levels of care, need to know and use as tools in the war against cancer.

This article provides a current overview of colorectal, breast, and prostate cancers. For each cancer, data related to incidence and prevalence are discussed, as well as nonmodifiable and modifiable risk factors. Information about detection and evidenced-based screening guideline recommendations is reviewed, with the most common and recent treatment modalities emphasized. Current clinical and treatment-related issues are discussed along with nursing care and implications for cancer care. Future directions for these 3 cancers are addressed also.

Lung cancer is the leading cause of cancer death worldwide. Tobacco use remains the single most important preventable cause of cancer and is responsible for 80% of all cases of lung cancer. Implementation of tobacco control measures, including preventing initiation and treating dependence, are pivotal to address the lung cancer epidemic. New evidence continues to emerge on the significant positive impact of incorporating tobacco dependence treatment within all lung cancer treatment protocols. Evidence and guidelines on how to implement these strategies exist and present an opportunity for nurses to make a difference in reducing suffering and preventing deaths from lung cancer.

Cancer therapeutics has been growing in an unprecedented fashion and has evolved rapidly in the past two decades. Specific gene mutation, protein dysfunction and dysregulation, intracellular signaling pathways, and immune modulation have been targeted. These therapeutic advances came largely because of improved understanding of the pathobiology of cancer at the genetic and molecular levels. This article addresses the need of novice nurses for cancer treatment–related information and evidence-based nursing care of patients diagnosed with cancer while undergoing novel and breakthrough therapeutics.

Cancer treatments usually have side effects of bone marrow depression, mucositis, hair loss, and gastrointestinal issues. Rarely do we think of skin side effects until patients have been treated successfully with epidermal growth factor receptor inhibitors (EGFRi). Those reactions include papulopustular rash, hair changes, radiation dermatitis enhancement, pruritus, mucositis, xerosis, fissures, and paronychia. This article discusses the common skin reactions seen when using EGFRi and presents an overview of skin as the largest and important organ of the body, including an overview of skin assessment, pathophysiology of the skin reactions, nursing care involved, and introduction to oncodermatology.

As cancer treatment shifts to a combination of oral and intravenous agents for systemic treatment, health care professionals must adapt with practice changes aimed at supporting patients and optimizing adherence. Moving toward a shared decision-making model or a personal systems approach is a potential mechanism to minimize barriers and enhance facilitators to oral treatment adherence. Additional research is needed to understand what works for patients and how health care providers can change systems and care strategies to support patients with the ultimate goal of improved patient care and outcomes.

Clinical trials are paramount to improving human health. New trial designs and informed consent issues are emerging as a result of genomic profiling and the development of molecularly targeted agents. Many groups and individuals are responsible for ensuring the protection of research participants and the quality of the data produced. The specialty role of the clinical trials nurse (CTN) is critical to clinical trials. Oncology CTNs have competencies that can help guide their practice; however, not all oncology clinical trials are supervised by a nurse. Using the process of engagement, one organization has restructured oncology CTNs under a nurse-supervised model.

The ever-increasing cancer care demand has posed a challenge for oncology nurses to deliver evidence-based, innovative care. Despite efforts to promote evidence-based practice, barriers remain and executives find it difficult to implement evidence-based practice efficiently. Using the successful experience of an Australian tertiary cancer center, this paper depicts 4 effective strategies for facilitating evidence-based practice at the organizational level—the Embedded Scholar: Enabler, Enactor, and Engagement (4 Es) Model—includes a 12-week evidence-based practice program that prioritizes relevant research proposed by clinical staff and endorses high-quality, evidence-based point-of-care resources.

Caregiving is a highly individualized experience. Although numerous articles have been published on caregiver burden from a variety of diagnoses and conditions, this article presents the unique features of caregiving in patients with brain metastases. Improved long-term survival, concerns about disease recurrence or progression, the cancer experience (initial diagnosis, treatment, survivorship, recurrence, progression, and end of life), and the increasing complexity of cancer treatments add to the demands placed on the caregivers of patients with brain metastases. Health care professionals must identify caregiver burden and administer the appropriate interventions, which must be as unique and individualized as the caregivers' experiences.

The clinical context for advanced cancer has changed in recent years, with extended survival rates and more diverse and complex cancer trajectories and symptomatology. Advances have been made in symptom management of advanced disease, and the contribution of palliative care is better understood. Palliative care is more likely offered earlier in the disease not just at end of life. This article discusses symptom management together with palliative care. Key features are greater appreciation of the complex and multidimensional nature of mechanisms underpinning co-occurring symptoms in advanced cancer patients, comprehensive and systematic symptom assessment, and individualized approaches to cancer management.

This article provides a synopsis of the status of cancer survivorship in the United States. It highlights the challenges of survivorship care as the number of cancer survivors has steadily grown over the 40 years since the signing of the National Cancer Act in 1971. Also included is an overview of various models of survivorship care plans (SCPs), facilitators and barriers to SCP use, their impact on patient outcomes, and implications for clinical practice and research. This article provides a broad overview of the cancer survivorship, including models of care and survivorship care plans.

Tracy Truant

There is growing evidence of inequities among people living with cancer. Aligning with nursing's social justice imperative, addressing these inequities is an integral, yet underdeveloped, aspect of the nurses' role. Understanding the social determinants of health, and the factors, contexts, and structures that influence individuals' opportunities for health, is an essential foundation for moving the health equity agenda forward. Oncology nurses can implement a two-pronged approach to further this agenda through strategies focusing on the direct care of individuals and communities, and addressing the root causes of inequity through leadership, policy influence, advocacy, education, and research.

NURSING CLINICS OF
NORTH AMERICA

THE CLINICS ARE AVAILABLE ONLINE!
Access your subscription at:
www.theclinics.com

NURSING CLINICS OF
NORTH AMERICA

FORTHCOMING ISSUES

June 2017
Fluids and Electrolytes
Joshua Squiers, Editor

September 2017
Geriatric Nursing
Sally Miller and Jennifer Kim, Editors

December 2017
Glucose Regulation
Celia Levesque, Editor

RECENT ISSUES

December 2016
Implications of Disaster Preparedness for Nursing
Deborah J. Persell, Editor

September 2016
Palliative Care
James C. Pace and Dorothy Wholihan, Editors

June 2016
Psychiatric Mental Health Nursing
Deborah Antai-Otong, Editor

ISSUE OF RELATED INTEREST

Critical Care Nursing Clinics of North America, December 2015
(Volume 27, Issue 4), Pages 433–572
Palliative Care in Critical Care
Tonja M. Hartjes, editor

Preface
Cancer Nursing Care in the Twenty-first Century

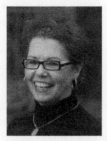

Margaret Barton-Burke, PhD, RN, FAAN
Editor

In 1971, President Nixon declared war on cancer by signing the National Cancer Act, establishing the National Cancer Institute at the National Institutes of Health. The National Cancer Act funded basic research and began the US clinical trials, drug development programs that are still in existence today. Subsequently the incidence of cancer in this country started dropping in 1990 and has continued to drop annually, along with mortality. Fast forward to the twenty-first century with the sequencing of the human genome in April 2003, moving our understanding of cancer away from the cellular to the molecular and genomic level. This important scientific breakthrough leads to new drug development targeting specific mechanisms and precision medicine. These scientific steps changed how we treat and care for patients with cancer. This issue brings these scientific innovations to nurses caring for patients with cancer. The articles are organized into clinical and contextual factors impacting cancer nursing care in the twenty-first century.

This issue begins with an overview of genetics, providing an understanding for the changes in cancer treatments and the role of the nurse. The next two articles focus on the cancers seen most frequently. They are colon, breast, prostate, and lung cancers. Of these four, lung cancer remains difficult to treat, thus making this article's focus on prevention of, rather than treatment for, lung cancer. These initial articles are followed by three articles that cover aspects of newer anticancer treatments based on molecular and genomic knowledge. Many of these newer agents are given in pill form and have an unusual skin side effect. Skin reactions are not usually seen when caring for the patient with cancer, but this article covers the biological basis for the reactions and highlights the emerging specialty of oncodermatology.

Dr Barton-Burke acknowledges funding support from MSK Cancer Center Support Grant/Core Grant (P30 CA008748).

Nurs Clin N Am 52 (2017) xiii–xiv
http://dx.doi.org/10.1016/j.cnur.2016.12.001
0029-6465/17/© 2016 Published by Elsevier Inc.

nursing.theclinics.com

All this new drug development is conducted using the clinical trials mechanisms, but nurses are taking a more active and important role in clinical trials. The article on clinical trials includes another specialty: that of the clinical research nurse. Clinical trials drive practice change based on the evidence. The article on evidence-based practice highlights one institution's experience. Newer knowledge and better treatments lead to patients with cancer surviving their disease. Cancer survivorship is illustrated in the following article with the discussion of cancer survivorship care plans. An unintended consequence of cancer care is caregiver burden, and the article about the patient with brain cancer highlights this oft overlooked topic. Finally, the idea of equity in cancer care is addressed in the final article of this issue.

This issue addresses cancer care in the twenty-first century, but it is important to note that the authorship represents cancer nurse leaders from around the globe, highlighting that cancer care is global as well.

Margaret Barton-Burke, PhD, RN, FAAN
Nursing Research
Memorial Sloan-Kettering Cancer Center
205 East 64th Street
Room 251 Concourse Level
New York, NY 10065, USA

E-mail address:
bartonbm@mskcc.org

Genetics and Genomics in Oncology Nursing

What Does Every Nurse Need to Know?

Julie Eggert, PhD, GNP-BC, AGN-BC, AOCN[a,b,*]

KEYWORDS

- Genetics and genomics • Clinical practice • Nurses • Hereditary cancer syndromes
- Cancer risk assessment • Cancer genetics

KEY POINTS

- Research shows nurses, including oncology nurses, need more education about genetic information that includes how to assess risk in an inherited cancer family history.
- Red flags for other genetic disorders, not just inherited cancers, need to be identified because they can be intensified with cancer treatments.
- Enhancing the skill of taking a 3-generation family history and creating a pedigree more easily identify a family pattern of cancers that can be transmitted to the next generation.
- Oncology nurses should update their knowledge of the central dogma of molecular biology (DNA to RNA to protein) to include the smaller RNA molecules and epigenetics.
- Oncology nurses are essential to the fight against many diseases of cancer. Embracing the knowledge of genetics/genomics enables providers at all levels to provide individualized quality care to patients and families with a cancer diagnosis.

INTRODUCTION

The need for the application of genetics in nursing education and practice was noted decades before the 2003 announcement of the sequencing and mapping of the entire human genome.[1] As early as 1962, Brantl and Esslinger[2] wrote about the implications for including genetics in nursing curricula. In 1984, Felissa Cohen[3] authored a book about genetics for nurses. This created a paradigm shift and offered traditional information about genetics in an easier to understand language that could be applied to nurses' clinical practice.

Conflict of Interest: None.
[a] School of Nursing, College of Behavioral, Social and Health Sciences, Clemson University, Clemson, SC 29634, USA; [b] Inherited Cancer Clinic, Bon Secours St. Francis Cancer Center, 104 Innovation Drive, Greenville, SC 29607, USA
* 111 Chesterton Court, Greer, SC 29650.
E-mail address: jaegger@clemson.edu

Background

Since 2003, there has been the development of publications describing core genetic and genomics competencies required of registered nurses.[4–7] Nursing faculty and new graduates of baccalaureate programs learned that *genetics* refers to the study of genes and their roles in inheritance. Genomics describes the complex study of all genes belonging to an individual, including how genes connect with other genes and interact with a person's environment (American Association of Colleges of Nursing [AACN], National Coalition for Health Professional Education in Genetics [NCHPEG], American Nurses Association [ANA], International Society of Nurses in Genetics [ISONG], and National Council of State Boards in Nursing). The support of and interest in these publications led to a movement for inclusion of more genetics and genomics undergraduate and graduate levels education and identified an overall lack of knowledge for registered nurses, including faculty in academia and those nurses practicing in the oncology specialty.

As a specialty, oncology nurses led the translation of genetics and genomics into clinical nursing practice. Several publications written by oncology nurses identify and describe core competencies for oncology nurses, including the *Statement on the Scope and Standards of Oncology Nursing Practice*,[8,9] with Jenkins'[10,11] publication using case studies to describe how oncology nurses can apply genetic/genomic competencies. These documents were important building materials for the practice model of genetics and genomics in oncology nursing depicted in **Fig. 1**.

In the practice model, the multiple levels of oncology nursing practice incorporating genetics and genomics are depicted as a structure built on deep and shallow foundations. The deep and solid structural foundation represents The ANA Nursing: Scope and Standards of Practice, the basis of nursing practice.[12] Like the structural foundation of a building, Nursing is built in the "strong soil" of research based evidence for effective clinical interventions.

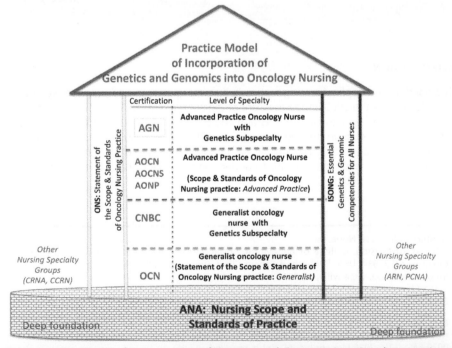

Fig. 1. Practice Model of Incorporation of Genetics and Genomics into Oncology Nursing.

Passing through all levels of the model on each side are two supporting structures that support and strengthen the ascending levels of oncology nursing practice (Generalist and Advanced Practice). In the model, the left supporting wall is the ONS Scope and Standards of Oncology Nursing Practice.[9] The supporting wall on the right is the Essential Genetic and Genomic Competencies for all nurses, distributing the Essentials across all practice settings (inpatient, infusion, ambulatory, and survivorship) including the multiple subspecialties in oncology nursing.[7] See **Box 1** for the history of preparation of the U.S. nursing workforce in genetics/genomics.

On these foundational documents guide and support the care settings of oncology nursing. The first level is the practice of the general oncology nurse (GON) with specialty in the direct care of patients in the hospital, ambulatory care, and infusion center areas. The second level is the GON with a genetics subspecialty, also supported by *Genetics and Genomics Nursing: Scope and Standards of Nursing Practice*.[13]

The upper 2 levels of the model depict building on the basics of oncology and genomics, while designating the expertise of the advanced practice oncology nurses (APONs) and APONs with a genetics subspecialty. All levels are associated with certifications to alert the public and other caregivers that they specialize in oncology nursing and have expert knowledge and experience in areas like navigation for various cancer diagnoses; and APON, with nurse practitioners, clinical nurse specialists, and, most recently, advanced practice nurses in genetics.[17,18]

Clinical practice for all levels is based on the *Statement on the Scope and Standards of Oncology Nursing Practice: Generalist and Advanced Practice*[9] and the *Essential genetic and genomic competencies for nurses with graduate degrees*.[9,13,18]

In 2014, "A Blueprint for Genomic Nursing Science"[19] contained a map of a strategic plan for nursing research in genetics and genomics. Although the map outlines a plan for research, it also contains a guide of outcomes that suggest direction for incorporation of genomics into clinical practice in nursing. See **Table 1** to review a comparison of clinical practice categories of literature addressing the nursing genomic science blueprint mapped to the NINR strategic research plan.

National Institute of Nursing Research Strategic Plan and Nursing Genomic Science Blueprint

Incorporation of genomics into oncology nursing practice requires an understanding of how to apply the documents discussed previously to clinical practice and the basics

---

Box 1
History of preparation of US nursing workforce in genetics/genomics

Education

1. Inclusion of genetic/genomics into *The Essentials of Baccalaureate Education for Professional Nursing Practice*[4]

2. Essentials of genetic and genomic nursing: competencies, curricula guidelines, and outcome indicators[5]

3. Inclusion of genetic/genomics into *The Essentials of Master's Education in Nursing*[14]

4. *Essential Genetic and Genomic Competencies for Nurses with Graduate Degrees*[15]

Research

1. National Institute of Nursing Research (NINR) Summer Genetics Institute[16]

2. NINR funding for institutional training grants, fellowships, and career development awards

Table 1
Comparison of clinical practice categories of literature (2010–2014) addressing the nursing genomic science blueprint mapped to National Institute of Nursing Research strategic research plan

NINR Strategic Plan Areas (SPA), A-D levels	Specific Nursing Research Categories	Blueprint Topic Areas of Genomic Nursing Science with Literature Articles 2010-14 and Areas Requiring More Research (Williams et al,[20] 2016)

A. Health promotion and disease prevention	1. Risk assessment	a. Biological plausibility
		   [a]See also SPA B2a
		b. Comprehensive screening opportunities (family history, identify risk level)—Needs Research
		c. Components of risk assessment (family history, risk levels of patients)
		   [a]See also SPA B2a
		d. Risk-specific healthcare decision making.
		   [a]See also SPA A3a-d

	2. Communication	a. Risk communication (interpretation, timing, risk reports to providers and client) b. Informed consent c. Direct-to-Consumer marketing & testing (knowledge & personal utility) [a]See also SPA A1a, c-d; SPA A3a-d

	3. Decision support	a. Informed consent
		b. Match of values/preferences with decision
		c. Risk perception/risk accuracy
		d. Effect of decision support on decision quality
		   [c]Patient populations included: hereditary breast or ovarian cancer; common chronic conditions such as hypertension; prenatal testing; ethnic communities' attitudes toward genomic testing and research
		   [a]See also SPA B2e

B. Advancing the quality of life	1. Family	a. Family context (family functioning, structure, family relationships and communication) [a]See also SPA B4a-d b. Ethical issues—Research needed c. Healthcare provider communications with families—Research needed

	2. Symptom Management	a. Biologic plausibility
		   [a]See Also SPA A1a, c-d
		b. Clinical utility—Research needed
		c. Personal utility—Research needed
		d. Decision making
		   [a]See also SPA A3a-d
		e. Effect of decision support on decision quality (eg, knowledge, personal utility)—Research needed
		f. Evidence based effective ness of approaches—Research needed

	3. Disease states (acute, common complex & chronic)	a. Genomic-based interventions that reduce morbidity and mortality [a]See also SPA A3 b. Gene-environments interactions (epigenetics, genotoxicity) c. Pharmacogenomics d. Evidence-based effectiveness of approaches
	4. Client self-management	a. Collecting and conveying information that informs self management b. Lifestyle behaviors

(continued on next page)

Table 1 (continued)		
NINR Strategic Plan Areas (SPA), A-D levels	**Specific Nursing Research Categories**	**Blueprint Topic Areas of Genomic Nursing Science with Literature Articles 2010-14 and Areas Requiring More Research (Williams et al,[20] 2016)**
		c. Environmental exposure and protection (eg, occupational)—Research needed
		d. Synergy of client and provider expectations (client family centered care
		e. Personal utility (positive effect on person's life)
C. Innovation [b]None noted in literature	1. Technology development	a. Incorporation of new technologies (eg, whole exome sequencing)—Research needed
		b. Ethics—Research needed
		c. Policy and guidelines to support applications—Research needed
		d. Applications (eg, clinical and analytic validity, and clinical utility)—Research needed
		e. Genomic bioinformatics—Research needed—Research needed
		f. Translation, dissemination, implementation—Research needed
		i. Use of technology in information delivery—Research needed
		ii. Performance improvement by provider (eg, point-of-care support)—Research needed
		iii. Resources that support genomic research (eg, registries of tools, best practices, nursing outcomes)—Research needed
	2. Informatics support systems	a. Data storage and use to facilitate research process and outcomes—Research needed
		b. Facilitate cross-generational sharing of genomic data (eg, family history, laboratory analyses)—Research needed
		c. Managing, analyzing, interpreting genomic information (eg, sequencing data)—Research needed
		d. Point-of-care decision support for client and healthcare provider—Research needed
		e. Common terminology and taxonomy
		f. Common formats for data—Research needed storage/exchange and queries—Research needed
	3. Environmental influences (physical social environments & policy context)	a. Evidence-based guidelines—Research needed
		b. Healthcare reform—Research needed
		c. Economics (eg, cost effectiveness)—Research needed
		d. Regulatory gaps and/or variability—Research needed

(continued on next page)

Table 1 *(continued)*		
NINR Strategic Plan Areas (SPA), A-D levels	Specific Nursing Research Categories	Blueprint Topic Areas of Genomic Nursing Science with Literature Articles 2010-14 and Areas Requiring More Research (Williams et al,[20] 2016)
D. Training	1. Capacity building [c]Excluded in literature review	a. Training future nursing scientists in genomics b. Preparing nursing faculty in genomics c. Education of current and future workforce in genomics (eg, d. Preparation of nurse scientists to lead interprofessional teams e. Preparation of clinical and administrative leaders to advance appropriate genomics/genetics integration into practice f. Innovative uses of biorepositories (eg, informed consent, result interpretation) g. Bioethics
	2. Education [c]Excluded in literature review	a. Optimal methods to train the existing nursing workforce in genomics b. Optimal methods to train the nursing leadership in genomics to support genomic translation, research and practice. c. Optimal methods to integrate nursing genomic competencies in basic-prelicensure and postlicensure in academic programs
	3. Health disparities	a. Racial, ethnic, socioeconomic, and cultural influences on disease occurrence and response to disease and treatment 　[a]See also SPA A1a, c, SPA A2a, SPA B2a, & SPA B2d b. Genomic health equity (access) c. Diseases that disproportionately affect specific groups 　[a]See also SPA B1a, SPA B4a-b & d-e d. Targeted therapeutics e. Overcoming misinformation and genomic "myths"
	4. Cost [b]None noted in literature	a. Cost effectiveness—Research needed b. Comparative effectiveness—Research needed c. Value—Research needed
	5. Policy [b]None noted in literature	a. Policy as context of science—Research needed b. Research to inform policy—Research needed
	6. Public education [b]None noted in literature	a. Health literacy—Research needed b. Genomic literacy—Research needed

[a] Other categories are cross-linked with this category content.
[b] Lack of literature identified based on inclusion criterion.
[c] Literature excluded based on definitions for inclusion (eg, at least 10 citations to meet "good" article impact).
　Data from Williams J, Tripp-Reimer T, Daack-Hirsch S, et al. Five-year bibliometric review of genomic nursing science research. J Nurs Scholarsh 2016;48(2):179–86.

of genetic/genomic knowledge for implementation. Oncology nurses are part of the the team of fighters organizing against cancer.[21] For current and future oncology clinical practice, all of the team members will find it necessary to implement the genetic/genomic tool kit, especially how to communicate the basics of DNA, RNA, proteins (the central dogma), and epigenetics apply in the clinical setting and research protocols.[22] Multiple educational resources are listed in **Box 2**.

HEALTH PROMOTION AND CANCER PREVENTION
Risk Assessment

Promotion of health and prevention of disease includes risk assessment, a key skill in genetics and genomics. A few studies tested registered nurses' use of knowledge about genetics and genomics in clinical practice.[34–37] Results of the studies indicated a lack of knowledge of how to use basic skills, such as the collection of a complete 3-generation family health history or construction of an accurate pedigree.[36] These basic skills should also include the ability to understand the patterns of inheritance and to identify the individuals within a family that are at highest risk for the genetic disorder and potential health compromise. There are concerns the practicing nurses in the study could not generalize the individual's risk status to make an informed referral to genetics professionals. The ability to explain risks and benefits for the initiation of genetics services is an important skill in clinical practice, one identified as a competency for newly graduated baccalaureate registered nurses.[4,6,20,37,38] If at-risk families are not identified for referral, an opportunity for patient advocacy has been missed.

Other subspecialties (cardiovascular, renal disease, and mental illness) are known to have inherited diseases that could be affected by or associated with side effects of cancer treatments. If any of these diseases, such as cardiomyopathy, are reported in multiple generations of the family history, family members should be specifically assessed and diagnosed to provide oncology health care providers with information relevant to future treatments. Genetic testing may also yield important information. Recent literature suggests a thorough collection of family history of inherited cardiomyopathy, or other heart disease, could redirect choice in chemotherapy from

Box 2 Genetic/genomic educational resources for practicing oncology nurses		
Dolan DNA Learning Center[23]	Teaching images and aids with 2-D/3-D animations	www.dnalc.org
Genetics/Genomics Competency Center[24]	Instructional resources	http://www.g-2-c-2.org/
Genomic Medicine for Patients and the Public[25]	News topics for patients and the Public	https://www.genome.gov/19016903/
Global Genetics and Genomics Community[26]	Case studies	http://www.g-3-c.org
National Coalition for Health Professional Education in Genetics[27]	Family history	http://nchpeg.org/
National Human Genome Research Institute[28]	Online genetics education	www.genome.gov
Genetics Home Reference[29]	Genetic variation effects	https://ghr.nlm.nih.gov
The Genetics of Cancer[30]	Genetics of cancer topics	https://www.cancer.gov/about-cancer/causes-prevention/genetics
The Pharmgenetic Education Program[31]	Pharmacogenomic educational materials	http://pharmacogenomics.ucsd.edu
Online Mendelian Inheritance in Man[32]		http://www.ncbi.nlm.nih.gov/omim
Gene Tests[33]		http://www.ncbi.nlm.nih/gov/sites/GeneTests/

anthracycline to taxane regimens.[39,40] A recent meta-analysis found that methylation of CpG islands were significantly different between current smokers and former smokers versus never-smokers with potential for use as biomarkers and therapeutic targets for prevention or treatment of tobacco-related diseases.[41] This is an example of potential health promotion and disease prevention interventions that could advance the quality of life of patients and the families.

A review of family history is necessary for every new patient, to be updated annually for returning patients, especially cancer survivors.[42] While initially noting, updating, or reviewing the family history at the bedside or chairside, a nurse in any practice, especially oncology, should possess the ability to identify inherited cancer risk in at least 3 generations for the maternal and paternal side of the family and if the cancer occurred at an early age. These markers are an alert for action and or referral to a genetics specialist. One study discovered that some nurses thought only first-degree relatives needed to be included in a family history.[36] Another study found that over the previous 3 months less than 5% of nurses consistently questioned their patients for a complete family history. Staff nurses were among the group of responders that were least likely to always or often collect a family history.[19] This is a target area necessary for quality care of oncology patients.

After completion of a family history, drafting a pedigree helps registered nurses focus on patterns of inherited cancers and other related risk assessment concerns (history of blood clots) and the need for a genetic referral. Although identified as low-tech, a drawn pedigree is based on the science and art of the collection of an accurate family history.[43]

Pedigree construction is identified as a necessary competency by the ACCN (2008), recently found to be a competency deficiency of newly-graduated nurses and a competency not routinely used in clinical practice.[36] Of special concern is the identified low importance senior staff nurses place on pedigree construction. Perhaps this is due to a lack of knowledge of the importance of converting pertinent family history into a visual aid that will guide patient care of these families possessing genetic disease.[36,37,44] Having this visual guide enhances the possibility that red flags will be recognized in order to alert healthcare professionals to recognize a potential inherited cancer.[45]

Construction of a complete pedigree to be communicated with the health care team should include

- The designated proband
- A legend to communicate the meaning of all symbols (**Box 3**)[46]
- Identification of 1st-generation, 2nd-generation, and 3rd-generation family members in both paternal and maternal lineages
- Visualization of relationships between affected individuals in the family
- Date of pedigree construction/update and office visit[45,47–52]
- Limitations to quality pedigrees can be a problem for correct interpretation. It is important that each issue be considered and prevented if possible. Careful attention should be paid to
- Inaccurate family histories without verification by pathology reports, medical records, prior testing reports, or death certificates
- Lack of desire to explore family history
- Limited family history, which can include small family structure or limited male or female gender in a generation
- History of patient adoption
- Time required to construct the pedigree
- Lack of follow-up by provider to document pedigree in patient record for future reference[45,47,48]

Box 3
List of *The Essentials of Baccalaureate Education for Professional Nursing Practice, AACN*[4]

Professional responsibilities domain
- Recognize when one's own attitudes and values related to genetic and genomic science may affect care provided to clients
- Advocate for clients' access to desired genetic/genomic services and/or resources including support groups
- Examine competency of practice on a regular basis, identifying areas of strength as well as areas in which professional development related to genetics and genomics would be beneficial
- Incorporate genetic and genomic technologies and information into registered nurse practice
- Demonstrate in practice the importance of tailoring genetic and genomic information and services to clients based on their culture, religion, knowledge level, literacy, and preferred language
- Advocate for the rights of all clients for autonomous, informed, genetic-related and genomic-related decision making and voluntary action

Professional practice domain
  Nursing assessment: applying/integrating genetic and genomic knowledge
  - Demonstrates an understanding of the relationship of genetics and genomics to health, prevention, screening, diagnostics, prognostics, selection of treatment, and monitoring of treatment effectiveness
  - Demonstrates ability to elicit a minimum of 3-generation family health history information Constructs a pedigree from collected family history information using standardized symbols and terminology
  - Collects personal, health, and developmental histories that consider genetic, environmental, and genomic influences and risks
  - Conducts comprehensive health and physical assessments that incorporate knowledge about genetic, environmental, and genomic influences and risk factors
  - Critically analyzes the history and physical assessment findings for genetic, environmental, and genomic influences and risk factors
  - Assesses clients' knowledge, perceptions, and responses to genetic and genomic information
  - Develops a plan of care that incorporates genetic and genomic assessment information
  Identification
  - Identifies clients who may benefit from specific genetic and genomic information and/or services based on assessment data
  - Identifies credible, accurate, appropriate, and current genetic and genomic information, resources, services, and/or technologies specific to given clients
  - Identifies ethical, ethnic/ancestral, cultural, religious, legal, fiscal, and societal issues related to genetic and genomic information and technologies
  - Defines issues that undermine the rights of all clients for autonomous, informed, genetic-related and genomic-related decision making and voluntary action
  Referral activities
  - Facilitates referrals for specialized genetic and genomic services for clients as needed

Provision of education, care, and support
- Provides clients with interpretation of selective genetic and genomic information or services
- Provides clients with credible, accurate, appropriate, and current genetic and genomic information, resources, services, and/or technologies that facilitate decision making
- Uses health promotion/disease prevention practices that
  ○ Consider genetic and genomic influences on personal and environmental risk factors
  ○ Incorporate knowledge of genetic and/or genomic risk factors (eg, a client with a genetic predisposition for high cholesterol who can benefit from a change in lifestyle that decreases the likelihood that the genetic risk will be expressed)
- Uses genetic-based and genomic-based interventions and information to improve clients' outcomes
- Collaborates with health care providers in providing genetic and genomic health care

- Collaborates with insurance providers/payers to facilitate reimbursement for genetic and genomic health care services
- Performs interventions/treatments appropriate to clients' genetic and genomic health care needs
- Evaluates impact and effectiveness of genetic and genomic technology, information, interventions, and treatments on clients' outcome

Communication

Information from the family pedigree, as well as other assessment data, can be included when calculating level of risk for developing a cancer. Use of cancer risk calculation tools, such as the National Cancer Institute breast cancer risk assessment tool, the International Breast Cancer Intervention Study breast cancer risk program for families with a significant incidence of breast cancer, and the colorectal cancer risk assessment tool from the National Cancer Institute, should be used as appropriate and applied with national screening guidelines (NCI-BCRA; IBIS [Tyer-Cuzick]; NCI-C-CRA). Knowledge of evidence-based high-risk level for different inherited cancers to determine management guidelines is important for nurses in some clinical settings although not required for all. Germline genetic testing results or biomarkers may also be important components to include in a risk assessment. Available direct-to-consumer test results might be of value for inclusion in the risk result discussion. Incorporation of red flags or alerts into the electronic health record could identify a need for more information, a high-risk report, and/or a referral. Risk communication should include interpretation, timing of management interventions, and distribution of risk reports to the health care provider and patient.[20,38] Application of these genetic risk profiles can be used to direct surveillance for survivors with early detection and prevention strategies for those never diagnosed with cancer.[20,53]

In **Table 2**, examples of red flags for identification of common inherited disorders incorporates the mnemonic, *family genes*, to help identify alerts for any condition. A complete family history is the initial component in this red flag list.

Having a general idea of common adult conditions that suggest a genetic predisposition should be noted and patients referred to an advanced practice genetics nurse or a medical genetics professional.

A list of some common red flags associated with inherited cancers that oncology nurses, in ambulatory settings or hospital practice, need to recognize are included in **Table 2**. These alerts can be used when following-up with cancer survivors because guidelines of inherited cancer traits are frequently updated and may have only recently become included in the inherited cancer guidelines for detection prevention and risk reduction (**Table 3**).[27]

Although inherited cancers are rare, there are common physical assessment questions that can further reveal the markers of risk. These can be observed, and sometimes easily noticed, such as skin tags on the neck, axillary, and/or groin regions, by any level or subspecialty oncology nurse.[57–59] Notations of these observations should be included in the medical record.

Decision Support

Communication of accurate and understandable genetic and genomic information is important as cancer patients begin to consider their decision to participate in genetic testing. Approaching the informed consent process includes matching patient values and preferences with their decision and confirming their risk perception with the accuracy of calculated risk and requires trust, openness, and expression of support and

Table 2
Some examples of red flags for identification of common inherited disorders

Red Flags	What to Check For
Family History • Sibling or parents (1st degree relative) • Aunts & uncles or nieces & nephews (2nd degree relatives) • Grandparents or 1st cousins (3rd degree relatives	• Common adult conditions with two more close (1st, 2nd, or 3rd degree) family members who have been diagnosed with a disease (heart disease, cancer or dementia) at a young age. • Demonstrate pattern of inheritance (recessive, dominant, X-linked) • Look for shared genetics and environmental risk factors
Group of congenital anomalies	• Look for two or more. (Many people normally can have one, but two or more may indicate a genetic syndrome) • Be alert for anomalies of the teeth, eg, baby teeth at birth, baby teeth that are not replaced with adult teeth or multiple teeth. • Papillomatous papules in the mouth • Macrocephaly >58 cm women and 60 cm men
*E*xtreme or exceptional presentation of common conditions	• Recurrent miscarriage, even in two generations of a family. • Cancers in bilateral organs • Multiple primary cancers of different tissues • Early onset (than typically anticipated) cardio-vascular disease, cancer, or renal failure • Unusually severe reaction to infectious or metabolic stress
*N*eurodevelopmental delay in pediatric age group, growth problems or mental retardation	• Early onset dementia in adults
*E*xtreme or exceptional pathology	• Unusual tissue histology eg, pheochromocy-tyoma, acoustic neuroma, medullary thyroid cancer, multiple colon polyps, plexiform neu-rofibromas, multiple exostoses, most pediatric malignancies.
*S*urprising lab values	• Transferrin saturation of 65%, potassium of 5.5 mmol/L, & sodium of 128 mmol/> in an infant • Cholesterol of >500 mg/dL and unconjugated bilirubin of 2.2 mg/dL in otherwise healthy 25 y/o • Phosphate of 2 mg/dL and glucose of 35 mg/dL in 6-month-old child.
Additional Red Flags	
Dysmorphologies (unusual physical features)	• Many present at birth
Disease occurring in an individual of the less commonly affected sex	• Male breast cancer • Rheumatoid arthritis
Presence of disease without other risk factors	• Sudden unexplained death in an athletic 20 year old) hypertrophic cardiomyopathy) • Diabetes mellitus (hereditary chromotosis or myotonic dystrophy)

(*continued on next page*)

Table 2 (*continued*)	
Red Flags	**What to Check For**
Ethnicity associated with some genetic disorders	• Hemoglobinopathies (thalassemia, sickle cell anemia) in person of Mediterranean, African, Middle Eastern and South East Asian Ancestry • Breast and ovarian cancers associated with Ashkenazi Jewish ancestry • Diabetes with Native Americans
Consanguinity	• Union between two individuals related as second cousins or closer. This is viewed as desirable unions in certain Middle Eastern countries or parents in some religions like for their children to marry someone in the same religion
History of more than three unexplained miscarriages, still birth, childhood death, infertility or congenital anomalies (eg, heart defect, imperforate anus)	
Red flags of Cardiac Disease	
Arryhthmias	
Long QT syndromes	• Structurally normal heart, inherited vs. acquired, palpitations, syncope, risk for sudden cardiac death
Brugada	• More commonly in males in 3rd-4th decade of life, structurally normal heart, palpitaitons, syncope, risk for sudden cardiac death
Cardiomyopathies	
Hypertrophic	• Unexplained LVH, SOB, chest pain, palpitations, presyncope & syncope Risk for sudden cardiac death
Dilated	• Dilated & impaired contraction of LV, edema, SOB, fatigue & arrhythmias, risk for sudden cardiac death • Progressive fibrofatty replacement of the myocardium, palpitations, syncope, risk for sudden cardiac death
Arrythmogenic right ventricular dysplasia or cardiomyopathy	• An inherited disorder with structural and functional abnormalities of the right ventricle. It is associated with 11% of sudden cardiac death in young adults, 22% of cases among athletes and could be affected by chemotherapy such as adriamycin.
Marfan Syndrome and related disorders	• Aortic root dilation, dislocated eye lenses, and other systemic findings such thoracic aneurysm and dissections
Other • Clotting • Amyloid	

Abbreviation: SOB, shortness of breath.
Data from Refs.[54–56]

Table 3
Some examples of Red Flags associated with inherited cancers

Cancer or Feature	Signs & Symptoms for Genetic Counseling Referral	Syndrome & Gene for Consideration
Skin Cancers		
Basal cell carcinoma (BCC)	Jaw cysts beginning in the teens and at least 5 BCC's beginning in the 20's, abnormally protruding forehead (bossing), macrocephaly, and milia	Nevoid basal cell carcinoma syndrome (NBCCS) Gene = PTCH
Melanoma	Individual with personal history of or first-degree relative with: a. Three or more melanomas in same person b. Three or more cases or melanomas and/or pancreatic cancer.	Hereditary melanoma, familial atypical mole and malignant melanoma Gene = CDKN2A/ARF
	Personal history of or first-degree relative with a. Melanoma and astrocytoma in the same person b. One melanoma case and one astrocytoma case in two first-degree relatives.	Melanoma-astrocytoma syndrome Gene(s) = CDKN2, p14ARF, p14AF alone and perhaps ANRIL antisense noncoding RNA
Hematologic malignancies, brain/CNS tumors & colon tumors/ polyps	1. Rare childhood cancer predisposition syndrome with 4 main tumor types: hematologic malignancies, brain/CNS tumors, colorectal tumors, multiple intestinal polyps and other malignancies including embryonic tumors and rhabdomyosarcoma. a. Tumor(s) diagnosed prior to age 18 with any other criteria below: i. Café-au-lait macules and/or other signs of NF1, or hypopigmented skin lesions ii. Consanguinous parents iii. Family hx of colon cancer iv. Second primary cancer v. Sibling with a childhood cancer b. Medulloblastoma c. >10 cumulative adenomatous colon polyps in same person	Constitutional Mismatch Repair Deficiency (CMMRD) Autosomal recessive inheritance Genes = MLH1, MSH2, PMS2, APC, and NF1

Abbreviations: BCC, basal cell carcinoma; CNS, central nervous system; NBCCS, nevoid BCC syndrome; NF1, neufibromatosis type 1.
Data from Refs.[57–59]

resource suggestions. Race and ethnicity also need to be considered, because there are genetic mutations that are found or carried among certain races and ethnic groups. It is well known that the *BRCA1* and *BRCA2* mutations are common to the Ashkenazi Jewish population. A recent publication identifies a new Mexican founder mutation at *BRCA1* ex9-12del.[60]

When a patient receives a positive mutation result, it can cause pressure for a variety of decisions to be made by the family. These can include the need for testing of relatives. Personal decisions would include the use of chemoprevention medication with potential side effects versus scheduling a prophylactic bilateral mastectomy. Sometimes persons find themselves trying to defend a decision to avoid body-changing surgeries in order to prevent a disease they may never develop when they feel comfortable using the state-of-the art technologies for screening and surveillance. All these decisions require support by oncology nurses to educate, clarify, and listen to the patient/family as the various decisions are considered.

ADVANCING THE QUALITY OF LIFE
Family

Advancing quality of life for the family includes consideration of family functioning, structure, family relationships, and communication. Communication by a health care provider can enhance the quality of life for a patient and family, even at the end of life.[38] The family history of the disease is important; therefore, collecting family history, identifying risk, and conveying information assists in management of an inherited cancer risk and promotes quality of life. Sometimes family history about disease can be used to target education about the disease and an opening to discuss resources or lifestyle changes and modification of risky behaviors, such as smoking.[38]

Symptom Management

Precision medicine (PM) is a new term and concept in health care that designs treatment and diagnostics based on individual needs and genetics and genomics of patients. As PM continues to emerge as an approach to treat and prevent disease, it takes into account individual variability in genes, environment, and lifestyle.[29] The unique perspective of PM, promoted by President Obama, offers better tools for clinicians to interpret the complex mechanisms of disease that can affect a person's health and better predict individualized treatments that will be most effective. **Box 4** lists objectives of the PM initiative. The ultimate outcome of PM is to address all the rights for the treatment of 1 person instead of maneuvering a 1-size-fits-all approach.[61]

See **Box 5** for "The rights in patient care." If nurses can predict patient responses to their interventions based on genetic and genomic variability, the optimal outcome will more likely be due to the personalized intervention, not just a shot in the dark.[53] Tailoring nursing interventions based on PM can advance quality of life for individuals and families.[38]

For cancer patients currently receiving retreatment or survivors who have been out of treatment for years, cancer-related fatigue (CRF) continues to be a persistent, common, and distressing symptom. There are several biological studies with a focus on proteomics and inflammatory responses to psychological stress in cancer patients

---

Box 4
Objectives of the precision medicine initiative

- More and better treatments for cancer by accelerating the design and testing of effective tailored treatments for cancer

- Creation of a voluntary national research cohort of Americans who volunteer to participate in research

- Commitment to protecting privacy and security of data in the context of precision medicine

- Regulatory modernization to support development of new types of research and care protection network

- Public-private partnerships with existing research cohorts, patient groups, and the private sector to develop infrastructure needed to expand cancer genomics and to launch a voluntary million-person cohort

---

Box 5
The rights in patient care

- Right patient
- Right drug
- Right dose
- Right route
- Right time
- Right reason

---

and survivors.[62–64] Recently, 2 studies examined profiles of changes in gene sequences associated with activation and deactivation of genes and changes in cytokine and other protein levels, suggesting the genetic basis of CRF cancer and ultimately a better understanding of the symptom mechanism.[53,65,66] A clearer understanding of the biology and genetics of CRF will enable the identification of new pharmacologic targets for CRF intervention.

Pharmacogenomics and targeted therapies

The goal of pharmacogenomics is to identify how a person's genes affect individual responses to drugs. Although historical drug treatment is 1-size-fits-all, there currently is minimal guidance to predict who will benefit versus those who will have life-threatening side effects.[67] PM may identify those at highest risk of developing specific health problems and those to target with presymptomatic counseling versus those who may receive little or no effect from health promotion activities. These outcomes may be predicted based on the genotype of the individual, positively enhance compliance in patients, improve finances in the family (plus overall health care costs), and ultimately prevent harmful exposure for genetically vulnerable patients.[53] Rehabilitation for oncology patients is an area of intervention that has been associated with reductions in stress and impact on coping plus positive immune responses. Over time, research studies identified the positive effects of exercise on resistance to fatigue, cardiorespiratory fitness, muscle strength, physical well-being, reduced anxiety and depression, and improved quality of life.[68] Oncology nurses need to understand the timing of actual biological and molecular effects of personalized medicine while considering the need for rehabilitation. If genotyping indicates 1 patient population can expect drug results whereas another might anticipate fewer results, there could be an impact on patient tolerance or outcomes related to the exercise therapy that would be important consider with the exercise prescription.[53] **Table 4** lists some targeted therapies and how associated genetic/genomic information could be addressed.

Disease States

Use of genetics and genomics in oncology has already had an effect on reducing morbidity and mortality in cancer. Community education and incorporation of discussion about genes and environmental interactions and even genomic interventions, such as personalized medicine, can have and is having an effect on cancer incidence, detection, treatment, and interventions. Measurement of effectiveness of approaches is important to monitor and document in publications, Internet Web sites, and clinical trials.[20,38,53]

Table 4 Targeted therapies		
Type	**Action**	**How to Address**
Histone deacetylase inhibitors[69]	Add acetyl tails to histone and nonhistone targets	• Monitor complete blood cell counts, signs and symptoms of infection, bleeding, fatigue, diarrhea, nausea, vomiting, anorexia weight loss, and constipation. • Implement interventions to decrease specific clinical problems. • Family for disease prevention.
Biotherapy		
Biologic response modifiers		
Granulocyte colony-stimulating factor	Stimulate production of neutrophils	• Treat with acetaminophen. • Monitor for splenic rupture, acute respiratory distress syndrome, allergic reactions, generalized erythema, and flushing. • Educate that pain is typically associated with bone marrow sites. • Acetominophen
Granulocyte-macrophage colony-stimulating factor	Stimulate production of neutrophils, monocytes macrophages, basophils, and eosinophils	• Cold compress • Monitor signs and symptoms.
Erythropoietin	Stimulate production of red blood cells	• Treat symptoms. • Educate that occurs typically with 1st administration only.
Thrombopoietin	Stimulate production of platelets	• Monitor for signs and symptoms. • Educate family/patient what to monitor for and when to call report.
Proteins		
Peptibody protein		
Interferons		
Interleukins		
Immunomodulatory agents		
Thalidomide Lenalidomide		• Educate patients about black box warnings, including signs and symptoms. • Monitor for 5q myelodysplastic syndrome deletions and potential neutropenia and thrombocytopenia.

(continued on next page)

Table 4 (continued)		
Type	**Action**	**How to Address**
Monoclonal abs		• Educate patients and family about type of ab and how they target receptors, ligands, or growth factors associated with the various cell types.
Hematologic		
Solid tumor		
Epidermal growth factor receptor family Immune checkpoint inhibitors[71]	• Abs block the programmed death-1; checkpoint, to inhibit T-cell activation	• Educate about most common side effects of fatigue, decreased appetite, and diarrhea. • Monitor carefully for lung microbes and potential for infections in patients with chronic obstructive pulmonary disease and acute pneumonia.
Vaccines		Still under development
Intracellular targeted therapies		Still under development
Small molecules		
TKIs	• 20 Types • Inhibits tyrosine kinase-mediated signaling	• Educate about oral administration. • Carefully review prescribed and over-the-counter medications. • Use teaching tools available from ONS and other organizations.
TKIs for hematologic malignancies		• Monitor for side effects and provide supportive measures. • Educate family about interventions, such as tonic water for bone pain or hand and foot cramps.
TKIs for solid tumors		• Educate about avoidance of grapefruit products and ethyl alcohol.
Dual inhibitors of kinase binding sites		• Educate about commonly used drug interactions (pharmacogenetics/personalized medicine).
Inhibitors of multiple signaling pathways	• Block signaling of ≥3 pathways	• Educate about commonly used drug interactions (pharmacogenetics/personalized medicine).
Signaling pathway inhibitors		• Educate about pharmacogenomics.

(continued on next page)

Table 4 (continued)		
Type	Action	How to Address
Proteasome inhibitors	• Block function of proteasomes causing apoptosis of malignant cells	• Educate about neuropathy and potential safety precautions.
Telomerase inhibitors	• Target telomerase • Allow chromosome ends to shorten	Currently in clinical trials with lipid delivery system and vaccines

Abbreviations: Ab, antibody; TKI, tyrosine kinase inhibitor.
  Data from Refs.[69–72]

Client Self-management

The consequences of cancer such as the emotional experiences associated with the diagnosis of cancer, the impact on the life of the patient and family and effects of treatment are areas of expertise to be shared by oncology nurses at all levels. The inclusion of genetic information into the lives of patients adds a new and changing dimension to the issues that need to be addressed with the direction or support of the oncology nurse. This can include concerns for perceived risk of life-threatening, life-shorting disease and how to deal with the self-management of day-to-day care issues, information needs, stress, or coping demands.[20,44,53]

Collecting and sharing information that supports self-management is important for patients and families.[20,38,44,53]

Some of the resources in **Box 2** can be used directly or revised for patient education. Keeping the genetics component as simple as possible, without being disrespectful, is important to help patients and families believe the targeted problem is manageable. This includes educational-level assessments of appropriate information for elders without genetic education foundation, immigrants from other countries, or persons of other religions.

Family risk assessments that include culture and religion suggest a variety of lifestyle behaviors that can prevent or promote behavior. Both diet and exercise have guidelines supported by the American Cancer Society that suggest factors that might influence the development of certain cancers.[73,74]

Many elements from an individual's life history contain pieces of information pointing to potential environmental risk factors for gene and environment. It is well known that environmental exposures to carcinogens like asbestos or lead paint are associated with developing cancer at a later time.[75] Assessing for history of occupations, such as new carpeting warehouses (formaldehyde), textile mills (red dye and cotton dust), and even military service (agent orange or mustard gas), is important when discussing germline (de novo and inherited) or somatic mutations and the development of cancer(s).[74,76]

Incorporating a discussion about how changes from the environment might alter the DNA sequence requires an understanding of epigenetics. Simply, chemicals cause epigenetic changes that can alter the DNA molecule and the histones it is wrapped around. Because DNA is transcribed to RNA and the messenger RNA translated into amino acids and protein, the protein production can be stopped or modified., if incorrect information is received. Some chemicals are attached like tails to the wrapped DNA and include methyl (CH_3) and acetyl (CH_3CO) groups. The CH_3 group binds to the nucleotide cytosine and assists with silencing, or turning off, the genes. This silencing occurs because the CH_3 groups bind to DNA and prevent the gene transcription machinery from forming and expressing a protein. Other chemical changes, like CH_3CO, can alter the histone structure and cause the gene to turn on or off, depending on the change.[77] For example, if DNA methylation exists on a gene involved in controlling proper cell division, this could lead to the silencing of that gene and subsequent uncontrolled cell reproduction, common to cancer. These chemical modifications can change over time in response to age, environment/lifestyle, and disease state. Any discussion with a patient/family needs to include the emphasis that the known inheritance patterns of DNA sequence can be inherited from generation to generation, but there are still questions as to whether the epigenetic modifications are inherited in successive generations.[78]

Innovation

Technology and development

New technologies associated with genetics and genomics have already had an impact on prevention and treatment in oncology. Since 1992, identification of gene mutations has gone from 1 gene at a time, including pieces of genes; to next-generation sequencing, where panels 10 to 40 or more genes are analyzed at 1 time; to whole genome testing, complete sequencing of an individual's entire length of DNA, whether it forms proteins or not; and now to whole-exome sequencing with sequencing of approximately 20,000 genes that are translated into proteins.[45]

During genetic testing oncology nurses (usually one with specialized knowledge in inherited genetics) need to be able to explain the differences, translate information to help patients and families make knowledgeable decisions during the informed consent process and provide psychological support after receiving results. This may be more important than having a patient understand the technical details of the testing process.[79,80] Dissemination of the information to referring health care providers and assisting with implementation of the management plan are imperative. One piece of information from whole-exome sequencing that can cause distress is incidental findings (IFs), where a healthy person can receive unexpected information about a potentially devastating diagnosis. It is suggested that patients be given information about the indication for genetic testing first; this can be followed-up with information about IFs second.

Prior to testing, patients should be asked if they want to know all results, or only those that have clinically actionable steps.[81] The rationale for such discussions is based on the potentially overwhelming amount of genomics information available about testing for disease/s that may be associated with a result that is not known to be pathogeneic or benign; a variant of unknown significance. Not every oncology nurse can know everything about their specialty. It is important that oncology nurses recognize their boundaries of knowledge and refer to another colleague with expertise in a particular area. For instance, if a 27-year-old patient receives a report for a positive *BRCA2* mutation, an uninformed provider may suggest immediate removal of ovaries because there is an associated high risk for developing ovarian cancer. In reality, the evidence-based guidelines suggest oophorectomy may not need to occur until the patient is over 40 years of age. This is because *BRCA2* mutation associated ovarian cancers tend to occur 8 to 10 years later than patients diagnosed with *BRCA1* mutations.[82] The implications of an uninformed decision could include 13 or more years of postmenopausal symptoms and a potential decision that leads to a life without children. An informed nurse could promote a discussion about the current guidelines, their implications and options for the future.

Genomic bioinformatics is a new area important to oncological patient care but relatively unknown to nurses. In 2014, the Institute of Medicine created a report focusing on the use of genomic sequencing information to facilitate health care decision making.[83] Whole-genome sequencing offers extensive data that need to be organized into registries or studies that could support guideline development. For oncology nurses, the clinical annotation of genetic data will facilitate improved quality of care and new insights about outcomes that are based on precision medicine.

The Cancer Learning Intelligence Network for Quality (CancerLinQ) is an initiative implemented by the American Society of Clinical Oncology to compile, analyze, and annotate clinical information on patients in almost any setting, in real time.[84] CancerLinQ is a unique approach that allows doctors, and hopefully all health care providers, an opportunity to immediately compare their care against guidelines and the care of their peers. This information includes treatments, side effects, and personalized insights to gather patterns in patient characteristics. Oncology nurses could add to CancerLinQ database with insights on symptoms, such as fatigue, depression, or pain, to begin to put together common data elements to allow different and better research questions in the future and evaluate how 1 symptom can vary in intensity, trajectory, or management across different cancers, the life span, gender, ethnicities, or cultures.[85] Oncology nurses at all levels of care can contribute and use information about patterns of care for best practices for their oncology patients. With access to biomarkers and other laboratory values, this approach could help explain the fundamental mechanism of a troubling symptom, such as weight gain in some breast cancer patients or depression after stem cell transplant.[85,86]

Informatics and support systems

Support systems, such as the electronic health record, have contributed to organized data storage and facilitated the research process. There is still much to be gained, however, in developing tools for cross-generational sharing of genomic data, such as family history and pedigree construction. These fundamental areas could improve the management, analysis, interpretation, and use of genomic information for point-of-care decision support for patients and health care providers.[20,38] Oncology Nursing Society (ONS) publications and patient care products, such as the *Putting Evidence into Practice*[87] resources, could be used as a foundation of common terminology, a taxonomy to enable the development of common formats for data storage/exchange, and queries that could be linked to genomic information.[19,20,85,87] Ultimately, these could link peer-to-peer informatics queries and discussions of common data elements that could promote the development of personalized medicine.

Training

Genetics education resources

Oncology is a rapidly changing specialty, especially with the integration of personalized medicine. The development and incorporation of genetic/genomic information and technologies into oncology patient care require continuous updating for individual registered nurses and the existing nursing workforce. Educational strategies to remain current include a variety of educational approaches, such as incidence-based literature; journal clubs; online courses; organizational Web courses, such as those offered by ISONG (International Society of Nurses in Genetics) or the ONS; and even traditional conferences. When considering continuing education and further professional education, registered nurses need to consider the impact of genetics/genomics on their oncology practice and/or projected research program.

Graduate nursing programs offering specific genetic/genomic content or incorporating this content in an oncology career and program of research highlight the changing scientific environment that includes molecular science and should be considered for capacity building.[10,20,38,44,53] **Box 2** contains a list of educational resources for individualized learning, updating knowledge, identifying Web sites for patient/family education, and developing a curriculum that can be used to educate the existing oncology nursing workforce — those who lack genetics education in their basic program.[88]

SUMMARY

Multiple studies emphasize the importance of genomics in nursing, the need to educate nurses about ways to include genetics/genomics into practice, and the need to incorporate genomics into nursing research. Some studies report nurses' knowledge and ways to incorporate genetics/genomics into practice. Several investigators document the limited or lack of curriculum about genetics/genomics in grade school, high school, biology courses for college preparation, and nursing educational courses.[88–90] In addition to basic education, Calzone and colleagues[38] suggest awareness campaigns, continuing education courses, leadership persuasion, policy review, and development to encourage nurses at the bedside to integrate genomics into practice. This author has attempted to identify genomic information that oncology nurses, at all levels of care, need to know and use as tools in the fight to conquer cancer.

REFERENCES

1. National Human Genome Research Institute. An overview of the human genome project. 2015. Available at: https://www.genome.gov/12011238/an-overview-of-the-human-genome-project/an-overview-of-the-human-genome-project/. Accessed October 9, 2016.
2. Brantl V, Esslinger P. Genetics implications for the nursing curriculum. Nurs Forum 1962;1:90–100.
3. Cohen FL. Clinical genetics in nursing practice. Philadelphia: J.B. Lippincott; 1984.
4. American Association of Colleges of Nursing, 2008. The Essentials of Baccalaureate Education for Professional Nursing Practice, AACN.
5. American Association of Colleges of Nursing, 2009. The Essentials of Baccalaureate Education for Professional Nursing Practice Faculty Tool Kit, AACN.
6. National Coalition for Health Professional Education in Genetics [NCHPEG], 2007.
7. American Nurses Association [ANA] and the International Society of Nurses in Genetics [ISONG], 2012.
8. Brant J, Wickham R. Statement on the scope and standards of oncology nursing practice. Pittsburgh (PA): ONS; 2004.
9. Brant J, Wickham R. Statement on the scope and standards of oncology nursing practice: Generalist and advanced practice. Pittsburgh (PA): Oncology Nursing Society; 2013.
10. Jenkins J. Essential genetic and genomic nursing competencies for the oncology nurse. Semin Oncol Nurs 2011;27(1):64–71.
11. Understanding building construction. n.d. Available at: http://www.understand construction.com/types-of-foundations.html. Accessed October 9, 2016.
12. Nursing's social policy statement: the essense of the profession. ANA 3rd edition. Silver Spring (MD): Nursesbooks.org.
13. International Society of Nurses in Genetics and the American Nurses Association. Genetics and genomics nursing: scope and standards of nursing practice. Silver Spring (MD): American Nurses Association; 2006.
14. AACN, 2011.
15. ANA, 2012.
16. NINR-Summer Genetics Institute. 2000.

17. American Association of Colleges of Nursing (n.d.). Advanced Genetics Nursing Certification eligibility criteria. Available at: http://www.nursecredentialing.org/ Advanced-Genetics-Eligibility. Accessed December 6, 2016.
18. Greco KE, Tinley S, Seibert D. Essential genetic and genomic competencies for nurses with graduate degrees. Silver Spring (MD): American Nurses Association and International Society of Nurses in Genetics; 2012.
19. Calzone K, Jenkins J, Bakos A, et al. A blueprint for genomic nursing science. J Nurs Scholarsh 2014;45(1):96–104.
20. Williams J, Tripp-Reimer T, Daack-Hirsch S, et al. Five-year bibliometric review of genomic nursing science research. J Nurs Scholarsh 2016;48(2):179–86.
21. Springer M. Breast cancer survivors: a tribe of warrior women. Birmingham (United Kingdom): Crane Hill Publishers; 1996.
22. Crick F. Central dogma of molecular biology. Nature 1970;227(5258):561–3.
23. Dolan DNA Learning Center. Available at: www.dnalc.org. Accessed October 4, 2016.
24. Genetics/Genomics Competency Center for Education (G2C2). Available at: http://www.g-2-c-2.org/. Accessed October 4, 2016.
25. Genomic Medicine for Patients and the Public. Available at: https://www.genome. gov/19016903/. Accessed October 4, 2016.
26. Global Genetics and Genomics Community. Available at: http://www.g-3-c.org. Accessed October 4, 2016.
27. National Coalition for Health Professional Education in Genetics. Available at: http://nchpeg.org/. Accessed October 4, 2016.
28. National Human Genome Research Institute. Available at: www.genome.gov. Accessed October 4, 2016.
29. Genetics Home Reference: The genetics of cancer. Available at: http://ghr.nlm. nih.gov. Accessed October 4, 2016.
30. National Cancer Institute: About cancer. Available at: https://www.cancer.gov/ about-cancer/causes-prevention/genetics. Accessed October 4, 2016.
31. The PharmGenEdProgram. Available at: http://pharmacogenomics.ucsd.edu. Accessed October 4, 2016.
32. Online Mendelian Inheritance of Man. Available at: http://www.ncbi.nlm.nih.gov/ omim. Accessed October 4, 2016.
33. Gene Tests. Available at: http://www.ncbi.nlm.nih/gov/sites/GeneTests/. Accessed October 4, 2016.
34. Anderson C, Alt-White A, Schaa K, et al. Genomics for nursing education and practice: measuring competency. Worldviews Evid Based Nurs 2015;12(3): 165–75.
35. Coleman B, Calzone K, Jenkins J, et al. Multi ethnic minority nurses knowledge and practice of genetics and genomics. J Nurs Scholarsh 2014;46(4):235–44.
36. Calzone K, Jenkins J, Yates J, et al. Survey of nursing integration of genomics into nursing practice. J Nurs Scholarsh 2012;44(1):428–36.
37. Skirton H, O'Connor A, Humphreys A. Nurses' competence in genetics: a mixed method systematic review. J Adv Nurs 2012;68(11):2387–98.
38. Calzone K, Jenkins J, Culp S, et al. Introducing a new competency into nursing practice. J Nurs Regul 2014;5(1):40–7.
39. Shipman K, Arnold I. Case of epirubicin-incduced cardiomyopathy in familial cardiomyopathy. J Clin Oncol 2011;29(18):e537–8.
40. Jones S, Holmes FA, O'Shaughnessy J, et al. Docetaxel with cyclophosphamide is associated with an overall survival benefit compared with doxorubicin and

cyclophosphamide: 7-year follow-up of US Oncology Research Trial 9735. J Clin Oncol 2009;27:1177–83.

41. Joehanes R, Just A, Marioni R, et al. Epigenetic signatures of cigarette smoking. Circ Cardiovasc Genet 2016;9:436–47.

42. Berliner JL, Fay AM, Cummings SA, et al. NSGC practice guideline: risk assessment and genetic counseling for hereditary breast and ovarian cancer. J Genet Couns 2013;22:155–63.

43. Venne V, Scheuner M. Securing and documenting cancer family history in the age of the electronic medical record. Surg Oncol Clin 2015;24(4):639–52.

44. Camak D. Increasing importance of genetics in nursing. Nurse Educ Today 2016; 44:86–91.

45. Mahon S. The three-generation pedigree: a critical tool in cancer genetics care. Oncol Nurs Forum 2016;43(5):655–60.

46. Bennett RL, French KS, Resta R, et al. Standardized human pedigree nomenclature: Update and assessment of the recommendations of the National Society of Genetic Coun- selors. J Genet Couns 2008;17:424–33.

47. Lu KH, Wood ME, Daniels M, et al. American Society of Clinical Oncology expert statement: collection and use of a cancer family history for oncology providers. J Clin Oncol 2014;32:833–40.

48. Schaa K. Assessing patients with a genetic "eye": family history and physical assessment. In: Kasper C, Schneidereith TA, Lashley F, editors. Lashley's essentials of clinical genetics in nursing practice. 2nd edition. New York: Springer Publishing Company, LLC; p. 191–214.

49. Breast Cancer Risk Assessment Tool. 2011. Available at: https://www.cancer.gov/bcrisktool/. Accessed September 23, 2016.

50. IBIS Breast Cancer Risk Evaluation Tool. 2016. Available at: http://www.ems-trials.org/riskevaluator/. Accessed September 23, 2016.

51. Colorectal Cancer Risk Assessment Tool. 2014. Available at: https://www.cancer.gov/colorectalcancerrisk/#. Accessed September 23, 2016.

52. Whelan A, Ball S, Best L, et al. Genetic red flags: clues to thinking genetically in primary care practice. Prim Care 2004;31:497–508, viii.

53. Munro C. Individual genetic and genomic variation: a new opportunity for personalized nursing interventions. J Adv Nurs 2014;71(1):35–41.

54. NCHPEG (n.d.) Genetic Red Flags. Available at: http://www.nchpeg.org/index.php?option=com_content&view=article&id=59&Itemid=75. Accessed December 6, 2016.

55. Stepniak I, Trojanowski T, Drelich-Zbroja A, et al. Cowden syndrome and the associated Lhermitte-Duclos disease—case presentation. Neurol Neurochir Pol 2015;49(5):339–43.

56. NCCN Guidelines For Detection, Prevention, & risk reduction. Available at: https://www.nccn.org/professionals/physician_gls/f_guidelines.asp#detection. Accessed September 24, 2016.

57. Riley B, Culver J, Skrzynia C, et al. Essential elements of genetic cancer risk assessment, counseling, and testing: updated recommendations of the National Society of Genetic Counselors. J Genet Couns 2011;21(2):151–61.

58. Hampel R, Bennett R, Buchanan A, et al. A practice guideline from the American College of Medical Genetics and Genomics and the National Society of Genetic Counselors: referral indications for cancer predisposition assessment. Genet Med 2014;17:70–87.

59. Baudhuin L. Mayo Medical Labs Hot Topics: multi-gene panel testing for inherited cardiovascular disorders. 2015. Available at: http://www.mayomedical

laboratories.com/articles/hot-topic/2015/06-15-cardiovascular-disorders/index.html. Accessed December 6, 2016.

60. Weitzel J. Prevalence and type of BRCA mutations in Hispanics undergoing genetic cancer risk assessment in the southwestern United States: a report from the clinical cancer genetics community research network. J Clin Oncol 2013;31(2): 210–6.

61. Institute of Safe Medication Practices (ISMP). The five rights: a destination without a map. Available at: http://www.ismp.org/newsletters/acutecare/articles/20070 125.asp. Accessed September 23, 2016.

62. Minton O, Stone PC. Review: the use of proteomics as a research methodology for studying cancer-related fatigue: a review. Palliat Med 2010;24:310–6.

63. Bower JE, Ganz PA, Aziz N, et al. Inflammatory responses to psychological stress in fatigued breast cancer survivors: relationship to glucocorticoids. Brain Behav Immun 2007;21:251–8.

64. Minton O, Stone P. Cancer related fatigue: mechanisms, assessment and treatment in older people. Rev Clin Gerontol 2011;21:255–66.

65. Lyon DE, McCain NL, Pickler RH, et al. Advancing the biobehavioral research of fatigue with genetics and genomics. J Nurs Scholarsh 2011;43:274–81.

66. GHR. Pharmacogenomics. 2016. Available at: https://ghr.nlm.nih.gov/primer/ genomicresearch/pharmacogenomics. Accessed September 24, 2016.

67. Genetics Home Reference (GHR). Precision medicine. Available at: https://ghr. nlm.nih.gov/primer/precisionmedicine/definition. Accessed September 17, 2016.

68. Bouillet T, Bigard X, Brami C, et al. Role of physical activity and sport in oncology: Scientific commission of the National Federation Sport and Cancer CAMI. Crit Rev Oncol Hematol 2015;94(1):74–86.

69. Rubin K. Understanding immune checkpoint inhibitors for effective patient care. Clin J Oncol Nurs 2015;19(6):709–17.

70. Davis P, Douglas T, Gilbert C, et al. Side effects of cancer therapy. In: Polovich M, Olsen M, LeFebvre KB, editors. Chemotherapy and biotherapy guidelines and recommendations for practice. 4th edition. Pittsburgh (PA): Oncology Nursing Society; 2014. p. 25–47.

71. Brahmer J, Pardoll D. Immune checkpoint inhibitors: Making immunotherapy a reality for the treatment of lung cancer. Cancer Immunol Res 2013;1(2):85–91.

72. Eggert J, Lapka D, Franson P. Precision Medicine: biologics and targeted therapies. Chapter 10. In: Eggert J, editor. Cancer basics. 2nd edition. Pittsburgh: Oncology Nursing Societ7; 2017.

73. American Cancer Society (ACS): Diet and activity factors that affect risks for certain cancers. 2016. Available at: http://www.cancer.org/healthy/eathealthy getactive/acsguidelinesonnutritionphysicalactivityforcancerprevention/acs-guide lines-on-nutrition-and-physical-activity-for-cancer-prevention-dietand-activity. Accessed October 10, 2016.

74. Vineis P, Wild CP. Global cancer patterns: cause and prevention. Lancet 2014; 383:549–57.

75. National Cancer Institute: About cancer: environmental carcinogens and cancer risk. 2015. Available at: https://www.cancer.gov/about-cancer/causes-prevention/ risk/substances/carcinogens. Accessed October 9, 2016.

76. Occupational Safety and Health: Safety and health topics-Cotton dust. n.d. Available at: https://www.osha.gov/SLTC/cottondust/index.html. Accessed October 10, 2016.

77. Virani S, Colacino J, Kim J, et al. Cancer epigenetics: a brief review. ILAR J 2012; 53(3–4):359–69.

78. Heard E, Martienssen R. Transgenerational epigenetic inheritance: myths and mechanisms. Cell 2014;157(1):95–109.
79. Mahon S. Whole exome sequencing: the next phase of genetics care. Oncol Nurs Forum 2016;43(2):249–52.
80. Amendola LM, Lautenbach D, Scollon S, et al. Illustrative case studies in the return of exome and genome sequencing results. Per Med 2015;12:283–95.
81. Roche MI, Berg JS. Incidental findings with genomic testing: Implications for genetic counseling practice. Curr Genet Med Rep 2015;3:166–76.
82. NCCN: BRCA related breast and ovarian cancer syndrome. 2017. Available at: https://www.nccn.org/professionals/physician_gls/pdf/genetics_screening.pdf. Accessed October 8, 2016. BRCA-A page 1 of 2.
83. Institute of Medicine: Assessing genomic sequencing information for health care decision making. Available at: https://books.google.com/books?hl=en&lr=&id=mImcBAAAQBAJ&oi=fnd&pg=PT18&dq=Assessing+genomic+sequencing+information+for+health+care+decision+making–workshop+summary+2014&ots=dnADFPYbSJ&sig=_l1su-VoJIFpfi06X_VUkHvIOw4#v=onepage&q=Assessing%20genomic%20sequencing%20information%20for%20health%20care%20decision%20making–workshop%20summary%202014&f=false. Accessed October 9, 2016.
84. ASCO CancerLinQ. Available at: http://cancerlinq.org/. Accessed October 9, 2016.
85. Corwin EJ, Berg JA, Armstrong TS, et al. Envisioning the future in symptom science. Nurs Outlook 2014;62:346–51.
86. Ziegler A, Koch A, Krockenberger K, et al. Personalized medicine using DNA biomarkers: a review. Hum Genet 2012;131(10):1627–38.
87. ONS: Putting Evidence into Practice. Available at: https://ons.org/practice-resources/pep. Accessed October 9, 2016.
88. Beamer LC, Linder L, Wu B, et al. The impact of genomics on oncology nursing. Nurs Clin North Am 2013;48(4):585–626.
89. Peterson SK, Rieger PT, Marani SK, et al. Oncology nurses' knowledge, practice, and education needs regarding cancer genetics. Am J Med Genet 2001;98(1):3–12.
90. Prows C, Glass M, Nichol N, et al. Genomics in nursing education. JNS 2005;37(3):196–202.

The Big 3

An Updated Overview of Colorectal, Breast, and Prostate Cancers

Jeanine Gordon, MSN, RN, OCN, NE-BC*,
Erica Fischer-Cartlidge, MSN, CNS, CBCN, AOCNS,
Margaret Barton-Burke, PhD, RN, FAAN

KEYWORDS

- Colorectal cancer • Breast cancer • Prostate cancer

KEY POINTS

- Cancer is a serious public health issue responsible for 1 of every 4 deaths in the United States.
- Among new cancers, colorectal, breast, and prostate are 3 of the most commonly diagnosed cancers.
- As we learn more about cancer cellular mechanisms, treatment for these cancers are changing and these changes are delineated in this article.

INTRODUCTION

Cancer is a serious public health issue responsible for 1 of every 4 deaths in the United States. In 2016, it was estimated that 1,685,210 new cancer cases were diagnosed and there were 595,690 cancer-related deaths in the United States.[1] Among these, colorectal, breast, and prostate are 3 of the most commonly diagnosed cancers. As the population continues to grow and age, more people will be diagnosed with and/ or living with the sequelae of cancer treatment. It is important that nurses in all clinical settings have basic knowledge about the most common cancers and are kept abreast of the current trends in oncology patient care.

This article provides an update and overview of colorectal, breast, and prostate cancers. For each cancer, data related to incidence and prevalence are discussed as well as nonmodifiable and modifiable risk factors. Information about detection and evidenced-based screening guideline recommendations is reviewed, with an emphasis on the most common and recent treatment modalities. Finally, nursing care and clinical practice implications are summarized at the end of the article.

Dr Barton-Burke acknowledges funding support from MSK Cancer Center Support Grant/Core Grant (P30 CA008748).

Nursing, Memorial Sloan Kettering Cancer Center, 1275 York Avenue, New York, NY 10065, USA
* Corresponding author.
E-mail address: Gordonj1@mskcc.org

STAGING

For all cancers, understanding staging is essential. Stage is the strongest predictor of survival and drives treatment planning. It is linked to screening, because screening may result in early stage cancer diagnosis, thus improving treatment outcomes. Accurate staging is critical for appropriate patient management.[2] The tumor, node, metastasis (TNM) staging system of the American Joint Committee on Cancer is the standard for all cancers. Some cancers use additional staging and grading systems. For example, the International Union against Cancer is used to stage colorectal cancer (CRC) and the Gleason score is used grade prostate cancer and plan treatment after diagnostic workup.

In the TNM system, the designation "T" refers to the local extent of the untreated primary tumor at the time of the diagnosis and initial workup. The designation "N" refers to the status of the lymph nodes, and "M" refers to distant metastatic disease.[3] In this article, **Table 1** presents the staging systems for colorectal, breast, and prostate cancers.

COLORECTAL CANCER

Colon and rectal cancers are often paired together and are referred to as CRC because they have similar characteristics and treatment. CRC usually originates from polyps lining the colon or rectum. The epithelial tissue and mucosal lining of the colon have many secreting glandular structures in which benign tumors form. These precancerous polyps are called adenomatous polyps or adenomas. Hyperplastic polyps and inflammatory polyps are more common, but are not precursors to cancer. CRC begins in the innermost layers of the lining of the large intestine and can grow through the various layers of the colon and into blood vessels or lymph vessels, thereby spreading to other organs and the lymph nodes.[4] **Fig. 1** provides a more detailed picture of those surrounding tissues.

Incidence

The American Cancer Society (ACS) estimates that there are 95,270 new cases of colon cancer and 39,220 new cases of rectal cancer in the United States in 2016. The lifetime risk of developing CRC is about 1 in 21 (4.7%) for men and 1 in 23 (4.4%) for women. CRC is the third leading cause of cancer-related deaths in the United States when men and women are considered separately. Combining both groups, CRC is the second leading cause of cancer-related death and expected to cause approximately 49,190 deaths in 2016.[5] The incidence of CRC has decreased since the mid 1980s by about 3.3% to 4% per year. This trend is thought to be owing to decreased risk factors such as smoking and improved prevention by removing polyps during routine colonoscopy and before they become cancerous.[6]

Risk Factors

Risk factors can be modifiable and nonmodifiable. Modifiable risk factors mean just that—if one changes certain behaviors their risk of getting cancer may be lower. In CRC, these include obesity/being overweight, decreased physical activity, smoking, diet, and alcohol use. It is suggested that there are several ways to modify risk for CRC, including increasing the intensity and duration of physical activity, limiting the intake of red and processed meat, consuming recommended levels of calcium, ensuring a sufficient vitamin D status, eating more vegetable and fruits, avoiding obesity and central weight gain (middle of the body), and avoiding excess alcohol consumption.[7] Nonmodifiable risk factors include age, race, ethnicity, a personal or family history of colon cancer or polyps, a history of inflammatory bowel disease, and diabetes.

Because cancer is a disease of aging, individuals over age 50, as well as African Americans, are at greater risk of developing CRC.[4] The incidence and mortality rates

Table 1
Staging of colorectal, breast, and prostate cancers

Cancer	Stage 0	Stage I	Stage II	Stage III	Stage IV
Colorectal	This is called cancer in situ. The tumor cells are only in the mucosa, or the inner lining, of the colon or rectum.	The tumor has grown through the mucosa and has invaded the muscular layer of the colon or rectum. It has not spread into nearby tissue or lymph nodes.	**IIA** The tumor has grown through the wall of the colon or rectum and has not spread to nearby tissue or to the nearby lymph nodes. **IIB** The tumor has grown through the layers of the muscle to the lining of the abdomen, called the visceral peritoneum. It has not spread to the nearby lymph nodes or elsewhere. **IIC** The tumor has spread through the wall of the colon or rectum and has grown into nearby structures. It has not spread to the nearby lymph nodes or elsewhere	**IIIA** The tumor has grown through the inner lining or into the muscle layers of the intestine and spread to 1 to 3 lymph nodes, or to a nodule of tumor in tissues around the colon or rectum that do not seem to be lymph nodes but has not spread to other parts of the body. **IIIB** The tumor has grown through the bowel wall or to surrounding organs and into 1 to 3 lymph nodes or to a nodule of tumor in tissues around the colon or rectum that do not seem to be lymph nodes, but it has not spread to other parts of the body. **IIIC** The tumor of the colon, regardless of how deep it has grown, has spread to 4 or more lymph nodes but not to other distant parts of the body.	**IVA** The tumor has spread to a single distant part of the body, such as the liver or lungs. **IVB** The tumor has spread to more than 1 part of the body.

(continued on next page)

Table 1
(continued)

Cancer	Stage 0	Stage I	Stage II	Stage III	Stage IV
Breast	Disease that is only in the ducts and lobules of the breast tissue and has not spread to the surrounding tissue of the breast. It is also called noninvasive cancer or in situ.	I The tumor is small, invasive, and has not spread to the lymph nodes or only has microscopic amounts of cancer found in the lymph nodes. These cancers are 20 mm or less (2 cm) in size.	II Breast tumor is between 20 mm (2 cm) and 50 mm (5 cm) in size and may or may not have spread to the axillary lymph nodes. Stage II cancers may be larger tumors with no spread to the lymph nodes or smaller tumors with cancer that has spread to 3 or less axillary lymph nodes but not to distant parts of the body.	IIIA The tumor of any size has spread to 4 to 9 axillary lymph nodes, but not to other parts of the body. Stage IIIA may also be a tumor larger than 50 mm that has spread to 1 to 3 lymph nodes. IIIB The tumor has spread to the chest wall or caused swelling or ulceration of the breast or is diagnosed as inflammatory breast cancer. It may not have spread to the lymph nodes under the arm, but it has not spread to other parts of the body. IIIC A tumor of any size that has not spread to distant parts of the body but has spread to 10 or more axillary lymph nodes.	The tumor can be any size and has spread to other organs, such as the bones, lungs, brain, liver, distant lymph nodes, or chest wall.

| Prostate | No evidence of disease. | Tumor is found in the prostate only, usually during another medical procedure. It cannot be felt during the DRE or seen on imaging tests. A stage I cancer is usually made up of cells that look more like healthy cells and is usually slow growing. | This stage describes a tumor that is too small to be felt or seen on imaging tests. Or, it describes a slightly larger tumor that can be felt during a digital rectal examination. The tumor has not spread outside of the prostate gland, but the cells are usually more abnormal and may tend to grow more quickly. A stage II tumor has not spread to lymph nodes or distant organs. | The tumor has spread beyond the outer layer of the prostate into nearby tissues. It may also have spread to the seminal vesicles. | This stage describes any tumor that has spread to other parts of the body, such as the bladder, rectum, bone, liver, lungs, or lymph nodes. |

Abbreviation: DRE, digital rectal examination.

Data from American Cancer Society. What is colorectal cancer? Available at: http://www.cancer.org/acs/groups/cid/documents/webcontent/003096-pdf.pdf; and National Comprehensive Cancer Network Guidelines for Data from NCCN Clinical Practice Guidelines in Oncology (NCCN Guidelines) Prostate Cancer. Available at: http://www.nccn.org/patients. Accessed July 3, 2016.

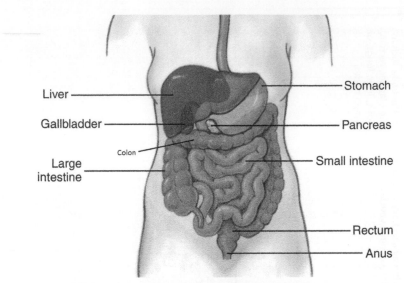

Fig. 1. Anatomy of the colon and rectum. (*From* Applegate EJ. The anatomy and physiology learning system. 4th edition. Philadelphia: Saunders; 2011.)

of CRC are decreasing among all age groups over 50 years. Yet, the incidence and mortality are increasing in younger individuals for whom screening is limited and key symptoms may go unrecognized.[8] Currently, research is being conducted to confirm if factors such as night shift work and previous treatment for certain cancers impact an individual's risk of developing CRC.[4]

Screening and Detection

Screening for CRC prevents cancer through the detection and removal of precancerous growths, as well as detecting cancer at an early stage when treatment is more effective. Screening reduces CRC mortality both by decreasing the incidence of disease and by increasing the likelihood of survival.[5] The US Preventive Services Task Force (USPSTF) recommends screening using high-sensitivity fecal occult blood testing, sigmoidoscopy, and/or colonoscopy beginning at age 50 years and continuing until age 75 years.[7] A summary of screening recommendations and intervals for CRC can be found in **Table 2**.

Genetics play a major role in CRC. Thirty percent of patients with CRC have a family history of CRC.[9] High-risk individuals are those with a family history of colorectal polyps or CRC, a history of inflammatory bowel disease, or a genetic syndrome such as familial adenomatous polyposis or hereditary nonpolyposis CRC. These individuals may require earlier or more frequent screenings.[10]

Early in the course of CRC, individuals may be asymptomatic or signs and symptoms may be vague like abdominal pain, flatulence, and minor changes in bowel movements with or without rectal bleeding. This is in contrast with the signs and symptoms of late cancer, which include severe pain that is sacral or sciatic in origin, anorexia and weight loss, jaundice, pruritus, ascites, hepatomegaly, and renal impairment.[11]

Treatment

Surgery

Surgery is the main treatment option for early stage tumors. The type of surgery used depends on the stage, location, and goal of the operation. A polypectomy involves

Table 2
US Preventive Services Task Force colorectal cancer screening guidelines

		Recommended Screening Guidelines		
Cancer Type	Diagnostic Examination	Age	Frequency	Comments
Breast	Mammogram	40–44	Option to begin annually	No clinical breast examination for breast cancer screening among average-risk women at any age.
		45–54	Annually	
		55–74	Biennially	
		≥75	Biennially until ≤10 y left of life expectancy	
Colon	High sensitivity guaiac-based fecal occult blood test	≥50	Annually[b] OR	
	Fecal immunochemical test		Annually[b] OR	
	Stool DNA test		Every 3 y[a] OR	
	Flexible sigmoidoscopy		Every 5 y[a] OR	
	Colonoscopy		Every 10 y OR	
	Double-contrast barium enema		Every 5 y[a] OR	
	CT "virtual" colonography		Every 5 y[a]	
Prostate	PSA Digital rectal examination	50 (average risk). 45 (High risk -African American or men with first degree relative diagnosed before 65 y of age). 40 (higher risk - more than 1 first-degree relative diagnosed before 65 y of age).	Biennially for PSA of <2.5 ng/mL Yearly for PSA level ≥2.5 ng/mL	If a man has a high PSA level and a biopsy of prostate does not show cancer, a prostate cancer gene 3 (PCA3) test may be done, which measures amount of PCA3 in urine.

Abbreviation: PSA, prostate-specific antigen.
[a] If the test is positive, a colonoscopy should be done.
[b] The multiple stool take-home test should be used. One test done in the office is not enough. A colonoscopy should be done if the test is positive.
Data from US Preventive Services Task Force. Breast cancer: screening. Available at: https://www.uspreventiveservicestaskforce.org/Page/Document/UpdateSummaryFinal/breast-cancer-screening1 and US Preventive Services Task Force, Final Recommendation Statement Colorectal Cancer: Screening; and US Preventive Services Task Force, Final Recommendation Statement Colorectal Cancer: Screening. Available at: https://www.uspreventiveservicestaskforce.org/Page/Document/Recommendation StatementFinal/colorectal-cancer-screening2; and American Cancer Society. Test for Prostate Cancer. Available at: http://www.cancer.org/cancer/prostatecancer/detailedguide/prostate-cancer-diagnosis. Accessed August, 2016.

removal of a polyp from the colon or rectum and is usually done during colonoscopy; a local excision removes superficial cancers and surrounding tissues; and a partial or total colectomy is a more advanced surgery removing a portion or the entire colon. Depending on the location of the cancer, some CRC operations involve a temporary or permanent colostomy to aid in waste elimination.[12]

Radiation therapy

Radiation therapy for rectal cancer may be used before surgery to decrease tumor size. Both colon and rectal cancer patients who are not surgical candidates can receive radiation to help control the disease, related symptoms, and areas of metastasis. At times, radiation therapy is administered concurrently with chemotherapy to enhance the effectiveness of both treatments. Radiation therapy or chemotherapy administered to patients who have undergone primary treatment, usually potentially curative surgical resection, is referred to as adjuvant therapy. Adjuvant treatment increases long-term survival, essentially by treating any micrometastases that remain after surgery.

Radiation poses significant toxicity potential to the cells of the gut owing to the rapid turnover of mucosal cells. Potential side effects of radiation include enteritis, diarrhea, nausea, vomiting, and flank pain.[13] The side effects of radiation can become worse as treatment continues and, therefore, requiring frequent and thorough assessment and intervention.

Systemic therapy

In CRC, chemotherapy is administered to patients if their disease recurs or metastasizes to other areas of the body. Standard first-line chemotherapy for metastatic colon cancer consists of 2 primary regimens: FOLFOX (5-FU, leucovorin, and oxaliplatin) or FOLFIRI (5-FU, leucovorin, and irinotecan). Adding bevacizumab (Avastin), a monoclonal antibody that cuts off nutrient supplies to the tumor by suppressing blood vessel growth (antiangiogenesis) may help to improve survival when added to either treatment regimen. Cetuximab (Erbitux) and panitumumab (Vectibix), both monoclonal antibodies targeting epidermal growth factor receptor, have been shown to improve survival when administered with multiagent chemotherapy. However, these antibodies are only effective in patients whose tumors possess certain cellular markers or characterisitics.[14]

Patients with metastatic CRC receiving an antiangiogenic agent in combination with chemotherapy may experience toxicities related to both chemotherapy and the antiangiogenic agent.[15] Clinical trials established the usefulness of antiangiogenic agents combined with new drugs in prolonging the survival of patients with advanced disease.[16] The complexity of the angiogenesis process presents a pathway with multiple cellular targets that can be disrupted and therefore decrease, slow, or stop cancer growth. Newer agents, such as ziv-aflibercept (Zaltrap) and regorafenib (Stivarga), increase the chance for successful angiogenesis inhibition resulting in tumor death.[17]

Future Directions

The scientific understanding of CRC is expanding with a focus on genetics, immunology, and newer targeted treatments. Immunotherapy, also called biologic therapy, is a type of cancer treatment designed to boost the body's natural defenses to fight the cancer. Immunotherapy is a promising area of cancer research that has delivered effective new treatments that, in some patients, achieve curelike responses. Progress specific to CRC immunotherapy has been limited; however, some new agents are being studied currently in early phase clinical trials and include viruses, vaccines, and cell therapy.[18]

BREAST CANCER

Breast cancer occurs when cells from the ducts or lobules of the breast (**Fig. 2**) become malignant, replicate, and spread outside their tissue of origin. Breast cancer is predominantly a disease of women; however, 1% of men develop breast cancer annually as well. When cancer cells invade beyond the original gland or duct, the

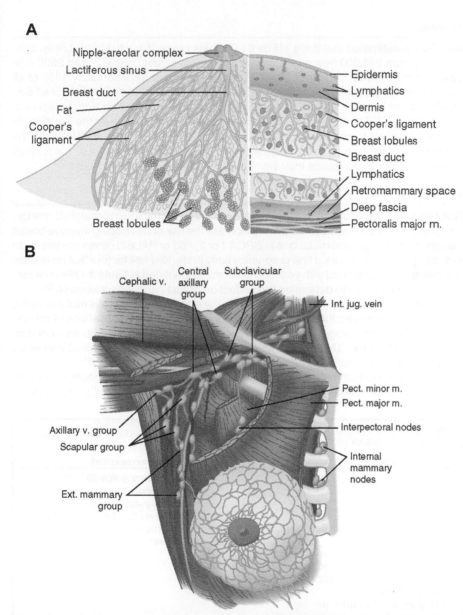

Fig. 2. Anatomy of the breast and regional lymph nodes. (*A*) Breast anatomy. The cutaway on the right illustrates the tissue layers. The breast is supported by deep fascia and muscle. (*B*) The axillary anatomy, showing lymph node drainage and the vascular supply. (*From* Donegan WL, Spratt JS. Cancer of the breast. Philadelphia: WB Saunders; 1988; with permission.)

tumor is considered invasive; if it is caught before this occurs, it is called in situ. Invasive breast cancer is classified into subtypes based on the presence of receptors found in and on the surface of the cell, these biomarkers include estrogen and progesterone receptor expression and HER2 amplification. When breast cancer cells do not express these biomarkers, it is called triple negative breast cancer.[19]

Incidence

In 2016, it is estimated that there will be 61,000 new cases of in situ female breast cancer, more than 246,000 new cases of invasive female breast cancer,[19] and 2600 new cases of male breast cancer.[20] These statistics represent approximately 14% of all new cancer diagnoses in the United States.[21] Although 89% of those diagnosed survive 5 years or longer, there are more than 40,000 individuals who die from breast cancer annually.[19–21] The incidence of breast cancer remained stable over the last decade except for a slight increase in incidence in African American women. In the 1970s, the lifetime risk of developing breast cancer was 1 in 11, whereas today it is 1 in 8 for all women. Both of these trends may be related to increased screening rates.[20]

Risk Factors

Risk factors for breast cancer are the subject of much epidemiologic research. Some behaviors and characteristics are known to increase the risk of developing invasive breast cancer, such as a genetic mutations in BRCA 1 or 2, P53 or PALB2; others are known to decrease risk, for example, a first pregnancy early in life. Key risk factors that have been established and confirmed with years of research are identified in **Table 3**. Other risk factors are being studied to determine their effect on breast cancer development.[20]

Over many years, research has focused on the effects of exogenous (not produced by the body) hormones throughout the lifecycle. The postmenopausal use of combination estrogen and progestin hormone replacement is associated with an increased risk for breast cancer. This risk increases the longer these drugs are used and when initiated near menopause.[22–24]

Studies suggest that high-dose estrogen and progesterone contraceptives initiated before age 20 or before a first pregnancy can increase the risk of breast cancer.

Table 3
Risk factors for breast cancer

Known to Increase Risk	Known to Decrease Risk
Smoking	First pregnancy ≤ age 20
Obesity	Breastfeeding >12 mo
Older age	Routine physical exercise
Increased breast density	Chemoprevention (ie, tamoxifen)
Menses ≤ age 11 or menopause ≥ age 55	Prophylactic mastectomy and salpingo-oopherectomy
First child birth ≥ age 35	
Radiation exposure between ages 10 and 30	
Diethylstilbestrol taken during pregnancy	
Germ line mutations (eg, BRCA 1, BRCA 2, P53, PALB2, PTEN)	
Alcohol intake of >1 drink per day	
Two or more first-degree relatives with breast cancer	
Breast cancer diagnosis before age 40	
Estrogen and progesterone replacement after menopause	
History of ductal carcinoma in situ or lobular carcinoma in situ	
Biopsy showing atypical ductal or lobular hyperplasia	

Data from American Cancer Society. Breast cancer facts & figures 2015-2016. Available at: http://www.cancer.org/acs/groups/content/@research/documents/document/acspc-046381.pdf. Accessed July 3, 2016.

However, risk begins to decrease after discontinuation of contraceptive use and returns to average after 10 years.[25,26] There is not enough research regarding newer agents including medroxyprogesterone acetate (Depo-Provera) and a levonorgestrel-releasing intrauterine device (Mirena) to establish a risk relationship to breast cancer.[20]

A link has also been established between increased breast density and an increased risk for breast cancer.[27] This information, combined with the fact that increased density impairs mammographic screening efficacy, led to new legislation requiring mammogram reports to include information on breast density, the impact on a patient's mammogram, and the potential benefit of additional screening examinations.[28] This does not mean that all patients with dense breasts should undergo additional testing, but reinforces that screening modalities are not one size fits all and should be chosen based on risk and individual characteristics.[29]

Screening and Detection

Screening for breast cancer is done using mammography, a radiographic image of the breast that looks for abnormal calcifications or other abnormalities such as densities or asymmetries. There are multiple recommendations from various organizations regarding when to initiate screening mammograms, the frequency, and when to discontinue (**Table 4**).[30–32] While recommendations are clarified, it is important that women have a discussion with their health care team about the appropriateness of mammography screenings for them. To prevent changes in insurance reimbursement for mammography while a consensus between organizations is reached, Congress called for third-party payers to reimburse based on the prior recommendations.[32]

Two new screening modalities have been approved recently by the US Food and Drug Administration (FDA): tomosynthesis, or 3-dimensional mammography, and contrast-enhanced spectral mammography. Tomosynthesis uses high-resolution radiographic images to create a 3-dimensional image of the breast,[33] whereas contrast-enhanced spectral mammography uses iodinated contrast injection to emphasize areas of suspicion, similar to an MRI but with decreased cost.[34] Both methods have the potential to decrease recall rates and increase detection of invasive cancers, particularly in women with dense breasts.[33,34] There is a 2-fold increase in radiation exposure with tomosynthesis, but it still falls below the FDA threshold for exposure.[33] Neither of these new options is available widely yet and insurance coverage for imaging varies.[33,34]

Table 4 Mammography screening guidelines for average-risk women			
Age (y)	USPSTF	ACS	ACR
40–44	Not recommended unless desired	Not recommended unless desired	Not recommended unless desired
45–49	Not recommended unless desired	Annually	Annually
50–54	Biennially	Annually	Annually
55–74	Biennially	Biennially	Annually or biennially
≥75	Not recommended	Biennially until ≤10 y left of life expectancy	Biennially until ≤10 y left of life expectancy

Abbreviations: ACR, American College of Radiology; ACS, American Cancer Society; USPSTF, US Preventive Services Task Force.
Data from Refs.[30–32]

Treatment

Breast cancer treatment is a multimodality approach that includes local and regional control of disease with surgery and/or radiation therapy as well as systemic control with chemotherapy, biotherapy, and/or hormonal therapy. Biomarkers play a significant role in the treatment plan but, as mentioned, the stage of the disease drives the plan of care and goal of treatment (**Table 5**).

Surgery: local and regional control

Surgical removal of the tumor is the primary treatment for women with stages I through III breast cancer. Breast-conserving surgery is usually a lumpectomy (removal of tumor and surrounding margin), whereas a mastectomy is the removal of the entire breast. The method used depends on many factors, such as tumor size, breast size, subtype of breast cancer, and patient preference.[20] The goal of breast surgery is removal of the tumor, leaving tumor margins without evidence of the breast cancer. Margins may be reexcised until there is no local evidence of the cancer and this is done to reduce the rate of local recurrence.[35]

Usually, surgical procedures are the first stage in a breast cancer treatment plan. If and when necessary, surgery is followed by systemic therapy. Systemic therapy can be either radiation or chemotherapy, and in many cases it is both. The use of radiation or chemotherapy after surgery is considered adjuvant treatment. Radiation therapy is used after breast-conserving therapy and in some high-risk individuals who undergo mastectomy.[20]

In certain clinical scenarios, the treatment plan includes completing surgery after chemotherapy. This is called neoadjuvant therapy. Indications for the use of neoadjuvant therapy include large inoperable tumors that cannot be completely removed because of size or location, cancers that cannot undergo breast-conserving surgery (eg, inflammatory breast cancer), cosmetic outcomes from surgery, or those who would benefit from delaying surgery such as with a contraindication for undergoing surgery such as pregnancy. The use of chemotherapy preoperatively does not change the risk of recurrence or overall survival.[36]

Surgical removal of axillary lymph nodes and sentinel lymph node biopsies (SLNB) add to the accuracy of staging a breast cancer. Sentinel lymph nodes are generally the first nodes where cancer cells spread once they leave the original tumor. An SLNB is used as a diagnostic tool in cases where there are no signs of lymph node involvement on either physical examination or imaging.[37]

Before 2010, the standard of care for anyone with a positive SLNB was a full surgical removal of axillary lymph nodes. New research related to overall survival suggests that some patients with T1 or T2 tumors choosing breast-conserving surgery and radiation therapy can avoid additional axillary surgery if SLNB does not yield 3 or more positive lymph nodes.[38] The use of SLNB results in fewer axillary lymph nodes being removed surgically and decreasing the rates of postoperative wound infections, lymphedema, seromas, and paresthesias.[39]

Table 5		
Breast cancer treatment approaches by stage		
Stage	**Treatment Strategy**	**Treatment Goal**
Early (stages I and II)	Surgery ± radiation → systemic	Cure
Locally advanced (stage III)	Systemic → surgery ± radiation ± additional Systemic	Cure and/or improved local control
Metastatic (stage IV)	Systemic ± radiation	Control/palliation

Systemic therapy

Many agents, chemotherapies, biotherapies, and endocrine therapies, are used in the treatment of breast cancer. These agents are used based on tumor characteristics like biomarkers, and whether these agents will be used as single agents or in combination is determined by the stage of disease.[37] Although various regimens exist for breast cancer, the National Comprehensive Cancer Network identified preferred regimens based on the strongest evidence. Preferred regimens for adjuvant, neoadjuvant, and metastatic breast cancer can be found in **Table 6**.

The 21st century, most notably the last 5 years, has included many drug discoveries affecting the systemic treatment of breast cancer. These findings are based on personalized medicine, wherein treatment plans are developed based on the individual's cancer subtype, biomarkers or other characteristics. This has changed the treatment paradigm, shifting away from cytotoxic chemotherapies toward biologic and targeted agents that act on molecular markers within the cancer cell.[38] Everolimus (Afinitor) and palbociclib (Ibrance) are oral agents used in combination with standard antiestrogen treatments. Adding everolimus to exemestane, a standard endocrine treatment regimen, improves effectiveness in individuals who become resistant to antiestrogen therapy.[40] Both palbociclib and everolimus also demonstrated the ability to lengthen time until disease progression.[40,41]

Groundbreaking discoveries in the treatment of Her2-positive breast cancer included trastuzumab (Herceptin) in 1998 and pertuzumab (Perjeta) in 2012. The addition of trastuzumab to standard chemotherapy decreases recurrence rates by 11.5% and improves overall survival by 8.8%. The addition of pertuzumab to trastuzumab and standard chemotherapy then demonstrated a 16-month increase in overall survival for patients with metastatic breast cancer.[42] Clinically, there is a 21% increase in cases where there is no residual cancer found when patients undergo surgery after receiving the treatment.[43]

In 2013, the first antibody–drug conjugate, ado-trastuzumab emtansine (Kadcyla), was approved by the FDA for Her2 6+ patients. This novel therapy binds a chemotherapeutic drug, DM1, a microtubule binding agents, to the biologic agent, trastuzumab. This delivery method protects the patient from the severe side effects of chemotherapeutic drug[44] while increasing progression-free survival by 3.2 months and overall survival by 5.8 months.[45,46]

Future Directions

The rate of scientific discovery in breast cancer is unprecedented. Researchers believe they are nearing conclusive findings on the link between obesity, inflammation,

Table 6
Breast cancer neoadjuvant/adjuvant regimens. NCCN preferred systemic treatments for breast cancer

Combinations for Her2-Negative Cancers	Combinations for Her2-Positive Cancers	Endocrine Treatments
DD AC →DD T	DD AC → THP	Anastrzole (Arimidex)
DD AC → weekly T	Docetaxel/carboplatin/H ± P	Letrzole (Femara)
Docetaxel/cyclophosphamide		Exemestane (Aromasin)
		Tamoxifen

Abbreviations: AC, doxorubicin/cyclophosphamide; CMF, cyclophosphamide/methotrexate/fluorouracil; DD, dose dense; H, trastuzumab; P, pertuzumab; T, paclitaxel.

Data from NCCN Clinical Practice Guidelines in Oncology (NCCN Guidelines) breast cancer. Available at: http://www.nccn.org/patients.

and breast cancer risk and those with triple negative breast cancer or who are BRCA positive may soon find hope for better disease control with a new class of agents, the poly adenosine diphosphate-ribose polymerase (PARP) inhibitors.[47] Like with CRC, immunotherapy shows promise with the study of ipilumimab in the breast cancer population,[48] and vaccine therapy clinical trials are ongoing.[46]

Bone health management has expanded beyond fracture prevention by treating osteopenia and osteoporosis. It now seems that the introduction of bisphosphonates may decrease metastases to the bone in early stage breast cancer. One study found that, when bisphosphonates are added to the treatment plan for postmenopausal women, there may be improved survival benefits.[49] Oncology teams are reviewing their current standard of care for bisphosphonate use and weighing the potential risks and benefits.

PROSTATE CANCER

Prostate cancer is cancer of the prostate gland. The prostate is a walnut-sized gland located at the base of the bladder and in front of the rectum. A gland found only in men, it creates the fluid that is a part of semen. Most prostate cancers are adenocarcinomas, originating from glandular cells. **Fig. 3** provides an illustration of the prostate gland.

Incidence

Prostate cancer is the most common cancer diagnosed in men in the United States and the second leading cause of cancer-related death. Prostate cancer, like most cancers, develops with age and its incidence is on the rise.[50] According to the ACS, in 2016 there were about 180,890 new cases of prostate cancer and 26,120 deaths from prostate cancer. The lifetime risk for a white man is 1 in 7, but there is a lifetime risk of 1 in 6 black men being diagnosed with prostate cancer. The majority of prostate cancers are diagnosed in men age 65 and older. After lung cancer, prostate cancer is the second leading cause of death in American men and approximately 1 in every 39 men will die from the disease.[51] Meanwhile, prostate cancer and CRC, along with lung cancer, are the major causes of death from cancer in black men.[52]

Prostate cancer occurs more often in black men than in white men. Black men have the highest death rate from prostate cancer of any racial or ethnic group. This difference reflects higher incidence rates among black men as well as variations in treatment patterns by race group.[52] Black men are also more likely to have advanced disease at the time of diagnosis. The reasons for these racial and ethnic differences are unclear. However, what is known is that black men are less likely to receive surgical treatment than their white counterparts with similar disease.

The National Comprehensive Cancer Network[50] estimates that the age-adjusted death rates are decreasing annually. The decrease in the death rate may be attributed to public awareness, with early detection and treatment or specific prostate cancer treatment. Unlike many other primary cancers, prostate cancer continues to be treated effectively by numerous modalities. Although prostate cancer is a serious cancer, most men do not die from this disease. According to the ACS,[51] there are more than 2.9 million men living with prostate cancer today.

Risk Factors

Prostate cancer has no specific presenting symptoms and the etiology of prostate cancer is not understood completely: The most common risk factor for prostate cancer is age. The known risk factors for prostate cancer are age, race/ethnicity,

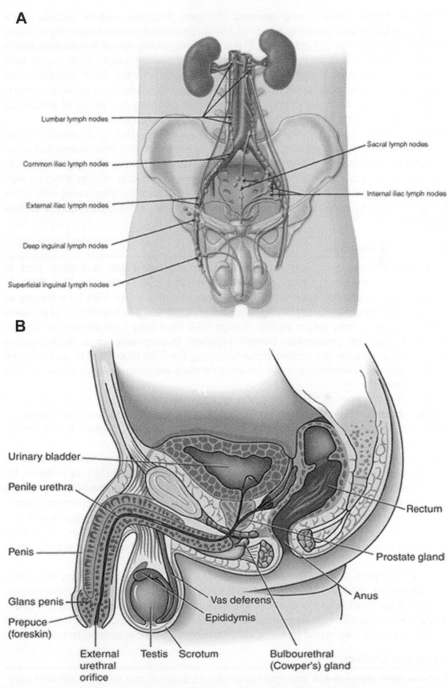

A

Lumbar lymph nodes

Common iliac lymph nodes

External iliac lymph nodes

Deep inguinal lymph nodes

Superficial inguinal lymph nodes

Sacral lymph nodes

Internal iliac lymph nodes

B

Urinary bladder

Penile urethra

Penis

Glans penis

Prepuce
(foreskin)

External
urethral
orifice

Testis   Scrotum

Vas deferens

Epididymis

Bulbourethral
(Cowper's) gland

Rectum

Prostate gland

Anus

Fig. 3. (*A*) Anatomy of the prostate and regional lymph nodes. (*B*) Male reproductive system. (*From* Warekois RS, Robinson R, editors. Phlebotomy. St Louis (MO): Saunders Elsevier; 2007; and Paulsen F. Pelvis and retroperitoneal space. In: Paulsen F, Waschke J, editors. Sobotta atlas of human anatomy. Fifteenth Edition. München: Elsevier/Urban-Fischer; 2011. p. 157–240.)

geography, family history, and genetic changes. Prostate cancer occurs more frequently in black and Caribbean men of African descent and less frequently in Asian American and Hispanic or Latino men.[52] It is most commonly found in men from North America, Europe, Australia, and the islands of the Caribbean. It is found less commonly in Asia, Africa, Central American, and South America. Most prostate cancers occur in men without a family history, although there may be a genetic component to this cancer. Men with Lynch syndrome and inherited mutations of BRCA1 or BRCA2 genes may be at higher risk of developing prostate cancer.[51]

Researchers found factors that may affect risk include lifestyle and heredity.[53] The role of diet, obesity, and smoking are inconclusive regarding the development of prostate cancer. However, there is a growing body of literature linking these 3 lifestyle factors to an overall increase in cancer risk.[51,52] The risk of prostate cancer is higher with a family history of the disease and men with a father or brother diagnosed with prostate cancer have a higher risk if the relative was diagnosed with prostate cancer before the age of 60.

Screening and Detection

The prostate gland produces prostate-specific antigen (PSA), a protein that at increased levels may be a sign of prostate cancer. The PSA test can identify clinically asymptomatic, nonlethal tumors.[54] Screening examinations like PSA level begins at age 50 unless there is a history of prostate cancer. If there is a family history of prostate cancer, screening may begin earlier. A high PSA level may indicate noncancerous conditions such as prostatitis, benign prostatic hyperplasia, or a false-positive reading. Although prostate cancer screening using the PSA blood test is controversial and the evidence is equivocal, most prostate cancers are diagnosed as a result of this screening test.[54]

The ACS recommends that men make an informed decision with their health care provider about whether to be screened for prostate cancer. The decision should be made after an explanation about the uncertainties, risks, and potential benefits of prostate cancer screening.

Different recommendations have been proposed by various organizations, such as the American Urological Association, the ACS, and the National Cancer Network for PSA. However, the most influential group, the United States Preventive Services Task Force, is reviewing the literature currently and updating their screening recommendation. Prostate cancers are generally slow growing but can be aggressive biologically. The ACS recommends annual digital rectal examination and PSA screening in men over the age of 50. Screening for men at higher risk should begin at age 45.[54]

Symptoms, such as frequent urge or inability to urinate, trouble starting or holding back urine flow, frequent pain or stiffness in the lower back, hips, or upper thighs, and painful ejaculation or trouble having an erection, may be associated with a prostate cancer diagnosis.[53] Other associated symptoms include blood in the urine, pain in the hips, back (spine), chest (ribs), or other areas from cancer spread to bones.[52]

Staging and Grading

As mentioned, stage is the strongest predictor of survival and drives treatment planning for prostate cancer. Stage determines the extent of spread of the disease and **Table 1** identifies the details for prostate cancer staging. However, grading for prostate cancer is a unique system called a Gleason score. The histologic grade of prostate adenocarcinomas is usually reported according to the Gleason scoring system. This system is an adjunct to tumor staging and helps in determining prognosis. The

Gleason score is calculated based on the dominant histologic grades, from grade 1 (well-differentiated) to grade 5 (very poorly differentiated).[52,53] The score is derived by adding the 2 most prevalent pattern grades using scores ranging from 2 to 10 (eg, Gleason score 3 + 4 = 7; or 4 + 3 = 7).[52] Just like in staging, the higher the score (number), the more aggressive the cancer.

Treatment

The treatment choices for prostate cancer include single or a combination of therapies ranging from patients being offered watchful waiting or active surveillance, minimally invasive surgery, radiation therapy including brachytherapy, cryotherapy, hormonal manipulation, and chemotherapy or investigational drugs administered in a clinical trial, including the use of vaccines.[53] Patients with localized disease, cancer confined to the prostate, may be treated with surgery to remove the prostate (radical prostatectomy), cryotherapy, or radiation therapy.

Men with prostate cancer that has spread outside the prostate, or who cannot undergo radiation therapy or surgery, and men whose cancer has recurred after surgery or radiation therapy may need chemotherapy, hormonal therapy, and/or radiation therapy.[50]

Watchful waiting or active surveillance

Watchful waiting is used to watch for any changes and hold off on more direct treatment while monitoring the tumor closely for signs of growth.[55] It is used for the diagnosis of early stage prostate cancer and is offered as an option for older males with comorbidities. Active surveillance, formerly called watchful waiting, is a choice for localized prostate cancer; the patient puts off treatment until test results show that the prostate cancer is growing or changing. Examinations every 3 to 6 months include digital rectal examination and PSA with or without a biopsy during this period. This treatment approach is warranted if there are noticeable clinical changes in the prostate gland.[50–52]

Radiation therapy

External beam radiation therapy (EBRT) may be administered in curative doses to treat men with early prostate cancer and may be an option for patients wishing to avoid surgery or who are not candidates for surgery.[53] Radiation therapy is useful in managing complications of advanced prostate cancer, including side effects such as hematuria, urinary obstruction, urethral obstruction, and pelvic pain. Radiation therapy is used for a variety of reasons. It is a possible treatment choice if the prostate cancer is only in the prostate, or if it has spread to organs and tissue near the prostate; the patient is using hormone therapy; the disease returns after treatment; or it is used to reduce symptoms of advanced prostate cancer.

Men with localized prostate cancer may be candidates for a form of targeted radiation therapy called brachytherapy, in which tiny radioactive seeds are implanted surgically into the prostate: low-level radiation from the seeds kills the cancer cells. Other forms of radiation therapy, such as 3-dimensional conformal radiation therapy using sophisticated computer technology to shape radiation beam to the contours of a tumor, and intensity-modulated radiation therapy, in target of the tumor with radiation beams of different intensities, are used to minimize the radiation dose to the nearby strong tissues.

Brachytherapy, also called interstitial radiation (seed treatment), is standard therapy for prostate cancer and involves the placement of radioactive seeds directly into the prostate. It may be used alone or combined with EBRT. Implants may be permanent or temporary and patients with early stage disease may be offered brachytherapy as a single modality therapy or in locally advanced disease as a boost to primary therapy. Patients with a localized relapse receive brachytherapy as salvage therapy.[53] Image-guided radiation therapy delivers radiation while taking pictures of the tumor. Stereotactic body radiotherapy uses precise, high-dose beams offering targeted EBRT. This EBRT may be administered in curative doses treating men with early prostate cancer and may be an option for patients wishing to avoid surgery or who are not candidates for surgery.[53]

Radiation therapy is useful in managing complications of advanced prostate cancer, including side effects such as hematuria, urinary obstruction, urethral obstruction, and pelvic pain. Radiation therapy is a choice if prostate cancer is localized or if it has spread to organs and tissue near the prostate gland. It may also be used if the patient is using hormone therapy or the disease has returned after treatment, and it is used to reduce symptoms of advanced prostate cancer.[50]

Cryotherapy is a treatment offered when radiation therapy does not work or fails. Cryosurgery freezes prostate tumor cells, killing the cancer. The side effects of cryotherapy include urinary retention, painful swelling, and penile paresthesia. Long-term side effects include erectile dysfunction, stress incontinence, fistulas, and blockage of the urethra with rectal scar tissue.[56]

Surgery

Prostate cancer surgery offers better clinical outcomes for clinical stage T1 or T2 prostate cancer when the disease is confined to the prostate gland. When the PSA level is less than 20 ng/mL and the Gleason score is 8, there is a better chance of cure. Surgery for prostate cancer is restricted to men who are healthy enough to tolerate a major operation with 10-year or more life expectancy.[56]

According to the Urology Care Foundation, radical prostatectomy is a surgical removal of the prostate, seminal vesicles, nearest parts of the vas deferens, nearby tissue, and some pelvic lymph nodes. Prostate cancer usually spreads first to the soft tissues around the prostate. Then, it spreads to the seminal vesicles, lymph nodes, bones, and other organs. There are 4 types of radical prostatectomy surgery: retropubic open radical prostatectomy, perineal open radical prostatectomy, laparoscopic radical prostatectomy and robotic-assisted laparoscopic radical prostatectomy, and transurethral resection of the prostate.

Retropubic open radical prostatectomy is the most common type of prostate surgery and allows the prostate gland to be removed with limited blood loss. The neurovascular bundles and erectile function are preserved. In a perineal open radical prostatectomy, cuts are made between the anus and scrotum to remove the prostate. This surgery is not a common surgical choice today.

State of the art laparoscopic radical prostatectomy and robotic-assisted laparoscopic radical prostatectomy are the newer treatment choices. Laparoscopic prostatectomy entails the removal of the prostate gland and associated structures, including the seminal vesicles and pelvic lymph nodes.[50] Radical prostatectomy involves the removal of the prostate gland, ejaculatory ducts, seminal vesicles, and possibly the lymph nodes. Prostatectomy may offer a cure if the cancer has not spread beyond the gland.[57]

Other surgical interventions include a pelvic lymph node dissection, focal therapy, and a transurethral resection of the prostate. A pelvic lymph node dissection removes lymph nodes from the pelvis and is recommended for T1 or T2 tumors. The pelvic lymph node dissection varies depending on the number of lymph nodes removed, but helps with staging the cancer.[50] Focal therapy is a minimally invasive technique for eliminating small tumors confined to the prostate that show no signs of being aggressive[56] and transurethral resection of the prostate treats symptoms of bladder outlet obstruction with evidence that a previously unsuspected cancer is present.

Systemic therapy

Hormone therapy Hormone therapy is also known as androgen deprivation therapy or androgen suppression therapy. Patients who are not surgical candidates or those wishing to avoid surgery may choose this therapy. The goal of hormone therapy is to change the hormonal milieu of the body by reducing the level of circulating androgens to castration levels, causing the death of androgen-dependent cells and inhibiting the growth of androgen-sensitive cells, which reduce the tumor size. It can provide many patients with symptom control and palliation. An orchiectomy or luteinizing hormone treatment combined with nonsteroidal antiandrogenic drugs additionally suppress male hormone effects on the growth of prostate cancer cells.[53,54]

Chemotherapy Systemic therapy is recommended when the prostate cancer cells have metastasized from the gland or if the tumor is aggressive but there is no metastatic disease. An increased PSA after surgery or radiation therapy is indicative of either remaining tumor or a recurrence of the original prostate cancer and additional treatment may be necessary. Systemic therapy includes 1 or more of the following: hormone therapy, chemotherapy, biologic approaches, and immunotherapy, including vaccines.[58] **Table 7** lists drugs used to treat prostate cancer.

Chemotherapy is usually reserved for patients with advanced or progressive disease. Many chemotherapy drugs, such as docetaxel (Taxotere) and cabazitaxel (Jcvtana) have been shown to help men live longer.[51] The National Comprehensive Cancer

Table 7
Drug treatment for prostate cancer

Generic Name	Brand Name	Type of Treatment
Abiraterone acetate	Zytiga	Hormone therapy
Bicalutamide	Casodex	Hormone therapy
Cabazitaxel	Jeviana	Chemotherapy
Degarellix	Finmagon	Hormone therapy
Diethylstilbestrol	—	Hormone therapy
Docetaxel	Taxotere	Chemotherapy
Enzalutamide	Xlandi	Hormone therapy
Flutamide	—	Hormone therapy
Goserelin acetate	Zoladex	Hormone therapy
Histrelin acetate	Varitas	Hormone therapy
Ketaconazole	Nizoral	Hormone therapy
Leurprolide acetate	Eligard, Lupron Depot, Lupron	Hormone therapy
Miloxantrone hydrochloride	Novanitrone	Chemotherapy
Nilutamide	Nilandron	Hormone therapy
Prednisone	—	Hormone therapy
Radium-223	Xofigo	Radiopharmaceutical
Sipuleucel-T	Provenge	Immunotherapy
Triptoreline pamoate	Trelstar	Hormone therapy

Data from NCCN Clinical Practice Guidelines in Oncology (NCCN Guidelines) prostate cancer. Available at: http://www.nccn.org/patients.

Network recommends docetaxel and cabazitaxel to treat advance prostate cancer, whereas mitozantrone hydrochloride is used for symptom relief.[50]

Vaccines

Vaccines, being used to treat and boost the immune system, help fight prostate cancer. One vaccine approved in April 2010 by the FDA for use in metastatic prostate cancer patients is sipuleucel-T (Provenge).[53,56] It is designed to stimulate an immune response to prostatic acid phosphatase, an antigen found on most prostate cancer cells. In clinical trials, sipuleucel-T increased survival for a certain type of metastatic prostate cancer by approximately 4 months. Sipuleucel-T is individualized by isolating immune system cells called dendritic cells from a patient's blood. The dendritic cells cultured with PA2024, a (prostatic acid phosphatase) granulocyte colony stimulating factor fusion protein create the active component of sipuleucel-T and are infused into the patient to attack prostate cancer cells.[53,56]

Future Directions

Several types of vaccines to treat prostate cancer are being tested in clinical trials. One example is PROSTVAC, which uses a virus that has been genetically modified to contain PSA. The patient's immune system should respond to the virus and begin to recognize and destroy cancer cells containing PSA. Early results with this vaccine have been promising, and a larger study is now under way.[59,60]

Other innovations in treatment include checkpoint and network inhibitors, high-intensity focused ultrasound, and vascular targeted photodynamic therapy. Immune checkpoint inhibitors are another development in cancer treatment, where cancer cells use checkpoints to avoid being attacked by the immune system. Newer drugs targeting these checkpoints hold promise as cancer treatments. In mouse models, network inhibitors destabilize the proteins that prostate cancer cells use to evade existing treatments. These drugs target a network of signals, not just 1 pathway. This type of drug activity is less likely to result in drug resistance. High-intensity focused ultrasound is a treatment gaining ground in prostate cancer treatment, as is vascular-targeted photodynamic therapy. In vascular-targeted photodynamic therapy, there is a destruction of blood vessels leading to the prostate tumors. By stopping the blood supply to the tumor, it should theoretically stop growing with eventual apoptosis. Finally, complementary and alternative medicine, now called integrative oncology, is gaining interest for prostate cancer and it is being studied to determine benefits.[50,61]

NURSING CARE AND IMPLICATIONS

A cancer diagnosis can be devastating. Nurses must be prepared to provide physical care as well as emotional support throughout the continuum. The period immediately after diagnosis is difficult because it requires various decisions to be made at a time when the patient may not have yet come to terms with the diagnosis. Nurses should be knowledgeable to provide information regarding the extent of the disease as defined by staging and grading and available treatment options. Treatment decision-making should be approached by explaining the rationale for the modality, as well as the risks, benefits, and side effects for each intervention. Patients receiving systemic therapy require nursing care to help manage the chemotherapy side effects such as nausea, vomiting, diarrhea, constipation, fatigue, neuropathy, mucositis, hand–foot syndrome, hypersensitivity reactions, and myelosuppression. Radiation therapy side effects increase as the patient is treated and may or may not resolve completely when treatment finishes. Side effects of radiation may include changes in the skin at the site being radiated, keeping in mind that any organ within the radiation field maybe impacted; an example is bowel alterations with prostate cancer radiation treatments. Additionally, general side effects like fatigue take prolonged periods of time to resolve and can be worsened if the patient is also receiving chemotherapy. Patients should be educated in advance, because it will have a major impact on their quality of life.

Cancer patients require ongoing nursing assessment and care during and after treatment. Survivorship nursing care is essential for those living beyond treatment to manage the long-term side effects and to assess for disease recurrence. Advanced stage patients may require palliative and hospice care as well as greater involvement of caregivers to ensure end-of-life wishes are known and followed. Many health care professionals will be involved throughout the patient's diagnosis; however, the nurses' role as educator, advocate, advisor, and coordinator of care is instrumental in the cancer journey. Although these issues can occur regardless of the cancer type, there are unique nursing care needs based on the type of cancer as well.

Colorectal Cancer

Surgery for CRC patients may require a temporary or permanent colostomy, which drastically impacts the patient's body image and requires the nurse to provide ongoing psychosocial support and education to learn how to live with and care for the device.

Newer systemic drugs called antiangiogenic agents can be given alone or concurrently with chemotherapy and have an unusual side effect profile, which requires different nursing management. Toxicities commonly associated with antiangiogenic agents include hypertension, proteinuria, wound healing complications, bleeding or hemorrhage, thromboembolic events, hypersensitivity reactions, and gastrointestinal perforation. Patients require education regarding the importance of monitoring blood pressure, oral antihypertensive adherence, and reporting signs and symptoms of headache and bleeding immediately.

Breast Cancer

With every treatment modality, and even the disease itself, comes the need for more advancement in supportive care. This is an area predominantly managed by nursing, with collaborative decision making across the team. Side effects of treatment vary by the agent that the patient is on and are rarely unique in breast cancer. Nurses must be informed of the potential side effects of treatment and should be able to differentiate between expected side effects and concerning adverse events.

Within this population of patients, a notable side effect is alopecia related to treatment. It impacts self-esteem, body image and may lead patients to elect a less effective treatment to avoid it.[61,62] An intervention being reconsidered to combat alopecia is scalp cooling. Although commonly used in Europe, it has been met traditionally with doubt and concern in the United States.[63] Recent research demonstrating efficacy, safety, and tolerability,[63] coupled with FDA approval of the first cooling cap system suggests its incorporation into the future of breast cancer treatment is imminent, with nurses leading the reform of practice and education of patients.

Lymphedema, severe swelling owing to a collection of protein-rich lymph fluid, can occur in the arm or hand on the side where a patient has had lymph nodes removed or in the chest wall after lumpectomy or mastectomy. Patients who have had an axillary dissections should avoid medical procedures such as intravenous sticks and injections on the affected side. Although the incidence of lymphedema is much lower in those who have had SLNB, patients may also choose to avoid use of that arm when possible. Education is an essential component of nursing care in this patient population. Information on self-care practices to minimize the risk of developing lymphedema such as maintaining a healthy weight, engaging in full body exercise, and avoiding trauma such as cuts, bites, or burns in the arm or chest wall should be provided. Patients should be advised to report signs of lymphedema such as visible swelling, a sensation of heaviness, or new tightness in jewelry or clothing.

Prostate Cancer

Nurses must remain up to date regarding the multiple treatment options available as well as the nursing care associated with the disease. Nurses must also be active in prostate cancer education, screening, and early detection programs. Interventions to decrease physical, emotional, psychological, social, and spiritual distress during and after treatment must be reviewed with the patient. In addition to the aspects of care already mentioned, it is important to realize the meaning of the prostate in relationship to sexuality. It is important to address and promote sexual functioning throughout prostate cancer treatment into survivorship.

Patients with advanced prostate cancer may experience a number of symptoms requiring nursing management. They may include cachexia and weight loss, bone pain, spinal cord compression, fractures of the long bones, leg or scrotal edema, coagulation disorders, and bladder or urethral obstruction. It is important that nurses take part in all aspects of the patient care as the incidence and prevalence of prostate cancer continue to increase. Early detection programs that target vulnerable populations, public education and programs, and patient advocacy need to continue to be a priority of nursing.

SUMMARY

As oncology care continues to evolve and the population continues to grow and age, it is imperative that all nurses develop a basic knowledge of common cancers, because they will likely be caring for these patients in nononcology settings. This preparation includes a general understanding of the incidence, prevalence, risk factors, staging, and treatment options for common cancers. This understanding coupled with knowledge of what is forthcoming can help nurses to anticipate trends and care needs for oncology patients. Being familiar with updated information can improve early cancer diagnosis, lead to prompt cancer treatment, and result in increased survival and decreased mortality for individuals with cancer. More knowledgeable nurses will ensure that oncology patients receive safe and efficient care regardless of the clinical setting in which they are receiving care.

REFERENCES

1. American Cancer Society (ACS). Cancer facts & figures 2016. Atlanta (GA): American Cancer Society; 2016.
2. Institute of Medicine National Research Council. Fulfilling the potential of cancer prevention and early detection. Washington, DC: The National Academies Press; 2003. p. 174–218.
3. Compton CC, Greene FL. The staging of colorectal cancer: 2004 and beyond. CA Cancer J Clin 2004;54:295–308.
4. American Cancer Society (ACS). Colorectal cancer. 2016. Available at: http://www.cancer.org/cancer/colonandrectumcancer/detailedguide/colorectal-cancer-what-is-colorectal-cancer. Accessed March 7, 2016.

5. American Cancer Society (ACS). Colorectal cancer facts & figures 2014-2016. Atlanta (GA): American Cancer Society; 2014. Available at: http://www.cancer.org/cancer/colonandrectumcancer/detailedguide/colorectal-cancer-key-statistics.

6. Siegel R, Ma JU, Zou Z, et al. Cancer statistics 2014. CA Cancer J Clin 2014;64: 9–29.

7. Kushi LH, Doyle C, McCullough M, et al, The American Cancer Society 2010 Nutrition and Physical Activity Guidelines Advisory Committee. American Cancer Society guidelines on nutrition and physical activity for cancer prevention: reducing the risk of cancer with healthy food choices and physical activity. CA Cancer J Clin 2012;62:30–67.

8. Ahnen DA, Wade SW, Jones WF, et al. The increasing incidence of young-onset colorectal cancer: a call to action. Mayo Clinic Proc 2014;89(2):216–24.

9. Colorectal cancer: screening. U.S. Preventive Services Task Force (USPSTF); 2014. Available at: http://www.uspreventiveservicestaskforce.org/Page/Document/RecommendationStatementFinal/colorectal-cancer-screening. Accessed March 7, 2016.

10. Lodewijk AA, Brosens LA, Offerhaus GJ, et al. Hereditary colorectal cancer: genetics and screening. Surg Clin North America 1996;95(5):1067–80.

11. Centers for Disease Control and Prevention (CDC). Colorectal (colon) cancer. 2014. Available at: http://www.cdc.gov/cancer/colorectal/basic_info/screening/index.htm. Accessed February 12, 2016.

12. Wilkes GM. Colon, rectal, and anal cancers. In: Yarbro C, editor. Cancer nursing principles and practice. Sudbury (MA): Jones and Bartlett; 2011. p. 1205–57.

13. Ellerhorn JDI, Cullinane CA, Coia LR, et al. Colon, rectal and anal cancers. In: Pazdur R, Coia LR, Hoskins WJ, et al, editors. Cancer management: a multidisciplinary approach. 10th edition. San Francisco (CA): Oncology Publishing Group; 2006. p. 350–75.

14. Cancer Research Institute. Cancer immunotherapy: colorectal cancer. 2015. Available at: http://www.cancerresearch.org/cancer-immunotherapy/impacting-all-cancers/colorectal-cancer. Accessed March 7, 2016.

15. Grenon NN. Managing toxicities associated with antiangiogenic biologic agents in combination with chemotherapy for metastatic colorectal cancer. Clin J Oncol Nurs 2013;17(4):425–33.

16. Cancer Research Institute. Two leading cancer nonprofits join forces to tackle colorectal cancer with immunotherapy. 2015. Available at: http://www.cancerresearch.org/news/2015/november/two-leading-cancer-nonprofits-join-forces-to-tackle-colorectal-cancer-and-immunotherapy#sthash.jufySfKd.dpuf. Accessed March 7, 2016.

17. National Comprehensive Cancer Network (NCCN). Colon cancer (version 2.2016). 2016.

18. McIntyre K. An oncology nurses' guide to new targeted agents for metastatic colorectal cancer. Clin J Oncol Nurs 2015;19(5):571–9.

19. Surveillance, Epidemiology, and End Results (SEER). SEER stat fact sheets: female breast cancer. National Cancer Institute; 2014. Available at: http://seer.cancer.gov/statfacts/html/breast.html. Accessed February, 2016.

20. American Cancer Society (ACS). Breast cancer facts & figures 2015-2016. American Cancer Society; 2015. Available at: http://www.cancer.org/acs/groups/content/@research/documents/document/acspc-046381.pdf. Accessed February, 2016.

21. American Cancer Society (ACS). Cancer statistics center: breast. American Cancer Society; 2016. Available at: http://cancerstatisticscenter.cancer.org/?_ga=1.7785 2243.630716104.1453487825#/cancer-site/Breast. Accessed February, 2016.

22. Beral V, Reeves G, Bull D, et al, Million Women Study Collaborators. Breast cancer risk in relation to the interval between menopause and starting hormone therapy. J Natl Cancer Inst 2011;103(4):296–305.

23. Chelbowski RT, Manson JE, Anderson GL, et al. Estrogen plus progestin and breast cancer incidence and mortality in the Women's Health Initiative Observational Study. J Natl Cancer Inst 2013;105(8):526–35.

24. Manson JE, Chebowski RT, Stefanick ML, et al. Menopausal hormone therapy and health outcomes during the intervention and extended poststopping phases of the Women's Health Initiative randomized trials. JAMA 2013;310(13):1353–68.

25. Beaber EF, Buist DS, Barlow WE, et al. Recent oral contraceptive use by formulation and breast cancer risk among women 20 to 49 years of age. Cancer Res 2014;74(15):4078–89.

26. Nelson HD, Zakher B, Cantor A, et al. Risk factors for breast cancer for women aged 40 to 49 years: a systematic review and meta-analysis. Ann Intern Med 2012;156(9):635–48.

27. Bertrand KA, Scott CG, Tamimi RM, et al. Dense and nondense mammographic area and risk of breast cancer by age and tumor characteristics. Cancer Epidemiol Biomarkers Prev 2015;24(5):798–809.

28. United States Senate. Health, Education, Labor, and Pensions Committee. 114th Congress, S.370. Breast density and mammography reporting act. 2015. Available at: https://www.congress.gov/bill/114th-congress/senate-bill/370. Accessed February, 2016.

29. Freer PE, Slanetz PJ, Haas JS, et al. Breast cancer screening in the era of density notification legislation: summary of 2014 Massachusetts experience and suggestion of an evidence-based management algorithm by multi-disciplinary expert panel. Breast Cancer Res Treat 2015;153(2):455–64.

30. Oeffinger KC, Fontham ET, Etzioni R. Breast cancer screening for women at average risk: 2015 guideline update from the American Cancer Society. JAMA 2015;314(15):1599–614.

31. US Preventive Services Task Force (USPTF). Breast cancer: screening. U.S. Preventive Services Task Force (USPTF); 2016. Available at: http://www.uspreventive servicestaskforce.org/Page/Document/UpdateSummaryFinal/breast-cancer-screening1?ds=1&s=breast. Accessed February, 2016.

32. American College of Radiology. USPSTF breast cancer screening recommendations could endanger women. American College of Radiology; 2016. Available at: http://www.acr.org/About-Us/Media-Center/Press-Releases/2016-Press-Releases/20160111-USPSTF-Breast-Cancer-Screening-Recommendations-Could-Endanger-Women. Accessed February, 2016.

33. Friedewald SM, Rafferty EA, Rose SL, et al. Breast cancer screening using tomosynthesis in combination with digital mammography in. JAMA 2014;311(24):2499–507.

34. Drukteinis JS, Mooney BP, Flowers CI, et al. Beyond mammography: new frontiers in breast cancer screening. Am J Med 2013;126(6):472–9.

35. Moran MS, Schnitt SJ, Giuliano AE, et al. Society of Surgical Oncology-American Society for Radiation Oncology consensus guideline on margins for breast-conserving surgery with whole-breast irradiation in stages I and II invasive breast cancer. J Clin Oncol 2014;32(14):1507–15.

36. Rastogi P, Anderson SJ, Bear HD, et al. Preoperative chemotherapy: updates of national surgical adjuvant breast and bowel project protocols B-18 and B-27. J Clin Oncol 2008;26(5):778–85.
37. National Comprehensive Cancer Network (NCCN). Breast cancer (version 1.2016). National Comprehensive Cancer Network (NCCN) guidelines (2016). 2015. Available at: http://www.nccn.org/professionals/physician_gls/pdf/breast.pdf. Accessed February, 2016.
38. US Food and Drug Administration (FDA). Precision (personalized) medicine. U.S. Food and Drug Administration; 2016. Available at: http://www.fda.gov/ScienceResearch/SpecialTopics/PersonalizedMedicine/. Accessed March, 2016.
39. Giuliano AE, Hunt KK, Ballman KV, et al. Axillary dissection vs no axillary dissection in women with invasive breast cancer and sentinel node metastasis: a randomized clinical trial. JAMA 2011;305(6):569–75.
40. Yardly DA, Noguchi S, Pritchard KI, et al. Everolimus plus exemestane in postmenopausal patients with HR(+) breast cancer: BOLERO-2 final progression-free survival analysis. Adv Ther 2013;30(10):870–84.
41. Finn RS, Crown JP, Lang I, et al. The cyclin-dependent kinase 4/6 inhibitor palbociclib in combination with letrozole versus letrozole alone as first-line treatment of oestrogen receptor-positive, HER2-negative, advanced breast cancer (PALOMA-1/TRIO-18): a randomised phase 2 study. Lancet Oncol 2015;16(1):25–35.
42. Swain SM, Baselga J, Sung-Bae K, et al. Pertuzumab, trastuzumab, and docetaxel in HER2-positive metastatic breast cancer. N Engl J Med 2015;372(8):724–34.
43. Gianni L, Pienkowski T, Im YH, et al. Efficacy and safety of neoadjuvant pertuzumab and trastuzumab in women with locally advanced, inflammatory, or early HER2-positive breast cancer (NeoSphere): a randomised multicentre, open-label, phase 2 trial. Lancet Oncol 2012;13(1):25–32.
44. Poon KA, Flagella K, Beyer J, et al. Preclinical safety profile of trastuzumab emtansine (T-DM1): Mechanism of action of its cytotoxic component retained with improved tolerability. Toxicol Appl Pharmacol 2013;273(2):298–313.
45. US Food and Drug Administration (FDA). FDA approves new treatment for late-stage breast cancer. U.S. Food and Drug Administration; 2013. Available at: http://www.fda.gov/newsevents/newsroom/pressannouncements/ucm340704.htm. Accessed February, 2016.
46. Krop IE, Kim SB, Gonzalez-Martin A, et al. Trastuzumab emtansine versus treatment of physician's choice for pretreated HER2-positive advanced breast cancer (TH3RESA): a randomised, open-label, phase 3 trial. Lancet Oncol 2014;15(7):689–99.
47. American Cancer Society (ACS). What's new in breast cancer research? American Cancer Society; 2014. Available at: http://www.cancer.org/cancer/breastcancer/overviewguide/breast-cancer-overview-new-research. Accessed February, 2016.
48. Page DB, Diab A, Yuan J, et al. Pre-operative immunotherapy with tumor cryoablation (cryo) plus ipilimumab (IPI) induces potentially favorable systemic and intratumoral immune effects in early stage breast cancer (ESBC) patients. J Immunother Cancer 2015;3(Suppl 1):O6.
49. Early Breast Cancer Trialists' Collaborative Group. Adjuvant bisphosphonate treatment in early breast cancer: meta-analyses of individual patient data from randomised trials. Lancet 2015;386(10001):1353–61.
50. National Comprehensive Cancer Network. Prostate Cancer (Version 3.2016). National Comprehensive Cancer Network (NCCN) Guidelines. Fort Washington

(PA): National Comprehensive Cancer Network; 2016. Available at: https://www.nccn.org/professionals/physician_gls/pdf/prostate.pdf.

51. American Cancer Society (ACS). Prostate cancer facts & figures 2014-2016. Atlanta (GA): American Cancer Society; Available at: http://www.cancer.org/cancer/prostatecancer/index. Accessed January 20, 2016.

52. American Cancer Society (ACS). Cancer facts & figures for African Americans 2016-2018. Atlanta (GA): American Cancer Society; 2016.

53. Dunn MW, Kazer WM. Prostate cancer overview. Semin Oncol Nurs 2011;27(4): 241–50.

54. National Cancer Institute (NCI) at the National Institutes of Health (NIH). Prostate cancer. 2016. Available at: http://www.cancer.gov/types/prostate. Accessed August, 2016.

55. Hegarty J, Bailey DE. Active surveillance as a treatment option for prostate cancer. Semin Oncol Nurs 2011;27(4):260–6.

56. Carroll PR, Parsons JK, Andriole G, et al. Prostate cancer early detection, version 1.2014. featured updates to the NCCN guidelines. J Natl Compr Cancer Netw 2014;12(9):1211–9 [quiz: 1219].

57. Small E. Prostate Cancer. In: Goldman L, Schafer A, editors. Goldman-Cecil Medicine. 25th edition. Philadelphia: Saunders Elsevier Publishing Company; 2015.

58. Lawson PA. Chemotherapy regimens. In: Gullatte MM, editor. Clinical guide to antineoplastic therapy: a chemotherapy handbook. 3rd edition. Pittsburgh (PA): ONS Publications; 2014. p. 525–9.

59. Maliska LS. Prostate cancer. In: Itano KJ, editor. Core curriculum for oncology nursing. 5th edition. St Louis (MO): Elsevier; 2016. p. 126–31.

60. Ferraldeschi R, Welti J, Powers MV, et al. Second-generation HSP90 inhibitor onalespib blocks mRNA splicing of androgen receptor variant 7 in prostate cancer cells. Cancer Res 2016;76:2731–42.

61. Roe H. Chemotherapy-induced alopecia: advice and support for hair loss. Br J Nurs 2011;20(10):S4–11.

62. Cigler T, Isseroff D, Fiederlein B, et al. Efficacy of scalp cooling in preventing chemotherapy-induced alopecia in breast cancer patients receiving adjuvant docetaxel and cyclophosphamide chemotherapy. Clin Breast Cancer 2015;15(5): 332–4.

63. US Food and Drug Administration (FDA). FDA allows marketing of cooling cap to reduce hair loss during chemotherapy. U.S. Food and Drug Administration; 2015. Available at: http://www.fda.gov/NewsEvents/Newsroom/PressAnnouncements/ucm476216.htm. Accessed February, 2016.

Lung Cancer and Tobacco

What Is New?

Stella Aguinaga Bialous, MSN, RN, DrPH[a],*, Linda Sarna, PhD, RN[b]

KEYWORDS

- Lung cancer • Tobacco • Smoking status • Smoking cessation • Addiction
- Relapse nursing intervention

KEY POINTS

- Lung cancer is the leading cause of cancer death worldwide.
- Tobacco use is the single most important preventable cause of cancer.
- Implementation of tobacco control measures, including preventing initiation and treating dependence, are pivotal to address the lung cancer epidemic.
- Tobacco dependence treatment improves lung cancer treatment outcomes and increases overall survival.
- All nurses need to ensure that patients with a diagnosis of lung cancer who use tobacco receive tobacco dependence treatment and support to quit.

INTRODUCTION

One of the key developments in lung cancer treatment is the accumulation of compelling evidence on the positive impact of quitting tobacco use at any point along the lung cancer care continuum, from prevention to screening and from treatment to palliative care. Nurses can play a pivotal role by ensuring that tobacco dependence is included in minimal, basic care. Nurses can also support system changes that facilitate access to tobacco dependence treatment to all patients with lung cancer. This article reviews the role of tobacco use in causing lung cancer and the implementation of tobacco-control policies and tobacco dependence treatment as key strategies to address the lung cancer epidemic.

BACKGROUND

Lung cancer is the leading cause of cancer death globally, responsible for an estimated 1.59 million deaths a year.[1] Lung cancer is the most common cancer with an estimated

a School of Nursing, University of California San Francisco, 3333 California Street, Suite 340, San Francisco, CA 94118, USA; b School of Nursing, University of California, Los Angeles, 2-256 Factor, 700 Tiverton Avenue, Los Angeles, CA 90095, USA
* Corresponding author.
E-mail address: stella.bialous@ucsf.edu

Nurs Clin N Am 52 (2017) 53–63
http://dx.doi.org/10.1016/j.cnur.2016.10.003
0029-6465/17/© 2016 Elsevier Inc. All rights reserved.

1.8 million new cases a year, 58% in low- and middle-income countries (LMIC).[2] Lung cancer is more common in men than women following the pattern of tobacco use in men and women, and between women in high-income countries (HIC), where lung cancer rates are high, and women in LMIC, where lung cancer cases are inreasing.[2] In the United States, lung cancer deaths surpassed breast cancer deaths, and it is the most common cause of cancer death among women but breast cancer cases are still higher.[3]

Lung cancer has been labeled a global epidemic after the mass production and marketing of cigarettes, as it was considered a rare disease 100 years ago.[4] Although the number of lung cancer cases remains higher among HIC when compared with LMIC, there is an increase in incidence in LMIC that parallels the increase in tobacco use in these countries.[5] One way to measure the burden of lung cancer is to assess the disability-adjusted life year (DALY). A DALY represent the years of life lost due to disease, disability, or premature death. The Council on Foreign Relations estimated a 100% to 200% increase in lung cancer–related DALYs in several LMIC, mostly in South and Southeast Asia and sub-Saharan Africa.[6]

There are several types of lung cancer, with the most common (85%) being non–small cell lung cancer. Advances in genetic mapping of these tumors are providing new avenues to better understand the cause of lung cancer and informing the development of targeted therapies that have promising results in improving overall survival rates of patients with lung cancer.[7–9]

Treatment and survival improvements were aided by improvement in screening strategies that permit detection in earlier stages of the disease.[10,11] The benefits of screening are amplified when combined with tobacco dependence treatment.[12,13] It is recommended that tobacco dependence treatment be provided to all smokers undergoing screening, regardless of screening results.[14]

Despite this progress, the 5-year survival rates for lung cancer remain low. It is estimated to be approximately 18% in the United States.[15] Access to screening and treatment is nonexistent for large segments of the population in HIC, especially those with low literacy, low access to health care, and low income, and for most people in LMIC. Thus, reducing tobacco use through prevention and cessation remains a major approach for reducing the global burden of lung cancer.

TOBACCO AND CANCER

Tobacco causes 16 types of cancer (**Box 1**); 30% of all cancer deaths, globally, are due to tobacco. Thus, tobacco use is the largest preventable cause of cancer. Cigarettes contain more than 60 substances that are known to be carcinogenic in humans. Tobacco use damages the p53 gene, being responsible for p53 mutations in lung cancer.[16] It is important to note that in addition to cancer, tobacco causes diseases in almost every organ of the body, particularly in the cardiovascular and respiratory systems.[17]

The causal link between smoking and lung cancer was established by the Doll and Hill seminal study of British male doctors published in 1954[4] and became widely known with the publication of the 1964 US Surgeon General Report "Smoking and Health."[17] The body of research confirming the link between tobacco and lung cancer continued to grow in subsequent decades. Tobacco companies knew about this link, through their own research, but decided to publicly question the validity of these scientific findings, funding additional research and launching a public relations campaign to allay consumers' fears related to tobacco use and lung cancer.[4]

A part of the tobacco industry campaign to reassure the public about smoking and health concerns was the launch of light and mild cigarettes, as well as filters,

| Box 1 |
Types of cancer caused by tobacco use
Nose
Mouth
Larynx
Pharynx
Esophagus
Lung
Liver
Stomach
Pancreas
Kidney
Bladder
Ureter
Ovaries
Colon and rectum
Cervix
Acute myeloid leukemia
Data from Quit Victoria. Available at: http://www.quit.org.au/reasons-to-quit/health-risks-of-smoking/16-cancers. Accessed May 25, 2016.

promoting these as a safer alternative to regular cigarettes.[17,18] In fact, these were not safer[17]; there is evidence that a significant increase in diagnosis of adenocarcinoma of the lung is a direct consequence of these products.[19,20] The impact of light cigarettes was particularly devastating to women, who were the target of the tobacco companies' marketing campaigns.[21]

Lung Cancer in Nonsmokers

Exposure to second hand tobacco smoke (SHS) is also a cause of lung cancer, and other diseases, in nonsmokers. There is no safe level of exposure to SHS. It is estimated that SHS was responsible for 7300 deaths a year from lung cancer form 2005 to 2009.[22]

It is important to note that a small percentage of lung cancer diagnoses affect never smokers. In the United States, it is estimated that it represents approximately 10% to 15% of all lung cancer diagnoses and 16,000 to 24,000 lung cancer deaths per year. It is estimated that 20% to 50% of these deaths are attributed to exposure to SHS and, therefore, tobacco related.[23]

TOBACCO USE CESSATION

The health benefits of quitting are numerous both in the short- and the long-term after cessation. All patients with cancer benefit from, and should be provided with, tobacco dependence treatment. Patients with cancer who quit smoking improve treatment outcomes and overall survival.[24] Strategies to ensure that they receive this intervention as an integral component of cancer treatment are emerging.[24] Patients with lung cancer may present a specific challenge. The stigma associated with lung cancer has been associated with delayed care and lower quality of life for these patients compared with patients with other cancer diagnoses.[25–27] It is pivotal that patients with lung cancer receive support to quit smoking.[28] Emerging research demonstrates the positive impact of quitting for patients with lung cancer who smoke, such as higher overall survival rates, and the risk of continuing to smoke, including an increased risk of all-cause mortality.[29]

Nicotine Addiction

Tobacco products contain nicotine, a powerfully addictive substance.[17] Most tobacco users initiate use during their teenage years and are addicted by the time they become young adults. Approximately 70% of smokers would like to quit; in the United States, for example, 65.9% of smokers made a quit attempt in 2013, although the rate varied by state, ranging from 56.2% to 76.4%[30] Tobacco use cessation is a process, with relapse being common. Nonetheless, repeated quit attempts must be encouraged, as quit attempts are a predictor of successful quitting.[31,32] Only 3% to 5% of smokers who quit without support from health care providers are still nonsmoking 12 months later. These rates significantly improve when health care providers consistently offer tobacco dependence intervention.[31]

A cancer diagnosis is not an antidote against nicotine addiction. Although some people quit on diagnosis, a significant proportion of patients continue to smoke after diagnosis or resume smoking after treatment.[28,33,34] Burris and colleagues[35] (2015) conducted a systematic review and found that more than 50% of patients used tobacco at the time of cancer diagnosis. Cooley and colleagues[36] (2007) described ongoing tobacco use among women with lung cancer.

TOBACCO DEPENDENCE TREATMENT

There are global and US evidence-based guidelines and resources to assist health care providers in delivering tobacco dependence treatment (**Table 1**). Essentially these guidelines recommend a combination of behavioral therapy and approved pharmacotherapy as the gold standard. Intervention is provided within a framework known as the 5 As: Ask about tobacco use, Advise users to quit, Assess willingness to quit, Assist in developing a quitting plan, and Arrange for follow-up, including through a referral to the telephone quit line (**Table 2**).[31] It is essential that all health care providers address tobacco use at every encounter, reinforcing the significant negative impact of tobacco per se and the importance of quitting. These guidelines have been available for 2 decades, although the rate of adoption into routine health care practice has been slow, including in cancer care settings.[24]

Electronic Cigarettes and Cessation

Throughout the years, a series of innovations in tobacco products have been introduced in the market with varying degrees of commercial success. The past decade saw the broad introduction, and growth, of electronic nicotine delivery devices, commonly known as electronic cigarettes or e-cigarettes (although several other type of tobacco products are available in electronic formulations, such as electronic water pipe and electronic cigars). These products currently represent 0.1% of the global tobacco market, but their market growth in the past 5 years has been exponential. In the United States, there has been serious concern over the increase in use among adolescents: from 2011 to 2015, the use of e-cigarette among high school students increased from 1.5% to 16%.[37] Although it is possible that these products are

Table 1
Resources and guidelines on tobacco dependence treatment for health care providers

Organization	Comments	Link
Agency for Healthcare Research and Quality Tobacco Use and Dependence Clinical Practice	Access to the full text of the Tobacco Dependence Treatment Guideline and supplemental materials for patients and for health care professionals	http://www.ahrq.gov/professionals/clinicians-providers/guidelines-recommendations/tobacco/index.html
Centers for Disease Control and Prevention	Materials for statewide cessation programs, many helpful for nurses, health care facilities, and patients	http://www.cdc.gov/tobacco/quit_smoking/cessation/
Center for Tobacco Research and Intervention, University of Wisconsin	Several guideline-based resources for health professionals, smokers, and workplaces	http://www.ctri.wisc.edu/
Ottawa Model for Smoking for Smoking Cessation	Resources that can be adapted for different settings, to assist in implementing system changes to ensure that tobacco dependence treatment is integrated into daily practice within health systems	http://ottawamodel.ottawaheart.ca
Rx for Change	Online training for health care professionals, including a module for cancer care providers	http://rxforchange.ucsf.edu/welcome.php
Smoking Cessation Leadership Center	Resources for clinicians and opportunities for training	http://smokingcessationleadership.ucsf.edu/
Tobacco Free Nurses	Resources for nurses, including cancer-specific webcasts on addressing tobacco dependence within oncology settings	http://www.tobaccofreenurses.org
WHO Framework Convention on Tobacco Control Article 14 Guideline	Guideline for the implementation of policies addressing tobacco dependence at a global level, endorsed by all countries that are parties to the WHO FCTC, an international treaty	
WHO train of trainers modules on tobacco dependence treatment	A series of toolkits to assist in implementation of system changes to incorporate tobacco dependence treatment in primary care and resources for patients and health care professionals	http://www.who.int/tobacco/quitting/en/

Abbreviations: FCTC, Framework Convention on Tobacco Control; WHO, World Health Organization.

Table 2	
The 5 As framework for tobacco dependence treatment	
Elements of the Framework	Comments
ASK	Every patient should be asked about tobacco use at every encounter. It is important to ensure that the question is asked repeatedly, because relapse is common. The C-TUQ offers appropriate, standardized questions to be used.
ADVISE	Every patient that smokes should hear from a nurse that quitting is the best thing you could do for your health. Review with patients the benefits of quitting after diagnosis.
ASSESS	Patients must be assessed for their willingness to quit. Many might not be ready (although they should still receive advice, as per the aforementioned ADVISE). Assess what their concerns with quitting might be and discuss strategies to overcome these concerns.
ASSIST	Patients will need help in developing a plan to assist them with their quit attempt. Personalized plans are ideal, and discussion of using FDA-approved medication in addition to behavioral counseling should be discussed. How to manage nicotine withdrawal is an important component of a quitting plan. Remind patients that relapse is part of the process and quit attempts are a sign of progress.
ARRANGE	Follow-up is an essential component of treatment. Referral to cessation services might be needed, and notations on charts are essential for follow-up in subsequent contacts with the cancer care system. For patients who quit when hospitalized, follow-up within a month after discharge significantly increases the chance of long-term abstinence. Nurses should refer patients to the telephone quit line (in the United States 1-800-QUIT NOW) for quit support after discharge.

Abbreviations: C-TUQ, Cancer Patient Tobacco Use Questionnaire; FDA, Food and Drug Administration.

less harmful than regular cigarettes, they are not harmless. Several of these products contain carcinogenic substances, including formaldehyde.[37] One study demonstrated that the risk associated with inhaling formaldehyde could be 5 to 15 times higher among users of certain types of e-cigarettes than the risk among long-term smokers.[38] It is unknown what proportion of patients with cancer use e-cigarettes. One British study surveyed members of the British Thoracic Oncology Group on their perception of e-cigarette use by patients with lung cancer.[39] It found that most physicians surveyed (81.4%) had patients ask questions about e-cigarettes. Respondents also reported that they perceived that a 25% to 50% or more of their patients used e-cigarettes. However, additional research is needed to assess e-cigarette use among patients with cancer. The International Association for the Study of Lung Cancer stated that given the lack of evidence on the safety and efficacy of e-cigarettes, its use is not recommended.[40]

Marketing claims, and some public health professionals, claim that e-cigarettes could be used to help smokers quit. As of May 2016, there is no sufficient evidence demonstrating their efficacy or safety as cessation devices.[41] A meta-analysis of published studies assessing e-cigarettes and cessation concluded that there is no evidence to support claims that these products are effective smoking cessation devices. In fact, this study concluded that e-cigarette use could be detrimental to quitting.[42]

In the United States, the Food and Drug Administration (FDA) has not approved e-cigarettes as part of tobacco dependence treatment; on May 2016, the FDA issued a set of rules to regulate the manufacture, sales, and marketing of e-cigarettes and other tobacco products.[43] Regulations in US, and several other countries' generally aim at protecting children and adolescents from the potential harm of e-cigarette use including addiction to nicotine, restrict marketing claims, and ensure that e-cigarettes use is restricted in smoke-free public spaces.

Tobacco Dependence Treatment and Cancer

As previously discussed, tobacco dependence treatment needs to be included as minimally acceptable care in oncology settings.[31] The American Society of Clinical Oncology (ASCO) published a guide to assist oncology health care providers in providing tobacco dependence treatment to patients.[44] It is based on the US guideline,[31] but it assists health care providers in oncology settings to tailor the message to the concerns and needs of patients diagnosed with cancer, for example, by framing the benefits of quitting with a focus on cancer-related outcomes (**Table 3**). The guide offers suggestions to integrate tobacco dependence treatment as part of routine care in cancer care. The ASCO guideline also includes assessment of tobacco use and treatment of dependence, including referral for additional counseling and services, one of the core measures in its Quality Oncology Practice Initiative.[45] Furthermore, the National Cancer Institute and the American Association for Cancer Research Cancer Patient Tobacco Use Assessment Task Force found that it is not acceptable that tobacco use has not been given due recognition in cancer clinical trials, particularly because of the known negative impact of continuing tobacco use for treatment outcome, prognosis, and survival. The task force recommended that, at a minimum, tobacco use be assessed at study entry and at the end of the protocol and treatment be provided in order to support quit attempts.[46]

TOBACCO CONTROL AND CANCER

There is ample evidence that comprehensive tobacco-control measures, such as creation of 100% smoke-free environments, increasing price and tax on tobacco,

Table 3
Tailoring the benefits of quitting to patients with cancer

Benefits of Quitting Tobacco	Impact of Continuing to Smoke
Improved outcomes from all forms of treatment	Continuing smoking negatively impacts the outcome of surgery, including wound healing and higher toxicity from chemotherapy and radiation therapy. It increases the risk of infection.
Reduce instances and severity of side effects	Continuing smoking worsened several treatment side effects, including mucositis, and leads to more surgery complications.
Improved overall survival rates	Patients who continue to smoke have higher odds of mortality from all causes and recurrence.
Improved quality of life	There are lower energy levels and a negative impact on breathing.
Better health	There are increased risks of cardiovascular and other lung diseases and an increased risk of another primary cancer and of a secondary cancer.

restricting or banning marketing, among other measures, are successful in reducing tobacco-related premature deaths.[47] A 2016 study estimated that a 10% drop in smoking could lead to $63 billion reduction in health care costs in the United States.[48] Research on the first 10 years of California's tobacco-control program demonstrates a 6% reduction in the incidence of lung cancer, equivalent to 11,000 fewer cases of lung cancer in that state.[49]

IMPLICATIONS FOR ONCOLOGY NURSING PRACTICE

The Oncology Nursing Society, the International Society of Nurses in Cancer Care,[50] and several other nursing organizations throughout the world have unequivocally called on nurses to heighten their engagement in tobacco control. With the available body and evidence and the resources available to nurses, the provision of tobacco dependence treatment to patients who smoke must become the basic standard of evidence-based practice. The accelerated implementation of electronic medical records might facilitate the integration of this intervention into nurses' workflow.[24] Nurses can enhance the referral of patients to toll-free telephone quit lines in order to ensure they receive ongoing support in their quit attempts. Tobacco dependence treatment content must be integrated into basic nursing education and included in oncology nursing certification and continuing education programs. Nurses have the potential to make a significant contribution to address the lung cancer epidemic; but unless they become engaged in, at a minimum, tobacco dependence treatment, they will not realize this potential. Although this may not be a new approach, it is certainly time for nurses to embrace it.

REFERENCES

1. Stewart BW, Wild CP, editors. World cancer report 2014. Lyon (France): International Agency for Research on Cancer/World Health Organization; 2014. p. 630.
2. International Agency for Research on Cancer. GloboCan 2012. Available at: http://globocan.iarc.fr/Pages/fact_sheets_cancer.aspx?cancer=lung. Accessed May 1, 2016.
3. American Lung Association. (2014) Lung cancer fact sheet. Available at: http://www.lung.org/lung-health-and-diseases/lung-disease-lookup/lung-cancer/learn-about-lung-cancer/lung-cancer-fact-sheet.html. Accessed May 1, 2016.
4. Proctor RN. The history of the discovery of the cigarette–lung cancer link: evidentiary traditions, corporate denial, global toll. Tob Control 2012;21:87–91.
5. Didkowska J, Wojciechowska U, Mańczuk M, et al. Lung cancer epidemiology: contemporary and future challenges worldwide. Ann Transl Med 2016;4(8):150.
6. Council on Foreign Relations. The emerging crisis: noncommunicable diseases. Available at: http://www.cfr.org/diseases-noncommunicable/NCDs-interactive/p33802?cid=otr-marketing_use-NCDs_interactive/#!/. Accessed May 1, 2016.
7. Malhotra J, Malvezzi M, Negri E, et al. Risk factors for lung cancer worldwide. Eur Respir J 2016;48(3):889–902.
8. Brennan P, Hainaut P, Boffetta P. Genetics of lung-cancer susceptibility. Lancet Oncol 2011;12(4):399–408.
9. Cancer Genome Atlas Research Network. Comprehensive molecular profiling of lung adenocarcinoma. Nature 2014;511:543–50.
10. Sorrie K, Cates L, Hill A. The case for lung cancer screening: what nurses need to know. Clin J Oncol Nurs 2016;20(3):E82–7.
11. Atwater T, Massion PP. Biomarkers of risk to develop lung cancer in the new screening era. Ann Transl Med 2016;4(8):158.

12. Pedersen JH, Tønnesen P, Ashraf H. Smoking cessation and lung cancer screening. Ann Transl Med 2016;4(8):157.
13. Tramontano AC, Sheehan DF, McMahon PM, et al. Evaluating the impacts of screening and smoking cessation programmes on lung cancer in a high-burden region of the USA: a simulation modelling study. BMJ Open 2016;6(2): e010227.
14. Fucito LM, Czabafy S, Hendricks PS, et al, Association for the Treatment of Tobacco Use and Dependence (ATTUD)/Society for Research on Nicotine and Tobacco (SRNT) Synergy Committee. Pairing smoking-cessation services with lung cancer screening: a clinical guideline from the Association for the Treatment of Tobacco Use and Dependence and the Society for Research on Nicotine and Tobacco. Cancer 2016;122(8):1150–9.
15. SEER stat fact sheets: lung and bronchus cancer. Available at: http://seer.cancer. gov/statfacts/html/lungb.html. Accessed May 1, 2016.
16. U.S. Department of Health and Human Services. How tobacco smoke causes disease: the biology and behavioral basis for smoking-attributable disease: a report of the surgeon general. Atlanta (GA): U.S. Department of Health and Human Services, Centers for Disease Control and Prevention, National Center for Chronic Disease Prevention and Health Promotion, Office on Smoking and Health; 2010.
17. U. S. Department of Health and Human Services. The health consequences of smoking-50 years of progress: a report of the surgeon general. Atlanta (GA): U.S. Department of Health and Human Services, Public Health Service, Office of the Surgeon General; 2014.
18. FDA consumer update. "Light" tobacco products pose heavy health risks. Available at: http://www.fda.gov/ForConsumers/ConsumerUpdates/ucm227360.htm. Accessed May 1, 2016.
19. Ito H, Matsuo K, Tanaka H, et al. Nonfilter and filter cigarette consumption and the incidence of lung cancer by histological type in Japan and the United States: analysis of 30-year data from population-based cancer registries. Int J Cancer 2011;128(8):1918–28.
20. Janssen-Heijnen ML, Coebergh JW, Klinkhamer PJ, et al. Is there a common etiology for the rising incidence of and decreasing survival with adenocarcinoma of the lung? Epidemiology 2001;12(2):256–8.
21. Sarna L, Bialous SA. Why tobacco is a women's health issue. Nurs Clin North Am 2004;39(1):165–80.
22. Centers for Disease Control and Prevention. Secondhand smoke (SHS) facts. Available at: http://www.cdc.gov/tobacco/data_statistics/fact_sheets/secondhand_ smoke/general_facts/. Accessed May 1, 2016.
23. Samet JM, Avila-Tang E, Boffetta P, et al. Lung cancer in never smokers: clinical epidemiology and environmental risk factors. Clin Cancer Res 2009;15(18): 5626–45.
24. Sarna L, Bialous SA. Implementation of tobacco control programs in oncology settings. Semin Oncol Nurs 2016;32(3):187–96.
25. Sriram N, Mills J, Lang E, et al. Attitudes and stereotypes in lung cancer versus breast cancer. PLoS One 2015;10(12):e0145715. Available at: http://dx.doi.org/ 10.1371/journal.pone.0145715. Accessed May 1, 2016.
26. Brown Johnson CG, Brodsky JL, Cataldo JK. Lung cancer stigma, anxiety, depression, and quality of life. J Psychosoc Oncol 2014;32(1):59–73.
27. Cataldo JK, Brodsky JL. Lung cancer stigma, anxiety, depression and symptom severity. Oncology 2013;85(1):33–40.

28. Cataldo JK, Dubey S, Prochaska JJ. Smoking cessation: an integral part of lung cancer treatment. Oncology 2010;78(5–6):289–301.

29. Parsons A, Daley A, Begh R, et al. Influence of smoking cessation after diagnosis of early stage lung cancer on prognosis: systematic review of observational studies with meta-analysis. BMJ 2010;340:b5569.

30. Lavinghouze SR, Malarcher A, Jama A, et al. Trends in quit attempts among adult cigarette smokers — United States, 2001–2013. MMWR Morb Mortal Wkly Rep 2015;64(40):1129–35.

31. Fiore M, Jaen C, Baker T, et al. Treating tobacco use and dependence: 2008 update—clinical practice guideline. Rockville (MD): U.S. Department of Health and Human Services, Public Health Service; 2008.

32. Zhu SH, Lee M, Zhuang YL, et al. Interventions to increase smoking cessation at the population level: how much progress has been made in the last two decades? Tob Control 2012;21(2):110–8.

33. Duffy SA, Khan MJ, Ronis DL, et al. Health behaviors of head and neck cancer patients the first year after diagnosis. Head Neck 2008;30(1):93–102.

34. Cooley ME, Sarna L, Kotlerman J, et al. Smoking cessation is challenging even for patients recovering from lung cancer surgery with curative intent. Lung Cancer 2009;66(2):218–25.

35. Burris JL, Studts JL, DeRosa AP, et al. Systematic review of tobacco use after lung or head/neck cancer diagnosis: results and recommendations for future research. Cancer Epidemiol Biomarkers Prev 2015;24(10):1450–61.

36. Cooley ME, Sarna L, Brown JK, et al. Tobacco use in women with lung cancer. Ann Behav Med 2007;33(3):242–50.

37. US Food and Drug Administration. Vaporizers, e-cigarettes, and other electronic nicotine delivery systems (ENDS). Available at: http://www.fda.gov/TobaccoProducts/Labeling/ProductsIngredientsComponents/ucm456610.htm. Accessed May 10, 2016.

38. Jensen RP, Luo W, Pankow JF, et al. Hidden formaldehyde in e-cigarette aerosols. N Engl J Med 2015;372:392–4.

39. Sherratt FC, Newson L, Field JK. Electronic cigarettes: a survey of perceived patient use and attitudes among members of the British thoracic oncology group. Respir Res 2016;17(1):55.

40. Cummings KM, Dresler CM, Field JK, et al. E-cigarettes and cancer patients. J Thorac Oncol 2014;9(4):438–41.

41. Malas M, van der Tempel J, Schwartz R, et al. Electronic cigarettes for smoking cessation: a systematic review. Nicotine Tob Res 2016;18(10):1926–36.

42. Kalkhoran S, Glantz SA. E-cigarettes and smoking cessation in real-world and clinical settings: a systematic review and meta-analysis. Lancet Respir Med 2016;4(2):116–28.

43. US Food and Drug Administration. Extending authorities to all tobacco products, including e-cigarettes, cigars, and hookah. Available at: http://www.fda.gov/TobaccoProducts/Labeling/ucm388395.htm. Accessed May 10, 2016.

44. American Society of Clinical Oncology. (2012) Tobacco cessation guide for oncology providers. Available at: https://www.asco.org/sites/new-www.asco.org/files/content-files/blog-release/documents/tobacco-cessation-guide.pdf. Accessed May 10, 2016.

45. American Society of Clinical Oncology. ASCO Institute for Quality. Available at: http://www.instituteforquality.org/. Accessed May 10, 2016.

46. Land SR, Toll BA, Moinpour CM, et al. Research priorities, measures, and recommendations for assessment of tobacco use in clinical cancer research. Clin Cancer Res 2016;22(8):1907–13.

47. Holford TR, Meza R, Warner KE, et al. Tobacco control and the reduction in smoking-related premature deaths in the United States, 1964-2012. JAMA 2014;311(2):164–71.
48. Lightwood J, Glantz SA. Smoking behavior and healthcare expenditure in the United States, 1992-2009: panel data estimates. PLoS Med 2016;13(5): e1002020.
49. Barnoya J, Glantz S. Association of the California tobacco control program with declines in lung cancer incidence. Cancer Causes Control 2004;15(7):689–95.
50. Bialous SA, Sarna L. ISNCC tobacco position statement. Cancer Nurs 2016; 39(1):80–1.

Changes in Cancer Treatment

Mabs, Mibs, Mids, Nabs, and Nibs

Joseph D. Tariman, PhD, RN, ANP-BC, FAAN

KEYWORDS

- Monoclonal antibody • Nanoparticle albumin-bound drug • Tyrosine kinase inhibitor
- Immunomodulatory drug • Proteasome inhibitor • Cancer therapeutics
- Targeted therapy • Nursing care

KEY POINTS

- Stay abreast on latest cancer treatments; cancer treatments have evolved from genocidal to specific cellular, molecular, and genetic targeting approaches (targeted therapies) to kill cancer cells.
- Manage the side effects of cancer treatments; this is essential to adherence and a successful completion of planned targeted therapy.
- Educate patients and their caregivers on treatment-related information to empower them in becoming active participants of the cancer journey.

Cancer therapeutics has changed at a rapid pace over the past two decades. Cancer treatment changes are undoubtedly driven by the recent advances in the understanding of cancer pathobiology, leading to molecular classifications of various cancer types instead of organ-based cancer classifications.[1] Scientific advances and discoveries have led to an improved therapeutic approach and eventually forged a new pathway to cure cancer, leaving behind the primitive genocidal and toxic approach of cancer treatment. Moreover, improved understanding of the pathobiology of cancer at the molecular and genetic levels catalyzed the rapid changes in cancer therapeutics, ushering in the era of targeted therapies. Since the Food and Drug Administration (FDA) approval of the first monoclonal antibody, rituxi*mab* (Mab) for non-Hodgkin lymphoma in 1997,[2] first proteasome inhibitor (PI), bortezo*mib* (Mib) for myeloma in 2003,[3–5] first immunomodulatory drug, lenalido*mide* (Mid) for myeloma in 2006,[6] first nanoparticle albumin-bound drug, nab-paclitaxel (Nabs) for breast cancer in 2005,[7,8] and first tyrosine kinase inhibitor (TKI), imati*nib* (Nib) for chronic myelogenous leukemia (CML) in 2001,[9] cancer therapeutics has been growing in an unprecedented

Disclosure: Nothing to disclose.
School of Nursing, DePaul University, 990 West Fullerton Avenue, Suite 3000, Chicago, IL 60614, USA
E-mail address: jtariman@depaul.edu

Nurs Clin N Am 52 (2017) 65–81
http://dx.doi.org/10.1016/j.cnur.2016.10.004
0029-6465/17/© 2016 Elsevier Inc. All rights reserved.

nursing.theclinics.com

fashion, targeting specific gene mutation, protein dysfunction and dysregulation, intra-cellular signaling pathways, and immune modulation to name a few.

In myeloma (cancer of plasma cells) alone, four new drugs with different classifica-tions and mechanisms of action have been approved by the FDA in 2015. This is an unprecedented, record-breaking year for drug approval for one type of cancer. These new drug approvals in 2015 included a Mib (ixazomib[10]), two Mabs (daratumumab[11] and elotuzumab[12]), and a histone deacetylase inhibitor (panobinostat).[13] In 2012, a second-generation Mib (carfilzomib)[14] and a third-generation Mid (pomalidomide[15]) were also granted FDA approval as treatment of myeloma. In patients diagnosed with myeloma, a plethora of treatment options provides hope and opportunities, but they come with clinical challenges for oncology nurses and all other oncology clini-cians in terms of meeting the educational needs and treatment preferences of patients diagnosed with cancer, especially when treatment options are equivocal.

Patients newly diagnosed with cancer require immediate treatment in certain cir-cumstances because of organ damage and these patients clearly have information needs related to disease, treatment, and side effects, which must be provided to patients and families to empower them throughout their cancer journey.[16] This article addresses the need of novice and experienced oncology nurses alike for treatment-related information and evidence-based nursing care of patients diagnosed with cancer throughout the cancer treatment continuum, emphasizing novel and break-through targeted cancer therapies.

MONOCLONAL ANTIBODIES

In 1986 the first commercially available Mab, orthoclone OKT3 (muromonab-CD3), was initially approved by the FDA for use in preventing kidney transplant rejection.[17] Twelve years later, the FDA approved rituximab as the first Mab for the treatment of B-cell lymphoma. Rituximab is a genetically engineered chimeric (murine-human) Mab directed against CD20 antigen found on the surface of normal and malignant B cells.[18,19] Rituximab attacks cancer cells after binding with CD20 B cells by a variety of mechanisms including cell cycle arrest; direct induction of apoptosis (program cell death); and sensitization to cytotoxic (cell killing) drugs, complement-dependent cyto-toxicity, and antibody-dependent cellular cytotoxicity.[20] **Fig. 1** illustrates the mecha-nism of actions of rituximab. Since its first approval in 1997, rituximab has been combined with various other chemotherapeutic or biologic agents in the treatment

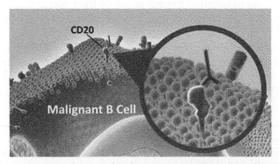

Fig. 1. Rituximab's mechanism of action: binds to CD20 receptor of B cells and once bound, the drug activates the immune system to attack the malignant B cells. (*From* National Cancer Insti-tute. Using the immune system in the fight against cancer: discovery of rituximab. Available at: https://www.cancer.gov/research/progress/discovery/blood-cancer. Accessed March 3, 2016.)

of B-cell lymphoma and other CD20-positive lymphoid neoplasms with excellent results leading to improved overall survival.[17,21]

There have been advances made in monoclonal antibodies. From the genetically
engineered chimeric murine-human Mab platform, scientists are now able to develop
fully humanized monoclonal antibodies, which have a better side effects profile, particularly ameliorating the severity of infusion-related allergic reactions from Mabs. Mabs
are now the fastest growing group of biotechnology-derived molecules in clinical trials
history targeting monoclonal cell receptors and ligands. Today, there are have more
than 30 Mabs approved for the treatment of various cancers and other medical conditions (**Table 1**).[22]

MIBS

Mibs is a term coined by oncology clinicians referring to a new class of targeted therapies called PIs. The PIs include first-generation bortezomib[23]; second-generation
carfilzomib[14]; and the first oral PI, ixazomib.[10] In 1998, Adams and colleagues[24] first
reported boronic acid dipeptides as potent inhibitors of the 20S segment of the
proteasome. The 20S proteasome is a key cellular component of the ubiquitin-
proteasome pathway that regulates the degradation of many cell cycle control proteins.[25] By 2003, bortezomib became the "first in class" potent and selective, but
reversible inhibitor of the 20S proteasome core approved by the FDA for the treatment
of patients with relapsed and refractory myeloma[3,26] and mantle cell lymphoma in
2006.[27] **Fig. 2** explains how bortezomib affects the process of cell cycle control.

Many patients with myeloma benefited from the rapid response from bortezomib,
but there were also many patients who did not respond to bortezomib, whereas other
patients eventually developed resistance. This phenomenon paved the way for the
development of other PIs with enhanced activity, such as the second-generation PI,
carfilzomib. Kuhn and colleagues[28] were among the first group of researchers to
report that the programmed cell death induced by carfilzomib was associated with
the activation of c-Jun-N-terminal kinase, mitochondrial membrane depolarization,
release of cytochrome c, and activation of intrinsic and extrinsic caspase pathways.
Carfilzomib received its FDA approval as a treatment of relapsed and refractory
myeloma in 2012 based on phase II clinical trial safety and efficacy data.[29–31]

Most recently, the first oral PI, ixazomib, was approved by the FDA.[10] Similar to its
parent compound bortezomib, ixazomib is also a boronic-based PI that is reversible.
Both bortezomib and ixazomib primarily target the chymotrypsin-like activity of the
20S proteasome core, leading to a blockade of cellular protein degradation pathway
and apoptosis (programmed cell death). However, there are differences between bortezomib and ixazomib. First, ixazomib has a shorter half-life (the time to it takes for its
plasma concentration to decline by 50%). Second, ixazomib demonstrated greater
tissue penetration when compared with bortezomib in preclinical study; overall ixazomib has shorter proteasome dissociation half-life and improved pharmacokinetics,
pharmacodynamics, and antitumor activity when compared with bortezomib.[32] Given
that ixazomib comes in oral formulation, its convenience and ease of therapy would
likely play a factor in patient preference for treatment among older adults diagnosed
with myeloma.[33] A second oral PI, oprozomib, is now undergoing phase II clinical trials
in patients with advanced solid tumors.[34]

MIDS

Immunomodulatory drugs (IMids or Mids) belong to a class of medications that enhances the ability of immune cells to kill abnormal cells, such as myeloma cells in

Table 1
A comprehensive list of monoclonal antibodies approved by the FDA

Generic Name	Trade Name	Antibody Format	Antigen Target	Year of Initial Approval and Indications
Muromomab	Orthoclone	Murine IgG2a	CD3	1986; allograft rejection in allogeneic renal transplantation
Abciximab	Reopro	Chimeric Fab	GPIIb/IIIa receptor	1993; prevention of cardiac ischemic complications
Rituximab	Rituxan	Chimeric IgG1κ	CD20	1997; non-Hodgkin lymphoma, chronic lymphocytic leukemia, and rheumatoid arthritis
Daclizumab	Zenapax	Humanized IgG1κ	IL-2Rα	1997; prophylaxis of acute organ rejection in renal transplants
Basiliximab	Simulect	Chimeric IgG1κ	IL-2Rα	1998; prophylaxis of acute organ rejection in renal transplantation
Palivizumab	Synagis	Humanized IgG1κ	RSV F protein	1998; RSV infection
Infliximab	Remicade	Chimeric IgG1κ	TNF-α	1998; Crohn disease and rheumatoid arthritis
Trastuzumab	Herceptin	Humanized IgG1κ	Her2	1998; breast cancer, gastric cancer
aGemtuzumab Ozogamicin	Mylotarg	Calicheamicin-humanized IgG4κ	CD33	2000; acute myeloid leukemia
Alemtuzumab	Campath	Humanized IgG1κ	CD52	2001; B-cell chronic lymphocytic leukemia
Ibritumomab Tiuxetan	Zevalin	Y^{90}-murine IgG1κ	CD20	2002; B-cell non-Hodgkin lymphoma
Adalimumab	Humira	Human IgG1κ	TNF-α	2002; rheumatoid arthritis and Crohn disease
Omalizumab	Xolair	Humanized IgG1κ	IgE	2003; moderate to severe persistent asthma
Tositumomab	Bexxar	I^{131}-murine IgG2aλ	CD20	2003; non-Hodgkin lymphoma
aEfalizumab	Raptiva	Humanized IgG1κ	CD11a	2003; moderate to severe plaque psoriasis
Cetuximab	Erbitux	Chimeric IgG1κ	EGFR	2004; head and neck cancer, colorectal cancer
Bevacizumab	Avastin	Humanized IgG1κ	VEGF-A	2004; colon cancer and various solid tumors

Natalizumab	Tysabri	Humanized IgG4κ	α4-integrin	2004; multiple sclerosis and Crohn disease
Ranibizumab	Lucentis	Humanized Fab	VEGF-A	2006; age-related macular degeneration
Panitumumab	Vectibix	Human IgG2κ	EGFR	2006; metastatic colorectal carcinoma
Eculizumab	Soliris	Humanized IgG2/4κ	C5	2007; paroxysmal nocturnal hemoglobinuria
Certolizumab Pegol	Cimzia	Pegylated humanized Fab	TNF-α	2008; Crohn disease and rheumatoid arthritis
Golimumab	Simponi	Human IgG1κ	TNF-α	2009; rheumatoid arthritis, psoriatic arthritis, and ankylosing spondylitis
Canakinumab	Ilaris	Human IgG1κ	IL-1β	2009; cryopyrin-associated periodic syndromes
Ustekinumab	Stelara	Human IgG1κ	IL-12/IL-23	2009; plaque psoriasis
Ofatumumab	Arzerra	Human IgG1κ	CD20	2009; chronic lymphocytic leukemia
Tocilizumab	Actemra	Humanized IgG1κ	IL-6R	2010; rheumatoid arthritis
Denosumab	Prolia	Human IgG2κ	RANK ligand	2010; postmenopausal women with risk of osteoporosis
Ipilimumab	Yervoy	Humanized	CTLA4	2011; melanoma
Pertuzumab	Perjeta	Humanized	Her2	2012; herceptin-2-positive metastatic breast cancer
Obinutuzumab	Gazyva	Humanized	CD20	2014; chronic lymphocytic leukemia, follicular lymphoma
Nivolumab	Opdivo	Humanized IgG4	PD-1, PD-L1, PD-L2	2014; melanoma; 2015; lung cancer, renal cancer
Elotuzumab	Empliciti	Humanized IgG1	SLAMF7	2015; multiple myeloma
Daratumumab	Darzalex	Humanized IgG1κ	CD38	2015; multiple myeloma

Abbreviations: C, complement; CD, cluster designation; CTLA, cytotoxic T-lymphocyte-associated protein; EGFR, epidermal growth factor receptor; GP, glycoprotein; Her, herceptin; IL, interleukin; PD-L, programmed cell death-ligand; RANK, receptor activator of nuclear factor kappa-B; RSV, respiratory syncytial virus; SLAMF7, signaling lymphocytic activation molecule F7; TNF, tumor necrosis factor; VEGF, vascular endothelial growth factor.

[a] Note: Gemtuzumab ozogamicin (Mylotarg) and efalizumab (Raptiva) have been withdrawn from the US market because of side effects and are no longer available in the United States.

Adapted from Li J, Zhu Z. Research and development of next generation of antibody-based therapeutics. Acta Pharmacol Sin 2010;31(9):1198–207.

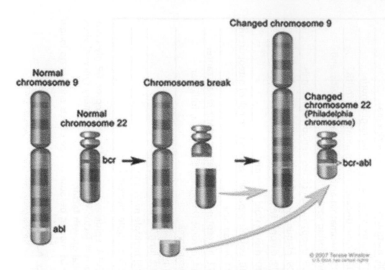

Fig. 2. The Philadelphia chromosome: the BCR (chromosome 22)-ABL (chromosome 9) gene fusion. (© 2007 Terese Winslow, U.S. Govt. has certain rights.)

the bone marrow. There are three well-known drugs under this classification and they are all approved for the treatment of patients diagnosed with myeloma. These drugs include thalidomide, lenalidomide, and pomalidomide.[35] The mechanisms of action of thalidomide,[36–40] lenalidomide,[39–44] and pomalidomide[40,41] are summarized in **Table 2**. Lenalidomide has been found to have a direct effect on myeloid cells with the del(5q) clone, which may contribute to its ability to induce cytogenetic responses in myelodysplastic syndrome with 5q deletion.[45] The FDA has approved lenalidomide as a treatment of myelodysplastic syndrome with 5q deletion in 2006[46] and mantle cell lymphoma in 2013.[47]

NIBS

A landmark discovery in genomics and leukemia treatment was confirmed when the BCR-ABL gene fusion (popularly called "Philadelphia chromosome"), which is present in 95% of CML cases, became a prime therapeutic target in CML.[48] In 1959, genetic researchers at Fox Chase Cancer Center in Philadelphia, Pennsylvania, discovered this first chromosome abnormality associated with cancer.[49] The translocated chromosome was later named Philadelphia chromosome to associate this seminal finding with the city where the discovery took place.

The BCR-ABL gene fusion is a phenomenon characterized by exchanges of bits of DNA from chromosome 9 (ABL) and chromosome 22 (BCR). These two DNA bits are translocated, hence it is called the BCR-ABL chromosomal translocation commonly expressed as t(9;22). This singular genetic mutation is the scientific underpinning behind CML overproduction of an enzyme called tyrosine kinase that stimulates malignant white blood cell growth.[48,50] **Fig. 2** illustrates how tiny bits of chromosomes 9 and 22 were translocated, forming the BCR-ABL fusion gene.

In 2001, a TKI imatinib mesylate (formerly STI571; Gleevec) was approved by the FDA for the treatment of Philadelphia chromosome–positive CML[51,52] and became the first Nib commercially available in the United States. Today, the BCR-ABL

Table 2 Mechanisms of action of immunomodulatory drugs			
Brand Name	**Generic Name**	**Mechanisms of Action**	**FDA-Approved Indications**
Thalomid	Thalidomide	Angiogenesis inhibition Direct inhibition of myeloma cell proliferation by inhibiting IL-6, a myeloma tumor growth factor 3-aminothalidomide, a thalidomide analogue, inhibits multiple myeloma through effects on the tumor and vascular compartment thereby synergistically curtailing tumor growth Depletes vascular endothelial growth factor receptors, such as neuropilin-1 and Flk-1 Modulates cytokines, particularly TNF-α Activates apoptotic pathways through caspase 8–mediated cell death Immune modulation: activates T cells to produce IL-2 augmenting the activity of NK-dependent cytotoxicity and suppresses nuclear factor-kappa B, a proinflammatory and a proliferative factor	Myeloma
Revlimid	Lenalidomide	Activates apoptotic pathways through caspase 8–mediated cell death Activates T cells to produce IL-2 and IFN-γ augmenting the activity of NK-dependent cytotoxicity Modulates immune system by suppressing proinflammatory and proliferative cytokines and activating T-cell proliferation Direct effect on the del(5q) clone, which may contribute to its ability to induce cytogenetic responses in myelodysplastic syndrome or myelodysplastic syndrome with 5q deletion 100–1000 times more potent than thalidomide; the dosing requirement is less	Myeloma Myelodysplastic syndrome with 5q deletion Mantle cell lymphoma
Pomalyst	Pomalidomide	Stimulates T-cell proliferation Enhances transcription factor T bet, which reverts Th2 cells to Th1 effector cells that are producers of IL-2, IFN-γ, and TNF-β, augmenting the activity of NK-dependent cytotoxicity Downregulates IFN regulatory factor 4, a downstream target of cereblon, which is a critical pathway of myeloma cell survival	Myeloma

Abbreviations: IFN, interferon; IL, interleukin; NK, natural killer cell; TNF, tumor necrosis factor.

abnormality is now considered the causative molecular abnormality of CML and the reversal of this genetic event through tyrosine kinase inhibition has been found to induce durable remissions in patients with CML.[53]

The initial discovery of imatinib as a single mutation TKI heralded an explosion of several other multitargeted TKIs. Second- and third-generations TKIs target multiple receptors including vascular endothelial growth factor receptor, rapidly accelerated fibrosarcoma kinase, mitogen-activated protein kinase/extracellular signal related

Table 3
Tyrosine kinase inhibitors (Nibs) and their targets approved by the FDA

Brand Name	Generic Name	Targets	Year of Initial FDA Approval and Indications
Gleevec	Imatinib mesylate	BCR-ABL PDGFR	2001 CML GIST ALL in children Myelodysplastic neoplasms Systemic mastocytosis Dermatofibrosarcoma protuberans Chronic eosinophilic leukemia
Tarceva	Erlotinib hydrochloride	EGFR	2004 Non–small cell lung cancer 2005 Pancreatic cancer
Iressa	Gefitinib	EGFR	2005 Non–small cell lung cancer
Nexavar	Sorafenib tosylate	VEGFR-2 RAF kinase PDGFR	2005 Renal cell carcinoma 2007 Hepatocellular cancer 2013 Thyroid cancer
Sprycel	Dasatinib	BCR-ABL Src-family protein kinases	2006 CML ALL
Sutent	Sunitinib malate	VEGFR-2 PDGFRb C-kit FLT3	2006 GIST Kidney cancer 2011 Pancreatic cancer
Tasigna	Nilotinib	BCR-ABL	2008 CML
Votrient	Pazopanib hydrochloride	VEGFR-1, -2, and -3, c-kit, and PDGF-R	2009 Advanced renal cell carcinoma 2012 Advanced soft tissue sarcoma
Caprelsa	Vandetanib	VEGFR2 EGFR	2011 Thyroid cancer
Iclusig	Ponatinib	BCR-ABL VEGFR Fibroblast growth factor receptor FLT3 TIE2	2012 CML ALL
Bosulif	Bosutinib	BCR-ABL Src-family protein kinases	2012 CML
Inlyta	Axitinib	VEGFR PDGFR	2012 Renal cell carcinoma

(continued on next page)

Table 3 (continued)			
Brand Name	Generic Name	Targets	Year of Initial FDA Approval and Indications
Mekinist	Trametinib	MEK MAPK/ERK RAS/RAF/MEK/ERK	2013 Metastatic melanoma
Tafinlar	Dabrafenib	BRAF MAP/ERK	2013 Metastatic melanoma
Gilotrif	Afatinib dimaleate	EGFR HER2 and HER4	2013 Non–small cell lung cancer
Cotellic	Cobimetinib	MAP2K1 ERK2 RAS/RAF/MEK/ERK	2015 Melanoma

Abbreviations: ALL, acute lymphoblastic leukemia; EGFR, endothelial growth factor receptor; ERK, extracellular signal related kinase; FLT, FMS-related tyrosine kinase; GIST, gastrointestinal stromal tumors; HER, herceptin; MAPK, mitogen-activated protein kinase; PDGFR, platelet-derived growth factor receptor; RAF, rapidly accelerated fibrosarcoma; VEGFR, vascular endothelial growth factor receptor.

kinase, and epidermal growth factor receptor–family kinases. TKIs are listed in **Table 3** with their FDA-approved indications.

IMPLICATIONS FOR PRACTICE

The roles of the oncology nurse during cancer therapy in contemporary oncology settings are varied. These roles include informant, educator, advocate, navigator, and outcomes evaluator roles. Additionally, oncology nurses monitor and manage side effects from treatment, provide psychological support, and help patients navigate complex health situations.[54] For nurses to monitor and manage side effects effectively, nurses must be familiar with the most common side effects associated with specific targeted therapy. **Table 4** provides the most common side effects associated with Mabs, Mibs, Mids, Nabs, and Nibs.

Patient education on disease and treatment side effects and early detection of the signs and symptoms of serious side effects are critical to treatment success. Involving patients and family members in the treatment decision making process could potentially lead to better satisfaction with treatment decisions, reduce decisional conflicts, and improve adherence to prescribed chemotherapy regimen.[55,56] The era of shared decision in oncology practice has begun. Oncology nurses must empower patients to express their treatment preferences and advocate for patients, particularly those patients who are unable to advocate for themselves because of the severity of their cancer status.[57–59]

A growing number of novel cancer treatments are now available in oral formulation.[60] The convenience of oral chemotherapies offers patients and families flexibility and less burden in making frequent clinic appointments for infusion. Given that patients no longer come to the clinic frequently with oral chemotherapies, the need for adequate patient and caregiver education on the safe handling of oral chemotherapy and early recognition of signs and symptoms of serious side effects are more critical than ever.[61] **Table 5** outlines the most common side effects from targeted therapies and self-care and side effects management strategies. The use of technology, such as electronic reporting of side effects by patients, must be encouraged whenever this technology is available.[62]

Table 4
Most common side effects associated with targeted therapies

Side Effects	Mabs	Mibs	Mids	Nabs	Nibs
Myelosuppression					
Anemia	●	●	●	●	●
Neutropenia	●	●	●	●	●
Thrombocytopenia	●	●	●	●	●
Gastrointestinal side effects					
Nausea	●	●	—	●	●
Vomiting	●	—	—	●	●
Diarrhea	●	●	●	●	●
Constipation	—	—	●	—	—
Thrombosis					
Deep vein thrombosis	—	—	●	●	● Ponatinib
Pulmonary embolism	—	—	●		
Infusion-related reactions	Likely during first infusion				
Fever	●	—	—	—	—
Chills or rigors	●	—	—	—	—
Itching	●	—	—	—	—
Hives	●	—	—	—	—
Bronchoconstriction	●	—	—	—	—
Flulike symptoms	●	—	—	—	—
Dermatologic toxicities					
Rash	●	—	●	—	●
Acne	—	—	—	—	●
Pruritus	—	—	—	—	●
Dry skin	—	—	—	—	●

Neurotoxicities			
Peripheral neuropathy	—	● Except lenalidomide	—
Cardiopulmonary Effects			
Bradycardia	—	● Specific to thalidomide	—
Hypotension	● Specific to bortezomib	—	●
Shortness of breath	● Specific to carfilzomib	—	●
QT prolongation	—	—	● Nilotinib
Abnormal electrocardiogram	—	●	—
Pleural effusion	—	—	● Dasatinib
Constitutional symptoms			
Fatigue	●	●	●
Body malaise	●	—	●
Headache	●	—	●
Muscle cramps	—	—	●
Other side effects			
Hemorrhage	● Bevacizumab	—	●
Fluid retention and edema	—	●	●
Congestive heart failure	—	—	●
Hepatic enzyme elevation	—	●	●

Table 5
Self-care and side effects management

Most Common Side Effects of Targeted Therapies	Self-Care and Side Effects Management	Clinical Pearls
Myelosuppression: anemia, neutropenia, thrombocytopenia	Monitor blood counts according to the individual drug's full prescribing information Use growth factors in a timely fashion Educate patients and caregivers on early signs and symptoms of infection Provide contact information of oncology care team members including weekend on-call telephone numbers Schedule blood products transfusion according to institutional protocol	Prevent severe neutropenia and sepsis by using recommended prophylactic growth factor
GI side effects: nausea, vomiting, diarrhea, or constipation	Instruct patient to keep a diary of GI side effects and to keep detailed information on frequency, severity, patterns, relieving factors of GI side effects Inform patient to communicate with the oncology care team any use of OTC drugs to relieve GI side effects as soon as possible Review with patients OTC drugs that may exacerbate GI side effects (eg, antacids with magnesium can cause diarrhea)	Avoid using OTC antidiarrheal agent in patients who recently completed a course of antibiotic therapy unless *Clostridium difficile* infection has been ruled out
Renal insufficiency	Instruct patient to avoid the use of nonsteroidal anti-inflammatory drugs, such as ibuprofen Educate patient on the importance of keeping well-hydrated during therapy	Monitor creatinine level closely and follow guidelines on holding or adjusting therapy dose if creatinine worsens during active therapy

PN	Monitor onset, severity, and progression of neuropathic toxicity before the next dose of therapy Follow the individual drug's full prescribing information on dose adjustment based on PN severity Advise patient to use complementary approaches, such as massage or acupuncture	No gold standard for tools in monitoring PN, but the consistent use of a well-validated PN monitoring tool is highly recommended
DVT or PE	Educate patients and caregivers on the signs and symptoms of DVT and PE Instruct patient to call 9-1-1 if sudden onset of chest pain or dyspnea occurs	Prevent DVT or PE using recommended prophylactic agents
Dermatologic toxicities (rash, urticaria, pruritus)	Educate patients and caregivers on high incidence of dermatologic side effects associated with Nibs and Mabs Follow skin toxicity evaluation protocol according to individual drug's full prescribing information Administer premedications and other preventive regimen for dermatologic toxicities	Pre-emptive skin treatment regimen can prevent development of severe form of dermatologic toxicities
Drug infusion reaction	Administer premedications according to individual drug's full prescribing information Monitor patient's vital signs including signs and symptoms of bronchoconstriction per institutional protocol Follow strictly the recommended rate of infusion at various time points of infusion	Stop infusion at the first sign of infusion reaction Administer recommended drugs for drug infusion reaction Resume infusion at a slower rate and monitor patient's vital signs per institutional protocol

Abbreviations: DVT, deep venous thrombosis; GI, gastrointestinal; OTC, over the counter; PE, pulmonary embolism; PN, peripheral neuropathy.

Access to oral chemotherapy is difficult for some patients. Patients who were pre-scribed oral chemotherapy may encounter issues with insurance coverage and high copays that could impact timely initiation of therapy and future adherence. Oncology nurses and all oncology practitioners must help patients resolve any obstacle to oral chemotherapy access.[63] An individualized approach to finding ways that promote ac-cess to oral chemotherapy must be in place to avoid delays in treatment.

SUMMARY

Cancer therapeutics has grown exponentially in the past several decades. The pinnacle of targeted therapies has been reached with great success, but cure remains elusive. Oncology nurses have the education, training, and skills to make significant contributions toward finding the cure for cancer by providing excellent nursing care throughout the cancer treatment continuum.

REFERENCES

1. Cortes J, Calvo E, Vivancos A, et al. New approach to cancer therapy based on a molecularly defined cancer classification. CA Cancer J Clin 2014;64(1):70–4.
2. Leget GA, Czuczman MS. Use of rituximab, the new FDA-approved antibody. Curr Opin Oncol 1998;10(6):548–51.
3. Tariman JD, Lemoine C. Bortezomib. Clin J Oncol Nurs 2003;7:687–9.
4. Richardson PG, Anderson KC. Bortezomib: a novel therapy approved for multiple myeloma. Clin Adv Hematol Oncol 2003;1(10):596–600.
5. Kane RC, Bross PF, Farrell AT, et al. Velcade: U.S. FDA approval for the treatment of multiple myeloma progressing on prior therapy. Oncologist 2003;8(6):508–13.
6. Celgene Corporation. Thalomid (thalidomide) [package insert]. Summit, NJ: Author; 2006.
7. Henderson IC, Bhatia V. Nab-paclitaxel for breast cancer: a new formulation with an improved safety profile and greater efficacy. Expert Rev Anticancer Ther 2007; 7(7):919–43.
8. Albumin-bound paclitaxel (Abraxane) for advanced breast cancer. Med Lett Drugs Ther 2005;47(1208):39–40.
9. Cohen MH, Moses ML, Pazdur R. Gleevec for the treatment of chronic myeloge-nous leukemia: US. Food and Drug Administration regulatory mechanisms, accel-erated approval, and orphan drug status. Oncologist 2002;7(5):390–2.
10. Shirley M. Ixazomib: first global approval. Drugs 2016;76(3):405–11.
11. McKeage K. Daratumumab: first global approval. Drugs 2016;76(2):275–81.
12. Markham A. Elotuzumab: first global approval. Drugs 2016;76(3):397–403.
13. Garnock-Jones KP. Panobinostat: first global approval. Drugs 2015;75(6): 695–704.
14. Herndon TM, Deisseroth A, Kaminskas E, et al. U.S. Food and Drug Administra-tion approval: carfilzomib for the treatment of multiple myeloma. Clin Cancer Res 2013;19(17):4559–63.
15. Elkinson S, McCormack PL. Pomalidomide: first global approval. Drugs 2013; 73(6):595–604.
16. Tariman JD, Doorenbos A, Schepp KG, et al. Information needs priorities in pa-tients diagnosed with cancer: a systematic review. J Adv Pract Oncol 2014; 2014(5):115–22.
17. Liu JK. The history of monoclonal antibody development: progress, remaining challenges and future innovations. Ann Med Surg (Lond) 2014;3(4):113–6.

18. Maloney DG, Grillo-Lopez AJ, White CA, et al. IDEC-C2B8 (Rituximab) anti-CD20 monoclonal antibody therapy in patients with relapsed low-grade non-Hodgkin's lymphoma. Blood 1997;90(6):2188–95.
19. Anderson DR, Grillo-Lopez A, Varns C, et al. Targeted anti-cancer therapy using rituximab, a chimaeric anti-CD20 antibody (IDEC-C2B8) in the treatment of non-Hodgkin's B-cell lymphoma. Biochem Soc Trans 1997;25(2):705–8.
20. Weiner GJ. Rituximab: mechanism of action. Semin Hematol 2010;47(2):115–23.
21. Storz U. Rituximab: how approval history is reflected by a corresponding patent filing strategy. MAbs 2014;6(4):820–37.
22. Li J, Zhu Z. Research and development of next generation of antibody-based therapeutics. Acta Pharmacol Sin 2010;31(9):1198–207.
23. Bross PF, Kane R, Farrell AT, et al. Approval summary for bortezomib for injection in the treatment of multiple myeloma. Clin Cancer Res 2004;10(12 Pt 1):3954–64.
24. Adams J, Behnke M, Chen S, et al. Potent and selective inhibitors of the proteasome: dipeptidyl boronic acids. Bioorg Med Chem Lett 1998;8(4):333–8.
25. Adams J. The proteasome: structure, function, and role in the cell. Cancer Treat Rev 2003;29(Suppl 1):3–9.
26. Adams J, Kauffman M. Development of the proteasome inhibitor Velcade (bortezomib). Cancer Invest 2004;22(2):304–11.
27. Fisher RI, Bernstein SH, Kahl BS, et al. Multicenter phase II study of bortezomib in patients with relapsed or refractory mantle cell lymphoma. J Clin Oncol 2006; 24(30):4867–74.
28. Kuhn DJ, Chen Q, Voorhees PM, et al. Potent activity of carfilzomib, a novol, irreversible inhibitor of the ubiquitin-proteasome pathway, against preclinical models of multiple myeloma. Blood 2007;110(9):3281–90.
29. Carfilzomib (Kryprolis) for multiple myeloma. Med Lett Drugs Ther 2012;54(1406): 103–4.
30. Siegel DS, Martin T, Wang M, et al. A phase 2 study of single-agent carfilzomib (PX-171-003-A1) in patients with relapsed and refractory multiple myeloma. Blood 2012;120(14):2817–25.
31. Jakubowiak AJ, Siegel DS, Martin T, et al. Treatment outcomes in patients with relapsed and refractory multiple myeloma and high-risk cytogenetics receiving single-agent carfilzomib in the PX-171-003-A1 study. Leukemia 2013;27(12): 2351–6.
32. Kupperman E, Lee EC, Cao Y, et al. Evaluation of the proteasome inhibitor MLN9708 in preclinical models of human cancer. Cancer Res 2010;70(5): 1970–80.
33. Tariman JD, Doorenbos A, Schepp KG, et al. Patient, physician and contextual factors are influential in the treatment decision making of older adults newly diagnosed with symptomatic myeloma. Cancer Treat Commun 2014;2(2–3):34–47.
34. Infante JR, Mendelson DS, Burris HA 3rd, et al. A first-in-human dose-escalation study of the oral proteasome inhibitor oprozomib in patients with advanced solid tumors. Invest New Drugs 2016;34(2):216–24.
35. Chang X, Zhu Y, Shi C, et al. Mechanism of immunomodulatory drugs' action in the treatment of multiple myeloma. Acta Biochim Biophys Sin (Shanghai) 2014; 46(3):240–53.
36. D'Amato RJ, Lentzsch S, Anderson KC, et al. Mechanism of action of thalidomide and 3-aminothalidomide in multiple myeloma. Semin Oncol 2001;28(6):597–601.
37. Yabu T, Tomimoto H, Taguchi Y, et al. Thalidomide-induced antiangiogenic action is mediated by ceramide through depletion of VEGF receptors, and is antagonized by sphingosine-1-phosphate. Blood 2005;106(1):125–34.

38. Leleu X, Micol JB, Guieze R, et al. Thalidomide: mechanisms of action and new insights in hematology. Rev Med Interne 2005;26(2):119–27 [in French].
39. Anderson KC. Lenalidomide and thalidomide: mechanisms of action–similarities and differences. Semin Hematol 2005;42(4 Suppl 4):S3–8.
40. Zhu YX, Kortuem KM, Stewart AK. Molecular mechanism of action of immune-modulatory drugs thalidomide, lenalidomide and pomalidomide in multiple myeloma. Leuk Lymphoma 2013;54(4):683–7.
41. Kotla V, Goel S, Nischal S, et al. Mechanism of action of lenalidomide in hemato-logical malignancies. J Hematol Oncol 2009;2:36.
42. Heise C, Carter T, Schafer P, et al. Pleiotropic mechanisms of action of lenalido-mide efficacy in del(5q) myelodysplastic syndromes. Expert Rev Anticancer Ther 2010;10(10):1663–72.
43. McDaniel JM, Pinilla-Ibarz J, Epling-Burnette PK. Molecular action of lenalido-mide in lymphocytes and hematologic malignancies. Adv Hematol 2012;2012: 513702.
44. Giagounidis A, Mufti GJ, Fenaux P, et al. Lenalidomide as a disease-modifying agent in patients with del(5q) myelodysplastic syndromes: linking mechanism of action to clinical outcomes. Ann Hematol 2014;93(1):1–11.
45. List A, Dewald G, Bennett J, et al. Lenalidomide in the myelodysplastic syndrome with chromosome 5q deletion. N Engl J Med 2006;355(14):1456–65.
46. New treatment for myelodysplastic syndrome. FDA Consum 2006;40(2):4.
47. National Cancer Institute. FDA approval for lenalidomide. 2013. Available at: http://www.cancer.gov/about-cancer/treatment/drugs/fda-lenalidomide#Anchor-MCL. Accessed March 20, 2016.
48. Lugo TG, Pendergast AM, Muller AJ, et al. Tyrosine kinase activity and transfor-mation potency of bcr-abl oncogene products. Science 1990;247(4946): 1079–82.
49. Nowell PC, Hungerford DA. Chromosome studies on normal and leukemic human leukocytes. J Natl Cancer Inst 1960;25:85–109.
50. Witte ON. Role of the BCR-ABL oncogene in human leukemia: fifteenth Richard and Hinda Rosenthal Foundation Award Lecture. Cancer Res 1993;53(3):485–9.
51. Kantarjian HM, Talpaz M. Imatinib mesylate: clinical results in Philadelphia chromosome-positive leukemias. Semin Oncol 2001;28(5 Suppl 17):9–18.
52. Cohen MH, Williams G, Johnson JR, et al. Approval summary for imatinib mesy-late capsules in the treatment of chronic myelogenous leukemia. Clin Cancer Res 2002;8(5):935–42.
53. Druker BJ, Guilhot F, O'Brien SG, et al. Five-year follow-up of patients receiving imatinib for chronic myeloid leukemia. N Engl J Med 2006;355(23):2408–17.
54. Tariman JD, Szubski KL. The evolving role of the nurse during the cancer treat-ment decision-making process: a literature review. Clin J Oncol Nurs 2015; 19(5):548–56.
55. Tariman JD, Berry DL, Cochrane B, et al. Preferred and actual participation roles during health care decision making in persons with cancer: a systematic review. Ann Oncol 2010;21(6):1145–51.
56. Kane HL, Halpern MT, Squiers LB, et al. Implementing and evaluating shared de-cision making in oncology practice. CA Cancer J Clin 2014;64(6):377–88.
57. Tariman JD, Doorenbos A, Schepp KG, et al. Older adults newly diagnosed with symptomatic myeloma and treatment decision making. Oncol Nurs Forum 2014; 41(4):411–9.
58. Haebler J. Shaping nurse leaders in policy and advocacy. Am Nurse 2013; 45(6):15.

59. Hanks RG. Sphere of nursing advocacy model. Nurs Forum 2005;40(3):75–8.
60. Esper P. Identifying strategies to optimize care with oral cancer therapy. Clin J Oncol Nurs 2013;17(6):629–36.
61. Schellens JH. Challenges of oral chemotherapy. Clin Adv Hematol Oncol 2005; 3(2):99–100.
62. Berry DL, Hong F, Halpenny B, et al. The electronic self report assessment and intervention for cancer: promoting patient verbal reporting of symptom and quality of life issues in a randomized controlled trial. BMC Cancer 2014;14:513.
63. Han D, Trinkaus M, Hogeveen S, et al. Overcoming obstacles in accessing unfunded oral chemotherapy: physician experience and challenges. J Oncol Pract 2013;9(4):188–93.

Dermatologic Reactions to Targeted Therapy

A Focus on Epidermal Growth Factor Receptor Inhibitors and Nursing Care

Margaret Barton-Burke, PhD, RN, FAAN[a],*,
Kathryn Ciccolini, RN, BSN, OCN, DNC[b], Maria Mekas, BSN, RN[b],
Sean Burke, BS[a]

KEYWORDS

- Skin reactions • EGFRi (epidermal growth factor receptor inhibitors)
- Oncodermatology

KEY POINTS

- Cancer treatments are changing.
- Treatments are targeting newer cellular mechanisms.
- Side effects to newer treatments differ from previous side effects.
- Skin reactions are some of the most problematic side effects to cancer treatments.
- There are now skin reactions to newer cancer therapies.

INTRODUCTION

Over the past decade, it has become important to incorporate dermatology into cancer care because skin reactions are one of the major reactions to newer anticancer therapies like epidermal growth factor receptor (EGFR) inhibitors (EGFRi). Overexpression of EGFR is strongly associated with the development of and progression in several cancers.[1–3] Agents that inhibit the EGFR pathway are (1) monoclonal antibodies (mAbs), such as cetuximab and panitumumab, and (2) small molecule inhibitors: erlotinib, gefitinib, afatinib, lapatinib.[4] Patients treated with EGFRi commonly

Dr Barton-Burke acknowledges funding support from MSK Cancer Center Support Grant/Core Grant (P30 CA008748).

[a] Department of Nursing Research, Memorial Sloan Kettering Cancer Center, 205 East 64th Street, Room 251 Concourse Level, New York, NY 10065, USA; [b] Department of Dermatology, Memorial Sloan Kettering Cancer Center, 16 East 60th Street, New York, NY 10022, USA
* Corresponding author.
E-mail address: bartonbm@mskcc.org

Nurs Clin N Am 52 (2017) 83–113
http://dx.doi.org/10.1016/j.cnur.2016.11.005
0029-6465/17/© 2016 Elsevier Inc. All rights reserved.

experience dermatologic side effects, including papulopustular rash, hair changes, radiation dermatitis enhancement, pruritus, mucositis, xerosis, fissures, and paronychia.[1] These side effects are important side effects related to new cancer treatments. This article presents the common skin reactions seen with EGFRi and presents an overview of skin assessment, pathophysiology, and nursing care. These side effects should be recognized early, diagnosed promptly, and treated before they affect patients' quality of life and mortality. This article also provides an introduction to the emerging cancer nursing specialty of oncodermatology.

PATIENT ASSESSMENT

Nurses play a key role in assessing, preventing, and managing patients with cancer treatment–related skin conditions. Understanding factors that comprise wound healing should be incorporated into nursing assessment and can be found in **Table 1**. **Table 2** outlines criteria for a basic skin assessment and common terminology to describe skin changes. When performing a skin assessment nurses must inspect and palpate the skin noting color, moisture, texture, morphology, and distribution. Using a grading system like the CTCAEv.4 (Common Terminology Criteria for Adverse Events Version 4.0) found in **Table 3** provides a consistent and standard way to assess and document skin and subcutaneous disorders.

Performing a comprehensive skin assessment and history includes assessment for patient and treatment-related factors (see **Table 1**). A detailed history from either the patient or caregiver includes questions about the onset of rash (date), initial presentation, progression of eruptions, alleviating and persisting factors, treatment history and outcomes along with a review of systems.[5]

The nurse needs to specify the affected area and can consider calculating body surface area using the Rule of Nines in **Fig. 1**. Obtaining a past medical, surgical, and social history is important, paying attention to past dermatologic conditions (ie, Herpes simplex virus, contact dermatitis) or allergies to medications. Reviewing a medication list including prescriptions (topical, oral, subcutaneous) and over-the-counter medications including complementary or alternative therapies is essential. The assessment should include dates of changes in prescription drugs and dosage, if indicated.

Table 1 Patient/treatment-related factors that compromise wound healing	
Patient-Related Factors	**Treatment-Related Factors**
Age	Medication
Compromised nutritional status	Medical treatments
Body type (extremes: obese vs extremely thin)	
Low performance status	
Location/site of injury	
Previous sun/radiation exposure	
Smoking	
Comorbidities (cardiovascular, pulmonary, renal & liver disease, lymphedema, autoimmune disorders, diabetes)	
Psychological distress	

Data from Haas M, Moore-Higgs GJ, editors. Principles of skin care and the oncology patient. Pittsburgh (PA): Oncology Nursing Society. 2010.

Table 2
Dermatologic assessment/history

Skin assessment/history	
Common Terminology	• Perform the skin assessment.
Macule — Small flat spot, up to 1 cm	○ Visually inspect and palpate the skin.
Patch — Flat spot 1 cm or larger	○ Describe the type of lesion, location, and distribution.
Papules — Up to 1 cm	○ Assess for signs and symptoms of infection.
Plaques — Elevated lesion 1 cm or larger	○ Take photographs to document the lesion and extent of involvement skin condition.
Vesicles — Up to 1 cm, filled with serous fluid	• Take a detailed history.
Bullae — 1 cm or larger filled with serous fluid	○ When did the skin reaction begin?
Pustule — A vesicle or bulla containing purulent fluid up to 1 cm	○ How long has the skin reaction been present?
Filled with pus (yellow proteinaceous fluid filled with neutrophils)	○ Does the skin itch?
Nodule — Knotlike lesion larger than 0.5 cm, deeper and firmer than a papule	○ Do you have pain?
	○ What did the reaction first look like?
	○ Has the skin reaction changed?
	○ Does the skin reaction subside and return?
	○ Review a list of all medication over a 2-mo period.
	○ Have you changed soap, detergents, lotions, and so forth, before you noticed the skin reaction?
	○ Is there any history of similar symptoms or a family member with drug allergies?
	○ Have you used or tried anything that seems to make the reaction better or worse?
	○ Do you have any other systems (ie, fever, malaise, pain, diarrhea)?
Review medications, including over-the-counter and complementary/alternative therapies	• Review all medications.
	○ Include the start date, if/when dose changed, and when drug was stopped over the past 2 mo. The drug timeline is extremely helpful.
	○ It is important to assess allergy history, including details of type of reaction.
Past medical and surgical history, including comorbidities, treatment, and nutritional status	• Take history, including recurrent HSV and infections.

Abbreviation: HSV, herpes simplex virus.

Data from Bickley LS, Szilagyi PG. Bates' guide to physical examination and history taking. Philadelphia: Wolters Kluwer Health/Lippincott Williams & Wilkins; 2013; and Johansen L. Skin assessment. Dermatol Nurs 2005;17:166.

Table 3
CTCAE V.4 grading scale

Skin and Subcutaneous Tissue Disorders

Adverse Event	Grade				
	1	2	3	4	5
Alopecia	Hair loss of <50% of normal for that individual that is not obvious from a distance but only on close inspection; may require different hair style to cover the hair loss; wig or hairpiece to camouflage not required	Hair loss of ≥50% normal for that individual that is readily apparent to others; requires wig or hairpiece if the patient desires to completely camouflage the hair loss; associated with psychosocial impact	—	—	—
Definition: It is a disorder characterized by a decrease in density of hair compared with normal for a given individual at a given age and body location.					
Body odor	Mild odor; physician intervention not indicated; self-care interventions	Pronounced odor; psychosocial impact; medical intervention required by patients	—	—	—
Definition: It is a disorder characterized by an abnormal body smell resulting from the growth of bacteria on the body.					
Bullous dermatitis	Asymptomatic; blisters covering <10% BSA	Blisters covering 10%–30% BSA; painful blisters; limiting instrumental ADL	Blisters covering >30% BSA; limiting self-care ADL	Blisters covering >30% BSA; associated with fluid or electrolyte abnormalities; ICU care or burn unit indicated	Death
Definition: It is a disorder characterized by inflammation of the skin characterized by the presence of bullae, which are filled with fluid.					
Dry skin	Covering <10% BSA and no associated erythema or pruritus	Covering 10%–30% BSA and associated with erythema or pruritus; limiting instrumental ADL	Covering >30% BSA and associated with pruritus; limiting self-care ADL	—	
Definition: It is a disorder characterized by flaky and dull skin; the pores are generally fine; the texture is a papery thin texture.					

	Grade 1	Grade 2	Grade 3	Grade 4	Grade 5
Erythema multiforme	Target lesions covering <10% BSA and not associated with skin tenderness	Target lesions covering 10%–30% BSA and associated with skin tenderness	Target lesions covering >30% BSA and associated with oral or genital erosions	Target lesions covering >30% BSA; associated with fluid or electrolyte abnormalities; ICU care or burn unit indicated	Death

Definition: It is a disorder characterized by target lesions (a pink-red ring around a pale center).

	Grade 1	Grade 2	Grade 3	Grade 4	Grade 5
Erythroderma	—	Erythema covering >90% BSA without associated symptoms; limiting instrumental ADL	Erythema covering >90% BSA with associated symptoms (eg, pruritus or tenderness); limiting self-care ADL	Erythema covering >90% BSA with associated fluid or electrolyte abnormalities; ICU care or burn unit indicated	Death

Definition: It is a disorder characterized by generalized inflammatory erythema and exfoliation. The inflammatory process involves >90% of the BSA.

	Grade 1	Grade 2	Grade 3	Grade 4	Grade 5
Fat atrophy	Covering <10% BSA and asymptomatic	Covering 10%–30% and associated with erythema or tenderness; limiting instrumental ADL	Covering >30% BSA; associated with erythema or tenderness; limiting self-care ADL	—	

Definition: It is a disorder characterized by shrinking of adipose tissue.

	Grade 1	Grade 2	Grade 3	Grade 4	Grade 5
Pain of skin	Mild pain	Moderate pain; limiting instrumental ADL	Severe pain; limiting self-care ADL	—	

Definition: It is a disorder characterized by marked discomfort sensation in the skin.

	Grade 1	Grade 2	Grade 3	Grade 4	Grade 5
Periorbital edema	Soft or nonpitting	Indurated or pitting edema; topical intervention indicated	Edema associated with visual disturbance; increased intraocular pressure; glaucoma or retinal hemorrhage; optic neuritis; diuretics indicated; operative intervention indicated	—	

Definition: It is a disorder characterized by swelling due to an excessive accumulation of fluid around the orbits of the face.

(continued on next page)

Table 3
(continued)

Skin and Subcutaneous Tissue Disorders

Adverse Event	Grade				
	1	2	3	4	5
Photosensitivity	Painless erythema and erythema covering <10% BSA	Tender erythema covering 10%–30% BSA	Erythema covering >30% BSA and erythema with blistering; photosensitivity; oral corticosteroid therapy indicated; pain control indicated (eg, narcotics or NSAIDs)	Life-threatening consequences; urgent intervention indicated	Death

Definition: It is a disorder characterized by an increase in sensitivity of the skin to light.

Pruritus	Mild or localized; topical intervention indicated	Intense or widespread; intermittent; skin changes from scratching (eg, edema, papulation, excoriations, lichenification, oozing/crusts); oral intervention indicated; limiting instrumental ADL	Intense or widespread; constant; limiting self-care ADL or sleep; oral corticosteroid or immunosuppressive therapy indicated	—	—

Definition: It is a disorder characterized by an intense itching sensation.

Purpura	Combined area of lesions covering <10% BSA	Combined area of lesions covering 10%–30% BSA; bleeding with trauma	Combined area of lesions covering >30% BSA; spontaneous bleeding	—	—

Definition: It is a disorder characterized by hemorrhagic areas of the skin and mucous membrane. Newer lesions appear reddish. Older lesions are usually a darker purple color and eventually become a brownish-yellow color.

					Death
Rash acneiform	Papules and/or pustules covering <10% BSA, which may or may not be associated with symptoms of pruritus or tenderness	Papules and/or pustules covering 10%–30% BSA, which may or may not be associated with symptoms of pruritus or tenderness; associated with psychosocial impact; limiting instrumental ADL	Papules and/or pustules covering >30% BSA, which may or may not be associated with symptoms of pruritus or tenderness; limiting self-care ADL; associated with local superinfection with oral antibiotics indicated	Papules and/or pustules covering any % BSA, which may or may not be associated with symptoms of pruritus or tenderness and are associated with extensive superinfection with IV antibiotics indicated; life-threatening consequences	Death

Definition: It is a disorder characterized by an eruption of papules and pustules, typically appearing in the face, scalp, upper chest, and back.

Rash maculopapular	Macules/papules covering <10% BSA with or without symptoms (eg, pruritus, burning, tightness)	Macules/papules covering 10%–30% BSA with or without symptoms (eg, pruritus, burning, tightness); limiting instrumental ADL	Macules/papules covering >30% BSA with or without associated symptoms; limiting self-care ADL	—

Definition: It is a disorder characterized by the presence of macules (flat) and papules (elevated). Also known as morbilliform rash, it is one of the most common cutaneous adverse events, frequently affecting the upper trunk, spreading centripetally and associated with pruritus.

Scalp pain	Mild pain	Moderate pain; limiting instrumental ADL	Severe pain; limiting self-care ADL	—

Definition: It is a disorder characterized by marked discomfort sensation in the skin covering the top and the back of the head.

Skin atrophy	Covering <110% BSA; associated with telangiectasias or changes in skin color	Covering 10%–30% BSA; associated with striae or adnexal structure loss	Covering >30% BSA; associated with ulceration	—

Definition: It is a disorder characterized by the degeneration and thinning of the epidermis and dermis.

Skin hyperpigmentation	Hyperpigmentation covering <10% BSA; no psychosocial impact	Hyperpigmentation covering >10% BSA; associated psychosocial impact	—	—

(continued on next page)

Table 3
(continued)

Skin and Subcutaneous Tissue Disorders

Adverse Event	Grade				
	1	2	3	4	5
Definition: It is a disorder characterized by darkening of the skin due to excessive melanin deposition.					
Skin hypopigmentation	Hypopigmentation or depigmentation covering <10% BSA; no psychosocial impact	Hyperpigmentation or depigmentation covering >10% BSA; associated psychosocial impact	—	—	
Definition: It is a disorder characterized by loss of skin pigment.					
Skin induration	Mild induration, able to move skin parallel to plane (sliding) and perpendicular to skin (pinching up)	Moderate induration, able to slide skin, unable to pinch skin; limiting instrumental ADL	Severe induration, unable to slide or pinch skin; limiting joint movement or orifice (eg, mouth, anus); limiting self-care ADL	Generalized; associated with signs or symptoms of impaired breathing or feeding	Death
Definition: It is a disorder characterized by an area of hardness in the skin.					
Skin ulceration	Combined area of ulcers <1 cm; nonblanchable erythema of intact skin with associated warmth or edema	Combined area of ulcers 1–2 cm; partial-thickness skin loss involving skin or subcutaneous fat	Combined area of ulcers >2 cm; full-thickness skin loss involving damage to or necrosis of subcutaneous tissue that may extend down to fascia	Any size ulcer with extensive destruction, tissue necrosis, or damage to muscle, bone, or supporting structures with or without full-thickness skin loss	Death
Definition: It is a disorder characterized by circumscribed, inflammatory, and necrotic erosive lesion on the skin.					
SJS	—	—	Skin sloughing covering <10% BSA with associated signs (eg, erythema, purpura, epidermal detachment and mucous membrane detachment)	Skin sloughing covering 10%–30% BSA with associated signs (eg, erythema, purpura, epidermal detachment and mucous membrane detachment)	Death

Definition: It is a disorder characterized by <10% total body skin area separation of dermis. The syndrome is thought to be a hypersensitivity complex affecting the skin and the mucous membranes.

	Grade 1	Grade 2	Grade 3	Grade 4	Grade 5
Telangiectasia	Telangiectasias covering <10% BSA	Telangiectasias covering >10% BSA; associated with psychosocial impact	—	—	—

Definition: It is a disorder characterized by local dilatation of small vessels resulting in red discoloration of the skin or mucous membranes.

	Grade 1	Grade 2	Grade 3	Grade 4	Grade 5
TEN	—	—	—	Skin sloughing covering ≥30% BSA with associated symptoms (eg, erythema, purpura, or epidermal detachment)	Death

Definition: It is a disorder characterized by >30% total body skin area separation of dermis. The syndrome is thought to be a hypersensitivity complex affecting the skin and the mucous membranes.

	Grade 1	Grade 2	Grade 3	Grade 4	Grade 5
Urticaria	Urticarial lesions covering <10% BSA; topical intervention indicated	Urticarial lesions covering 10%–30% BSA; oral intervention indicated	Urticarial lesions covering >30% BSA; IV intervention indicated	—	—

Definition: A disorder characterized by an itchy skin eruption characterized by wheals with pale interiors and well-defined red margins.

	Grade 1	Grade 2	Grade 3	Grade 4	Grade 5
Skin and subcutaneous tissue disorders: other, specify	Asymptomatic or mild symptoms; clinical or diagnostic observations only; intervention not indicated	Moderate; minimal, local, or noninvasive intervention indicated; limiting age-appropriate instrumental ADL	Severe or medically significant but not immediately life threatening; hospitalization or prolongation of existing hospitalization indicated; disabling; limiting self-care ADL	Life-threatening consequences; urgent intervention indicated	Death

Abbreviations: ADL, activities of daily living; BSA, body surface area; ICU, intensive care unit; IV, intravenous; NSAIDs, nonsteroidal antiinflammatory drugs; SJS, Stevens-Johnson syndrome; TEN, toxic epidermal necrolysis.
Data from NIH.

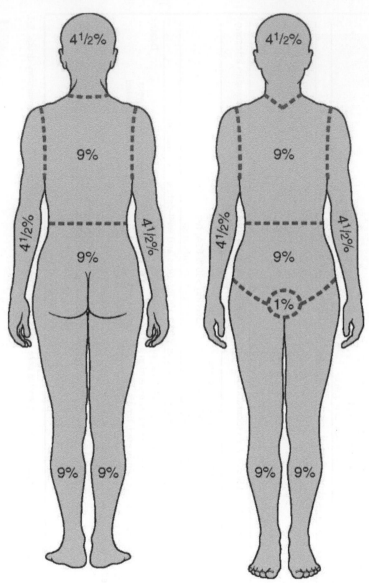

Fig. 1. Rule of Nines. (*From* Buck C. Next step: advanced medical coding 2012 edition textbook and workbook package. Philadelphia: W. B. Saunders; 2011. p. 223–76.)

PATHOPHYSIOLOGY AND CLINICAL PRESENTATION

EGFRs are primarily expressed in basal keratinocytes, the outer layers of hair follicles, eccrine sweat and pilosebaceous glands, and periungual tissues. Inhibiting EGF pathways in the skin results in arresting cell growth and migration, apoptosis, chemokine expression, and abnormal maturation and differentiation. The cellular cascade results in an inflammatory response with dermatologic manifestations, such as acneiform rashes, xerosis, pruritus, periungual inflammation, and hair and nail plate disturbance.

Acneiform rashes occur in up to 90% of patients on EGFRi. Rashes typically appear on the scalp, face, and upper body in sun-exposed areas within the first 2 weeks of starting therapy, peaking at 4 weeks.[6] The rash steadily declines by 6 to 8 weeks.[1] The rash first appears as erythema with a burning sensation as a result of an inflammatory cell release, vascular dilation, and increased permeability progressing to papules and pustules. The crusting of lesions occurs because of neutrophilic and keratinocyte debris, fibrin, and serum, indicating a noninfectious cause.[7] A prevalence of dermatologic infections has been reported in patients on EGFRi who are leukopenic.[4] It is important to note that acneiform rashes are confused with acne vulgaris but both are pathologically different from one another.

Severe rashes are more frequent with mAbs, such as cetuximab and panitumumab, than tyrosine kinase inhibitors (TKIs).[3] Yet EGFRi-induced rash has been reported to be an indication of treatment efficacy in some patients.[8] However, patients who underwent radiation therapy before starting EGFRi did not develop a rash during erlotinib therapy. But patients receiving EGFRi concomitantly with radiation are reported to have a higher incidence of high-grade radiation dermatitis.[1]

Xerosis is reported in up to 46.5% of patients receiving EGFRi within the first month of therapy and can be attributed to transepidermal water loss due to abnormal keratinocyte differentiation.[9] Pruritus often occurs concomitantly with xerosis following EGFRi administration with the highest incidence rate seen in cetuximab followed by erlotinib.[10] Paronychia occurs after 2 to 3 months of therapy. It is typically a sterile process but can become superinfected. Nail matrix inflammation occurs as a secondary process. Nonscarring alopecia can occur after 2 to 3 months of therapy initially presenting as patchy hair loss progressing into diffuse hair loss. This type of alopecia generally resolves after discontinuation of therapy.[1] The phases of skin changes and the pathophysiology are described in **Table 4**.

CLINICAL PRACTICE GUIDELINES

Despite the fact that most patients receiving EGFRi experience skin toxicities, there is a dearth of controlled studies, lacking strong level I evidence. In 2011, Lacouture and colleagues studied whether preemptive therapy could decrease the severity of panitumumab-related rash. They found that a grade 2 or higher rash and other skin changes were significantly reduced in patients who received daily moisturizer, sunscreen, topical hydrocortisone, and oral doxycycline for 6 weeks compared with a control group. Also, patients in the preemptive group reported less quality-of-life impairment than the control group. However, in 2016, Melosky and colleagues[11] conducted a prospective randomized study using prophylactic skin treatment of the prevention of erlotinib-induced skin rash. Patients receiving minocycline either prophylactically or reactively (after rash developed based on grade) were compared with those receiving no treatment unless there was a severe grade 3 rash. This study revealed a rash incidence of 84% but found no statistical difference between study arms. These two studies underscore the need for further research in this patient population.

Given the lack of evidence in the literature and the need for large-scale studies to define the best supportive care, there are a few clinical practice guidelines available for use with this patient population. The Multinational Association for Supportive Care in Cancer (MASCC)[12] and the Alberta Health Services[13] developed clinical practice guidelines for patients being treated with EGFRi. Both guidelines recommend that patients should receive individualized skin care management thus permitting the patient to receive maximum recommended EGFRi dose. The MASCC's skin toxicity

Table 4
Pathophysiology

Phase	Cellular Level Changes	Body Response	Goal of Treatment	Patient Information
Phase I: During weeks 0–1, there is erythema and edema like a sunburn. The patient feels a sunburnlike reaction (erythema, tenderness, slight swelling) on the face and areas that have previously been exposed to the sun.	EGFR inhibition in skin stops underlying keratinocytes from differentiating and migrating to skin surface to replace them, and they are arrested.	The body senses that these arrested replacement cells should not be there and, thus, causes them to undergo apoptosis or programmed cell death. The dead keratinocytes cause the release of chemokines, which recruit neutrophils to the area as part of the sterile, inflammatory response.	The goal is to preserve skin integrity, minimize discomfort, and prevent infection.	Key patient teaching includes (1) use skin cream with emollients to keep the skin from drying out; (2) avoid sun exposure, using a sunblock of SPF 30 or higher and protect skin with hat and clothes when out in the sun; (3) use a mild soap with active ingredients that reduce skin drying, such as pyrithione zinc (Head & Shoulders); (4) apply prescribed prophylactic skin creams; (5) report distressing tenderness, as pramoxine (lidocaine topical anesthetic) may help; (6) keep fingernails clean and trimmed.
Phase II: During weeks 1–3, papulopustules appear. The rash begins within 7–10 d of starting therapy and peaks in intensity in 2–3 wk and then gradually gets better.	This sterile inflammatory process results in death of the keratinocytes (apoptosis) and the formation of debris, which causes a popular rash on the skin.	At the same time, the skin is no longer fortified by healthy keratinocytes; thus, it thins and is unable to preserve water in the body, leading to skin dryness (xerosis) and itching.	The goal is to prevent infection, promote healing, and maximize comfort and coping during this time. See drug package inserts for specific information on holding or discontinuing drugs for severe dermatologic adverse effects.	

Phase III: During weeks 3–5, lesions crust.	The skin becomes drier (xerosis) with pruritus and the formation of telangiectasias (dilated capillaries in the skin).	The skin flakes and itches.	For flaking skin, keratolytics such as lactic acid, salicylic acid, or urea-containing topicals such as 12% ammonium lactate (Lac-Hydrin) or other exfoliating lotions can be helpful
Phase IV: During weeks 5–8, there are persistent dry skin, erythema, and other skin/hair changes.	EGFR blockade of the hair follicles and nail beds results in hair changes (hair thinning or alopecia on scalp but increased hair growth on the eyelids [trichomegaly] or face [hypertrichosis]).	The hair texture can change (changes in texture and strength). Paronychia (periungual inflammation) can develop with crusted lesions on nail folds and tenderness. Painful skin fissures on the fingers can develop.	It is important to assess eyelashes; if they are long, they can fold back and irritate the conjunctiva; refer to an ophthalmologist for redirection as needed (Borkar et al, 2013).

Abbreviation: SPF, sun protection factor.
Data from Lacouture ME. Mechanisms of cutaneous toxicities to EGFR inhibitors. Nature Reviews 2006;6(10):803–12.

guidelines can be found in **Table 5**. The guideline recommends prophylactic treatment in weeks 1 through 6 and week 8 when patients begin EGFRi therapy.[1]

Recommendations are based on level II evidence for prevention. Level II evidence consists of randomized trials that have low statistical power. Once treatment begins, the MASCC's skin toxicity guidelines recommend level IV evidence. Level IV evidence is considered weak evidence from descriptive and case studies. This level IV evidence includes topical hydrocortisone 1% cream, with moisturizer and sunscreen twice daily, and systemic doxycycline 100 mg by mouth twice daily or minocycline 100 mg daily if patients are in tropical areas, as minocycline is not photosensitizing.

IMPLICATIONS TO NURSING PRACTICE

Nursing care of patients receiving EGFRi therapy focuses on minimizing symptoms and helping patients maximize their quality of life. **Table 6** provides the nursing care and management, including the patient and caregiver education that is necessary for this patient population. Patient educational materials (**Table 7**) are available, such as "Skin Reactions to Targeted Therapies and Immunotherapy" (2016) by the American Society of Clinical Oncology,[14] available at http://www.cancer.net/navigating-cancer-care/side-effects/skin-reactions-targeted-therapies, or may be institution specific like the one found at https://www.mskcc.org/cancer-care/patient-education/skin-care-during-treatment-targeted-therapies.

The following is a more detailed description of the care for dermatologic problems that occur with new cancer treatments.

RASH

Treatment of EGFRi-induced rash[15] includes topical steroids, clindamycin 1% cream, and for, systemic treatment, doxycycline 100 mg by mouth twice daily or minocycline 100 mg daily. Treatment based on rash severity includes (1) grade 1: low to midpotency topical steroids, such as hydrocortisone or alclometasone cream 0.05% twice daily, and topical antibiotic, such as clindamycin gel 1% daily until rash resolution; (2) grade 2: low to midpotency topical steroid as discussed earlier and institute oral antibiotic (doxycycline 100 mg twice daily or minocycline 100 mg twice daily) for a minimum of 4 weeks, and continuing until rash resolves; (3) grade 3 or intolerable grade 2: consider EGFRi dose reduction per package insert or protocol as well as low to midpotency topical steroid and topical antibiotic as discussed earlier and oral doxycycline 100 mg twice daily for a minimum of 4 weeks, continuing until rash resolves. A methylprednisolone (Medrol) dose pack, high-potency topical steroid for the body, and low-dose isotretinoin may be considered.

PRURITUS

Pruritus management can be challenging and must be managed to prevent patients from scratching, resulting in secondary infections. The mainstay therapy for pruritus is topical corticosteroids using a midpotency agent, such as triamcinolone cream to the body and alclometasone to the face. If pruritus progresses, patients can switch to high-potency topical steroids, such as clobetasol. If patients' pruritus is refractory to topical corticosteroids, they may be placed on an alternative treatment, such as an immunomodulatory agent, like tacrolimus, or topical antidepressants, such as doxepin cream. Menthol-based moisturizers are used for antipruritic, nonpharmacologic therapy. Oral therapy for pruritus can include antihistamines, such as

Table 5
Multinational Association for Supportive Care in Cancer's grading tool for skin toxicities

Adverse Event	Grade 1	Grade 2	Grade 3	Grade 4
Papulopustular eruption (grading individually for face, scalp, chest or back)	1A: Papules or pustules <5 OR 1 area of erythema or edema <1 cm in size	2A: Papules or pustules 6–20 OR 2–5 areas of erythema or edema <1 cm in size	3A: Papules or pustules >20 OR more than 5 areas of erythema or edema <1 cm in size	—
	1B: Papules or pustules <5 OR 1 area of erythema or edema <1 cm in size AND pain or pruritus	2B: Papules or pustules 6–20 OR 2–5 areas of erythema or edema <1 cm in size AND pain, pruritus, or effect on emotions or functioning	3B: Papules or pustules >20 OR more than 5 areas of erythema or edema <1 cm in size AND pain, pruritus, or effect on emotions or functioning	—
Nail changes Nail plate	Onycholysis or ridging without pain	Onycholysis with mild/moderate pain; any nail plate lesion interfering with instrumental ADL	Nail plate changes interfering with self-care ADL	—
Nail changes Nail fold	Disruption or absence of cuticle OR erythema	Erythematous/tender/painful OR pyogenic granuloma OR crusted lesions OR any fold lesion interfering with instrumental ADL	Periungual abscess OR fold changes interfering with self-care ADL	—
Nail changes Digit tip	Xerosis AND/OR erythema without pain	Xerosis AND/OR erythema with mild/moderate pain or stinging OR fingertip fissures OR any digit: tip lesion interfering with instrumental ADL	Digit tip lesions interfering with self-care ADL	—

(continued on next page)

Table 5
(continued)

Adverse Event	Grade 1	Grade 2	Grade 3	Grade 4
Erythema	Painless erythema, blanching; erythema covering <10% BSA	Painful erythema, blanching; erythema covering 10%–30% BSA	Painful erythema, nonblanching; erythema covering >30% BSA	—
Pruritus	Mild OR localized, intermittent, not requiring therapy	2A: Moderate localized OR widespread intermittent AND requiring intervention 2B: Moderate localized OR widespread constant AND requiring intervention	Severe, widespread constant AND interfering with sleep	—
Xerosis	Scaling/flaking covering <10% BSA NO erythema/ pruritus/effect on emotions or functioning	2A: Scaling/flaking covering 10%–30% BSA + pruritus OR effect on emotions/ functioning 2B: Scaling/flaking + pruritus covering 10%–30% BSA AND effect on emotions/ functioning + erythema	3A: Scaling/flaking covering >30% BSA AND pruritus AND erythema AND effect on emotions/ functioning AND + fissuring/cracking 3B: Scaling/flaking covering >30% BSA AND pruritus AND erythema AND effect on emotions/ functioning AND fissuring/ cracking + signs of superinfection	—

Hair changes: scalp hair loss or alopecia	Terminal hair loss <50% of normal for that individual that may or may not be noticeable to others but is associated with increased shedding and overall feeling of less volume; may require different hair style to cover but does not require hairpiece to camouflage	2A: Hair loss associated with marked increase shedding and 50%–74% loss compared with normal for that individual; hair loss apparent to others, may be difficult to camouflage with change in hair style, and may require hairpiece 2B: Marked loss of at least 75% hair compared with normal for that individual with inability to camouflage except with a full wig OR new cicatricial hair loss documented by biopsy that covers at least 5% scalp surface area; may impact on functioning in social, personal, or professional situations	—
Hair changes: disruption of normal hair growth (specify): facial hair (diffuse, not just in male beard/mustache areas), eyelashes, eyebrows, body hair, beard and mustache hair (hirsutism)	Some distortion of hair growth but does not cause symptoms or require intervention	2A: Distortion of hair growth in many hairs in a given area that causes discomfort or symptoms that may require individual hairs to be removed 2B: Distortion of hair growth of most hairs in a given area with symptoms or resultant problems requiring removal of multiple hairs	—

(continued on next page)

Table 5
(continued)

Adverse Event	Grade 1	Grade 2	Grade 3	Grade 4
Hair changes: increased hair growth (specify): facial hair (diffuse, not just in male beard/mustache areas), eyelashes, eyebrows, body hair, beard and moustache hair (hirsutism)	Increase in length thickness and/or density of hair that the patient is able to camouflage by periodic shaving, bleaching, or removal of individual hairs	2A: Increase in length, thickness, and/or density of hairs that is very noticeable and requires regular shaving or removal of hairs in order to camouflage; may cause mild symptoms related to hair overgrowth 2B: Marked increase in hair density thickness and/or length of hair that requires either frequent shaving or destruction of the hair to camouflage; may cause symptoms related to hair overgrowth; without hair removal, inability to function normally in social, personal, or professional situations	—	—
Flushing	1A: Face OR chest, asymptomatic, transient 1B: Any location, asymptomatic, permanent	2A: Symptomatic on face or chest, transient 2B: Symptomatic on face or chest, permanent	3A: Face and chest, transient, symptomatic 3B: Face and chest, permanent, symptomatic	—
Telangiectasia	One area (<1 cm diameter) NOT affecting emotions or functioning	2A: 2–5 (1 cm diameter) areas NOT affecting emotions or functioning 2B: 2–5 (1 cm diameter) areas affecting emotions or functioning	More than 6 (1 cm diameter) OR confluent areas affecting emotions or functioning	—

Hyperpigmentation	One area (<1 cm diameter) NOT affecting emotions or functioning	2A: 2–5 (1 cm diameter) areas NOT affecting emotions or functioning 2B: 2–5 (1 cm diameter) areas affecting emotions or functioning	More than 6 (1 cm diameter) OR confluent areas affecting emotions or functioning	—
Mucositis Oral Anal	Mild erythema or edema and asymptomatic	Symptomatic (mild pain, opioid not required); erythema or limited ulceration, can eat solid foods and take oral medication (oral mucositis only)	Pain requiring opioid analgesic; erythema and ulceration, cannot eat solids, can swallow liquids (oral mucositis only)	Erythema and ulceration, cannot tolerate PO intake; requires tube feeding or hospitalization (oral mucositis only)
Radiation dermatitis	Faint erythema or dry desquamation	Moderate to brisk erythema; patchy moist desquamation, mostly confined to skin folds and creases; moderate edema	Moist desquamation other than skin folds and creases; bleeding induced by minor trauma or abrasion	Skin necrosis or ulceration of full-thickness dermis; spontaneous bleeding from involved site
Hyposalivation	Can eat but requires liquids, no effect on speech	Moderate/thickened saliva; cannot eat dry foods, mild speech impairment (sticky tongue, lips, affecting speech)	No saliva, unable to speak without water, no oral intake without water	—
Taste	Altered or reduced taste; no impact on oral intake	Altered or reduced taste affecting interest and ability to eat; no intervention required	Taste abnormalities, requires intervention	—

From Multinational Association of Supportive Cancer Care. Supportive care in cancer. 2016. Available at: http://www.mascc.org.

Table 6
Nursing management for skin conditions

Patient Problem	Nursing Management	Patient Education
Anxiety related to, diagnoses, treatment, prognosis	<ul><li>Assess the patients' level of understanding of the disease, treatment, and prognosis</li><li>Provide patients with opportunities to verbalize concerns and questions</li><li>Provide patients with understanding of what to expect</li><li>Assess patients' ability to cope and effective past coping strategies</li><li>Assess support systems</li><li>Assess for signs and symptoms of anxiety</li><li>Administer medications to decrease anxiety as ordered</li><li>Monitor changes in level of anxiety</li><li>Provide a calm reassuring environment</li></ul>	<ul><li>Instruct patients/caregivers:<ul><li>○ What to expect</li><li>○ Signs and symptoms of anxiety</li><li>○ What increases their anxiety</li><li>○ Strategies to minimize anxiety, including relaxation exercises, mediation, distraction</li><li>○ Ways to decrease environmental stimuli</li><li>○ When to notify a health care professional</li></ul></li></ul>
Fatigue	<ul><li>Assess for fatigue</li><li>Assess ability to perform ADLs</li><li>Assess for contributing factors: pain, emotional distress, sleep disturbances, anemia, nutritional status, and comorbidities</li><li>Screen for potential etiologic factors</li><li>Monitor blood counts (CBC, Hgb, and HCT)</li><li>Transfuse prn</li><li>Develop an exercise program appropriate to patients' condition</li><li>Encourage rest as needed</li><li>Consider physical therapy, nutrition, or psychosocial referral</li></ul>	<ul><li>Instruct patients regarding<ul><li>○ The signs and symptoms of fatigue</li><li>○ Practicing energy conservation, including setting priorities, planning and pacing activities, delegating, scheduling activity at peak energy time, napping, structured routine, and distraction</li></ul></li></ul>

| High risk for infection r/t alteration in skin | • Monitor blood counts (CBC with diff)
• Assess skin and wound site for drainage
• Monitor for signs and symptoms of infection
• Monitor vital signs
• Administer antibiotics, antifungals, antiviral, and antipyretic as ordered
• Monitor for CMV and reactivation of HSV, VZV

Obtain culture and sensitivity as ordered; if patients' wounds exhibit signs of infection or the wounds are not healing, a culture should be taken after obtaining an order. This culture would allow the team to identify the organism and the appropriate antibiotic to treat the infection. It is important to obtain a wound culture

Use the swab technique. The culture should be collected after the wound tissue is cleansed with a nonantiseptic sterile solution (ie, normal saline). | • Instruct patients/caregivers regarding
  ○ The signs and symptoms of infection/healing
  ○ The increased risk of infection
  ○ Wound care
  ○ When to notify the health care professional
  ○ Long-term steroid use with GVHD and the risk of infections |

(continued on next page)

Table 6
(continued)

Patient Problem	Nursing Management	Patient Education

Alteration in skin integrity, skin care/pruritus	• Perform skin assessment
	  ○ Visually inspect and palpate the skin
	  ○ Assess skin (all body sites) for color (pigmentation changes) temperature, moisture, texture, mobility, turgor, and skin lesions
	  ○ Describe the type of lesion, location, and distribution
	  ○ Evaluate for other symptoms
	  ○ Assess for pruritus
	  ○ Take photographs to document lesion and extent of involvement skin condition
	• May consider being treated in a highly specialized skin unit or burn unit
	• Ensure handwashing
	• Use aseptic techniques for wound care
	• Keep bullae intact
	• Use prescribed ointment or silver nitrate on open areas
	• Débride areas per orders
	• Wound/skin care consult
	• Monitor for signs and symptoms of infection
	• Obtain a culture if ordered if infection suspected and obtain results
	• Monitor vital signs
	• Administer antibiotics as ordered
	• Administer medications/treatments per orders, that is, antihistamine
	• Assess nutritional and hydration status
	  ○ Review diet
	  ○ Monitor fluid and electrolytes
	  ○ Administer IV fluid per orders
	• May consider increasing room temperature to 30°C–32°C especial for large amounts of epidermal detachment
	• May consider a blanket warm per orders
		• Instruct patients/caregivers on basic hygiene
		  ○ Handwashing technique and nail care
		  ○ Aseptic technique
		  ○ Avoid abrasive washing and gently pat dry when washing
		  ○ Signs and symptoms of infection
		  ○ Avoid exposing skin to extreme heat or cold
		  ○ Wear loose fitting clothing
		  ○ Avoid scratching skin
		  ○ Lubricate with prescribed skin emollients
		  ○ Test all new products on a small area of skin to rule out hypersensitivity reaction
		  ○ Prevent dry skin
		    ■ Use nonperfume emollients
		    ■ Avoid hot baths & frequent bathing
		• Instruct patient/caregiver on expected side effects and when to notify a healthcare professional

- Careful handling of skin
  - Minimize shearing force, especially moving or changing in patients' position (anti–shear handling)
  - No evidence to suggest best skin practice
  - Cleanse wounds and intact skin by irrigating with warm sterile water or normal saline applied emollient to the whole skin
  - No tape on skin
  - Keep nails short and clean
  - Use mittens as needed
  - Administer topical creams per orders
  - Apply a topical antimicrobial agent to sloughed areas per orders
  - Should avoid use of silver sulfadiazine until sulfonamides are ruled out as the cause
  - Use of appropriate dressing to reduce fluid/protein loss, decrease risk of infection, pain control, and may increase reepithelialization
  - Ideally blisters should be left in place and only punctured if necessary, allowing the blister roof to serve as a biological dressing
  - If bullae are prominent, blister fluid should be aspirated/expressed, thus, allowing blister roof to settle onto the dermis
  - Apply a dressing to collect exudates if indicated
  - Clinician may consider debridement
  - Limit trauma by avoiding use of sphygmomanometer cuffs, EKG leads, and adhesive dressings (use nonadherent dressings)
  - Mucosal involvement depends on degree of skin detachment
  - Oral care, see *mucositis*
  - Genital changes in female patients may lead to adhesions or strictures
    - May be treated with wet dressing or sitz baths

(continued on next page)

Table 6
(continued)

Patient Problem	Nursing Management	Patient Education
Alteration in comfort		

Pain	• Assess for pain, including location, intensity, quality, onset, duration, whether it is affecting ADL, aggravating and alleviating factors
	• Administer analgesics as ordered and assess patients' response
	  ○ Assess for side effects
	  ○ Assess effects on sleeping, coping, and ADL
	  ○ Implement strategies to prevent/reduce side effects (ie, bowel function or nausea & vomiting)
	  ○ Administer analgesics prn with special consideration for dressing changes, movement
	• Use nonpharmacologic strategies
	• Consider placing on a alternating pressure air mattress may help with pain
		• Instruct patients/caregivers
		  ○ To report pain and response to intervention
		  ○ Explain treatment plan and address patient concerns
		  ○ Monitor for potential side effects of interventions
		  ○ Teach other techniques
		    ■ Distraction
		    ■ Relaxation/guided imagery
		    ■ Prayers/meditation
		    ■ Counseling

Mucositis	• Perform oral and pain assessment
	  ○ Grade mucositis using CTCAEv4
	  ○ Grade 1: No oral lesions or discomfort
	  ○ Grade 2: Moderate pain; not interfering with oral intake; modified diet indicated
	  ○ Grade 3: Severe pain; interfering with oral intake
	  ○ Grade 4: Life-threatening consequences; urgent intervention indicated
	• Perform oral care
	  ○ Clean mouth with water or saline
	• Administer lidocaine rinse as ordered
	• Assess nutritional status
	• Maintain adequate nutrition
	• Apply moisture to lips 4–6 times per day
	• Assess for mouth dryness or thrush
	• Apply topical agents for pain
	• Consult with dietician or dentist as needed
		• Instruct patients/caregivers regarding daily oral hygiene
		  ○ Preventive measures (oral rinse with water, saline, baking soda rinse and avoid alcohol containing mouthwash)
		  ○ Encourage oral intake
		  ○ Encourage high-protein diet, soft bland diet
		  ○ Discourage smoking and alcohol
		  ○ Oral hygiene and care
		  ○ The importance of adequate nutrition

Eye involvement	• Consult with an ophthalmologist
	• Apply lubricant eye drops per orders, usually every 2 h
	• Ocular hygiene performed by special trained staff
	• Administer eye drops per orders
		• Instruct patients/caregivers regarding
		  ○ Eye care
		  ○ Hygiene
		  ○ Eye drops

Alteration in body images/sexuality	• Encourage patients to express feelings • Acknowledge patients may see their body differently • Discuss patients' concerns about sexuality and plan ways to manage the problem • Review potential side effects	• Instruct patients/caregivers regarding ○ Other methods of expression (hand-holding and hugs)

Psychosocial concerns	• Identify patients' nature/level of concerns/distress
	• Assess support and past coping skills
	• Allow patient to verbalize
	• Refer to social worker, counseling services, or chaplaincy care
	• Provide advocacy and education
	• Provide community resources
	• Teach coping strategies
		• Instruct patients/caregivers regarding
		  ○ Disease, treatment, side effects, symptom management
		  ○ Coping strategies
		  ○ Relaxation techniques

Rehabilitation focus	• Assess patients' ability to perform ADL and return to normal activities
	• Consider referrals, that is, physical therapy
	• Review need for equipment and/or supplies
	• Schedule follow-up appointments
		• Instruct patients/caregivers regarding
		  ○ The importance of follow-up care
		  ○ Exercises as prescribed by the physical therapist despite the discomfort that they may cause patients

Abbreviations: ADL, activities of daily living; CBC, complete blood count; CMV, cytomegalovirus; diff, differential; EKG, electrocardiogram; GVHD, graft-versus-host disease; HCT, hematocrit; Hgb, hemoglobin; HSV, herpes simplex virus; IV, intravenous; VZV, varicella zoster Virus.

Table 7
Patient education materials

Interventions to prevent hair loss and damage	Shampoo gently with a mild shampoo every 2 to 4 d. Use hair conditioner to make combing easier. Use SPF shampoos to prevent further damage. Sleep on satin or silk pillowcases.
Products to avoid	Avoid hair spray, hair dye, bleach, or permanents (perm). Avoid clips, barrettes, bobby pins, ponytail holders, or scrunchies. Avoid hair dryers, curlers, curling irons, or hair straightener. Avoid rubber bathing or swimming caps. Avoid braids, cornrows, and ponytails.
Symptoms requiring medical assistance	White patches in the mouth Bleeding of the gums Pain when swallowing that is not relieved with analgesics Fever
Sun protection	Wear sun protective clothing and use sunbrellas/wide-brim hats. Avoid the sun as much as possible. Purchase sunscreens that are titanium dioxide based, have no chemicals, and are broad-spectrum (UVA and UVB), at least 30 SPF. Apply sunscreen daily to any areas that may be exposed to the sun as part of daily routine.

Abbreviation: SPF, sun protection factor.

diphenhydramine, hydroxyzine, and cetirizine.[1] For refractory pruritus, γ-aminobutyric acid agonists oral antidepressants[10] and aprepitant have been used in clinic practice.

XEROSIS

Patients should be encouraged to use emollients twice daily and should be applied within 15 minutes of showering or bathing for better absorption. Lotions and creams are the easiest to apply; however, ointments provide the most water retention in the skin. Ointments such as over-the-counter petrolatum jelly are effective for treating cracked hands and feet. This treatment works best when patients apply the ointment at night with cotton glove and sock occlusion.

Xerosis may be prevented by (1) bathing with bath oils or mild moisturizing soap, tepid water, and following with regular moisturizing creams and (2) avoidance of extreme temperatures and direct sunlight. Management of mild/moderate xerosis uses (1) emollient creams that are packaged in a jar/tub without irritants; (2) occlusive emollients containing urea, colloidal oatmeal, and petroleum-based creams; (3) exfoliants for scaly or hyperkeratotic areas, such as ammonium lactate 12% or lactic acid cream 12%; (4) urea cream (10%–40%); (5) salicylic acid 6%; (6) zinc oxide (13%–40%); and, for severe xerosis, (7) medium- to high-potency steroid creams.[9]

Also, patients should be encouraged to avoid alcohol, fragrance, or dyed shower products; use alcohol-free emollient creams and hypoallergenic makeup; avoid over-the-counter acne medications, such as benzoyl peroxide, and scented laundry detergents; avoid sun exposure by using a broad-spectrum sunscreen, sun protection factor 30 or higher, when exposed to the sun; and stay hydrated at all times, as this will help prevent xerosis and pruritus.

PREVENTING INFECTION

Educating patients on how to prevent skin infections is another important responsibility of nurses caring for this patient population. Patients are educated on routine handwashing, general hygiene, and common sense practical interventions. Patients are instructed to wash their hands before and after eating, using the restroom, and applying topical medications. The routine of handwashing should last 30 seconds with increased attention to underneath the fingernails. Excoriations secondary to severe pruritus and scratching while sleeping and awake provide an entry of portal for bacteria that normally lives on the skin. Aside from prescribed medications to reduce pruritus, nurses can educate patients on ways to reduce excoriating, such as wearing bandages on the fingertips or cotton gloves at night.

NAIL CHANGES

Lacouture and colleagues[1] recommend prevention of paronychia by using diluted bleach soaks and avoiding irritants. Paronychia management involves topical corticosteroids or calcineurin inhibitors (level II evidence) and systemic tetracyclines, reserving antimicrobials when culture and sensitivity testing is known.

Patients are encouraged to practice proper nail care, such as regular nail filing and conservative nail clipping. Patients should avoid frequent use of nail polish remover as they contain harsh chemicals that may weaken the nail. Additionally, nail polishes containing formaldehyde or other harsh chemicals should also be avoided. Patients may use over-the-counter nail polishes or take a daily supplement, such as biotin or orthosilicic acid (BioSil), to aid in strengthening the nails. To avoid onycholysis, patients are encouraged to wear comfortable footwear, avoid shoes that are too small, and limit the wear of high-heeled shoes.

Prevention involves using protective footwear, avoiding friction with fingertips, toes, and heels; treatment if fissures develop involves (1) application of thick moisturizers or zinc oxide (13%–40%) cream; (2) painting the fissure with liquid glue or cyanoacrylate to seal cracks; (3) steroids or steroid tape, hydrocolloid dressings, topical antibiotics; and (4) bleach soaks to prevent infection (level III evidence).

ALOPECIA

Alopecia is a difficult side effect to manage related to anticancer therapy. Nurses must address the physical and emotional aspects of this untoward event. Patients should ask their institution for further resources, such as support groups or stores that offer discounts on wigs and hairpieces. It is important for patients to understand that hair thinning may also be the cause of nutrient insufficiency, genetics, stress, hormonal changes, hair treatments, or other medications. For this reason, nursing assessment is particularly important to determine the cause of alopecia.

Nurses may assess onset, associated symptoms (ie, pruritus, dysesthesia, flaking); past treatments; and contributing factors, such as vitamin D and iron deficiency, hypothyroidism, autoimmune conditions, stress (telogen effluvium), and family history. As with nail changes, patients may take over-the-counter supplements to improve and speed up hair growth, such as biotin and BioSil. BioSil stimulates collagen production, an important protein for hair, skin, nails, joints, and bones. They may also choose to use topical medications, such as minoxidil (ROGAINE). Nurses are relied on to set reasonable expectations for patients on treatment to increase hair growth. Increased hair growth may take up to 8 to 12 weeks for noticeable results. Compliance in taking daily vitamins and applying topicals is also crucial for their effectiveness.[16]

PATIENT EDUCATION

Patient and caregiver education is fundamental to keeping patients on treatment. They should be educated on signs and symptoms to report, that is, rash, implications of stopping the drug, and when to notify their health care provider. Patients and their caregivers should be educated to contact health care providers for early evaluation. Early recognition of side effects and prompt intervention is important. Patient and caregiver education includes explaining about the treatment, side effects, symptom management, and care strategies. Patients should receive written information about how to manage their skin reactions. Patients should be able to care for themselves, including skin care and other symptom-related issues. **Table 7** includes information on patient education.

ONCODERMATOLOGY: A SUBSPECIALTY OF ONCOLOGY NURSING

Oncology nurses require a knowledge base in terms of early recognition, accurate diagnosis, and management strategies for this unique patient population.[17,18] The study of dermatologic and mucocutaneous symptom management in oncology is increasing, attempting to understand the pathophysiologic mechanism along with appropriate preventive and management strategies for EGFR-related skin toxicities.[17] Nurses are beginning to specialize in oncodermatology, a specialty incorporating principles of both dermatology and oncology. This specialty treats patients with skin cancers, cutaneous lymphoma, dermatologic surgery, and supportive oncodermatology.[19,20]

Supportive care is defined as the prevention and management of cancer or treatment-related effects for patients, families, and caregivers throughout the cancer continuum.[12] Supportive care improves health-related quality of life and decreases treatment interruptions related to adverse events (AEs).[21,22] Yet there are barriers to supportive care, such as personal knowledge of supportive care, perceived value of supportive care, and practice and organizational issues of time, role-definition, and resources.[21] These barriers result in unmet needs for patients with cancer[23,24] in varying ways, such as physical, financial, educational, personal control, emotional, societal, and spiritual.[25,26]

Oncodermatology supportive care is associated symptom management and underscores the need to improve patient outcomes.[27,28] Gandhi and colleagues[29] reported unanticipated concerns of cancer survivors, such as irritated and dry skin, a burning sensation, and hair loss. Patients reported other skin effects as either being physically damaging or being a negative result of cancer treatment, that is, nail problems, including discoloration; a stinging sensation and cracking of the nails; rash; and a loss of skin elasticity. These studies highlight the importance of dermatologic precancer treatment counseling with effective dermatologic interventions throughout cancer therapy.[29]

The role of the oncodermatology nurse is evolving at comprehensive cancer centers, such as the Memorial Sloan Kettering Cancer Center. Much work needs to be done to confirm this role as a specialty. Ongoing work includes a scope and standards statement; specific competencies must be developed along with a role delineation study to determine certification or certificate requirements. Additionally, research is necessary for testing the efficiency of the currently used empirical treatments. Such research will build the body of knowledge in this growing specialty area. Further prospective research is required to elucidate the role and patient and health care team outcomes.[30,31]

As another example, in 2014, Ruiz and colleagues[32] conducted a 24-item online survey with 119 US oncologists treating patients with advanced renal cell carcinoma eliciting practice settings, AE management practice patterns and beliefs (including dermatologic-related AE), treatment barriers, and patient education. Within this study, the investigators noted that 43% of clinicians followed a comprehensive supportive care plan with only 46% evaluating the outcome of AE management. Interestingly, 70% of clinicians referred patients to nononcology specialists for unique AEs. However, the most common barriers found for consulting with other specialists were finding interested physicians (43%) and time constraints (40%), which the latter may have hindered treatment optimization for this patient population. Lastly, lack of clinician education in management of AEs was also cited as a barrier in treatment optimization. This study demonstrates the need to increase the concerted effort among oncologists and specialists in the approach to managing these untoward events, ensuring patient compliance, improving quality of life and unmet needs, and maximization of patient outcomes.

SUMMARY

Caring for oncodermatology patients provides many opportunities for nursing education and interventions. With new targeted cancer therapies, like EGFRI, management of the dermatologic component is as important as all other body systems. Side effects vary depending on the type of anticancer therapy and dose. Because of the mechanism of action of many anticancer therapies, hair, skin, and nails are particularly affected. Often times patients are hesitant to discuss dermatologic issues and it is important that nurses assess patients' largest organ: their skin. Patients need to consider this treatment as chronic therapy; the challenge to nurses is to help patients minimize and manage symptoms and to maximize quality of life.

ACKNOWLEDGMENTS

The authors thank Catherine Hydzik, MS, RN, AOCN, Clinical Nurse Specialist, Memorial Sloan Kettering Cancer Center for her intellectual ideas and stimulating thoughts on this topic.

REFERENCES

1. Lacouture ME, Anadkat MJ, Bensadoun R-J, et al. Clinical practice guidelines for the prevention and treatment of EGFR inhibitor-associated dermatologic toxicities. Support Care Cancer 2011;19:1079–95.
2. Lynch TJ, Kim ES, Eaby B, et al. Epidermal growth factor receptor inhibitor-associated cutaneous toxicities: an evolving paradigm in clinical management. Oncologist 2007;12(5):610–21.
3. Wilkes GM, Barton-Burke M. Oncology nursing drug handbook. Sudbury (MA): Jones and Bartlett Publishing; 2016.
4. Eilers RE, Gandhi M, Patel JD, et al. Dermatologic infections in cancer patients treated with epidermal growth factor receptor inhibitor therapy. J Natl Cancer Inst 2009;102(1):47–53.
5. The skin physical examination. Available at: http://www.siumed.edu/medicine/dermatology/student_information/skinphysicalexam.pdf. Accessed August 22, 2016.
6. Boone SL, Rademaker A, Liu D, et al. Impact and management of skin toxicity associated with anti-epidermal growth factor receptor therapy: survey results. Oncology 2007;72(3–4):152–9.

7. Lacouture ME. Mechanisms of cutaneous toxicities to EGFR inhibitors. Nat Rev Cancer 2006;6:803–12.

8. Wacher B, Nagrani T, Weinberg J, et al. Correlation between development of rash and efficacy in patients treated with epidermal growth factor receptor tyrosine kinase inhibitor erlotinib in two large phase iii studies. Clin Cancer Res 2007;13: 3913–21.

9. Valentine J, Belum VR, Duran J, et al. Incidence and risk of xerosis with targeted anticancer therapies. J Am Acad Dermatol 2015;72(4):656–67.

10. Fischer A, Rosen AC, Ensslin CJ, et al. Pruritus to anticancer agents targeting the EGFR, BRAF, and CTLA-4. Dermatol Ther 2013;26(2):135–48.

11. Melosky B, Anderson H, Burkes RL, et al. Pan Canadian rash trial: a randomized phase III trial evaluating the impact of prophylactic skin treatment regimen on epidermal growth factor receptor-tyrosine kinase inhibitor-induced skin toxicities in patients with metastatic lung cancer. J Clin Oncol 2016;34(8):810–5.

12. Multinational Association of Supportive Cancer Care. Supportive care in cancer. 2016. Available at: http://www.mascc.org.

13. Available at: http://www.albertahealthservices.ca/assets/info/hp/cancer/if-hp-cancer-guide-supp003-egfri-rash.pdf.

14. American Society of Clinical Oncology. 2016. Skin reactions to targeted therapy and immunotherapy. Available at: http://www.cancer.net/navigating-cancer-care/side-effects/skin-reactions-targeted-therapy-and-immunotherapy.

15. Lacouture ME, Wolchok JD, Yosipovitch G, et al. Ipilimumab in patients with cancer and the management of dermatologic adverse events. J Am Acad Dermatol 2014;71(1):161–9.

16. Duvic M, Lemak NA, Valero V, et al. A randomized trial of minoxidil in chemotherapy-induced alopecia. J Am Acad Dermatol 1996;35(1):74–8.

17. Balgula Y, Rosen ST, Lacouture ME. The emergence of supportive oncodermatology: the study of dermatologic adverse events to cancer therapies. J Am Acad Dermatol 2011;65(3):624–35.

18. Ciccolini KT, Skripnik Lucas A. Exploring the role of oncodermatology nursing. Poster session presented at the meeting of Dermatology Nursing Association Annual Convention. Indianapolis (IN), April 1, 2016.

19. Ciccolini KT, Skripnik LA. Spotlight on dermatology nursing. 2015. Available at: https://www.mskcc.org/blog/spotlight-dermatology-nursing.

20. Skripnik Lucas A, Ciccolini KT. Oncodermatology and the nursing specialist. 2016. Available at: http://nursing.onclive.com/contributor/kathryn-ciccolini-and-anna-skripnik-lucas/2016/02/oncodermatology-and-the-nursing-specialist.

21. Ristevski E, Breen S, Regan M. Incorporating supportive care into routine cancer care: the benefits and challenges to clinicians' practice. Oncol Nurs Forum 2011; 38(3):E204–11.

22. Scotté F. The importance of supportive care in optimizing treatment outcomes of patients with advanced prostate cancer. Oncologist 2011;17(Suppl 1):23–30.

23. Husain A, Barbera L, Howell D, et al. Advanced lung cancer patients' experience with continuity of care and supportive care needs. Support Care Cancer 2013; 21(5):1351–8.

24. Johannsen L. Skin assessment. Dermatol Nurs 2005;17(2):166.

25. Burg MA, Adorno G, Lopez EDS, et al. Current unmet needs of cancer survivors: analysis of open-ended responses to the American Cancer Society Study of Cancer Survivors II. Cancer 2015;121(4):623–30.

26. Burtness B, Anadkat M, Basti S, et al. NCCN management of dermatologic and other toxicities associated with EGFR inhibition in patients with cancer. J Natl Compr Canc Netw 2009;7(1):1–21.
27. Fitch MI, Steele R. Supportive care needs of individuals with lung cancer. Can Oncol Nurs J 2010;20(1):15–22.
28. Palmer SC, DeMichele A, Schapira M, et al. Symptoms, unmet need, and quality of life among recent breast cancer survivors. J Community Support Oncol 2016; 14(7):299–306.
29. Gandhi M, Oishi K, Zubal B, et al. Unanticipated toxicities from anticancer therapies: survivors' perspectives. Support Care Cancer 2009;18(11):1461–8.
30. Ciccolini K. CREAM principles: the advanced nursing role in the management of dermatologic adverse events to anticancer therapy [abstract]. J Adv Pract Oncol 2015;7(1):120–1.
31. Ciccolini K. CREAM: nursing principles for an oncodermatology clinic dedicated to managing dermatologic adverse events to anticancer therapy [abstract]. Support Care Cancer 2016;24(1):S2–249.
32. Ruiz JN, Belum VR, Creel P, et al. Current practices in the management of adverse events associated with targeted therapies for advanced renal cell carcinoma: a national survey of oncologists. Clin Genitourin Cancer 2014;12(5):341–7.

Oral Agents for Cancer Treatment

Effective Strategies to Assess and Enhance Medication Adherence

Laura A. Fennimore, DNP, RN, NEA-BC[a],*,
Pamela K. Ginex, EdD, RN, OCN[b]

KEYWORDS

- Oral cancer agents • Medication adherence • Assessment
- Shared decision-making

KEY POINTS

- A significant number of treatments for cancer are now being developed in oral form.
- Although oral treatment offers advantages to patients and providers, many challenges exist that must be addressed.
- Effective approaches to enhance medication adherence should include a focus on patient education, convenient care, and effective patient monitoring and follow-up.
- Patient-centered approaches, including shared decision-making and a personal systems model hold promise to support patients who are taking oral treatments for cancer.

INTRODUCTION

Over the last several decades, cancer treatment has shifted from primarily intravenous (IV) medications administered by a nurse to oral agents self-administered by the patient or caregiver. More than half of the newly approved cancer drugs are being developed in oral form.[1] These oral agents for cancer (OAC) range from endocrine and traditional cytotoxic therapy to drugs that target specific genetic mutations. Although OAC are often more manageable and convenient for patients, they pose challenges to effective drug delivery due to concerns about medication adherence. A common truth attributed to former U.S. Surgeon General C. Everett Koop is that drugs don't work for people who don't take them. As many cancer treatments shift from acute to chronic

Disclosure Statement: The authors have nothing to disclose.
[a] Acute and Tertiary Care Department, University of Pittsburgh School of Nursing, 3500 Victoria Street, Pittsburgh, PA 15261, USA; [b] Department of Nursing, Memorial Sloan Kettering Cancer Center, 205 East 64th Street, Concourse Level Room 251, New York, NY 10065, USA
* Corresponding author.
E-mail address: Laf36@pitt.edu

Nurs Clin N Am 52 (2017) 115–131
http://dx.doi.org/10.1016/j.cnur.2016.10.007
0029-6465/17/© 2016 Elsevier Inc. All rights reserved.

nursing.theclinics.com

care management, nurses need to help patients participate in shared decisions that determine whether or not this form of cancer treatment is right or best for them. This article presents information that oncology nurses should know about oral adherence to anticancer agents and offers evidence-based assessment tools and strategies aimed at helping patients.

BACKGROUND
The Shift to Oral Cancer Treatment

The rapidly increasing understanding of cancer pathophysiology along with molecular and genetic changes at the cellular level has led to the development of oral medications to treat many types of cancer. This trend toward using OAC has led to an increase in both the number of OAC prescribed and the number of patients taking these drugs.[2-4] This paradigm shift has increased the burden and responsibility for patients and caregivers. In the past, a patient receiving IV therapy would come to a health care facility for treatment where they would have the opportunity to discuss any issues, symptoms, or side effects with their physician or nurse. With the shift toward oral treatments, patients are now managing their treatment at home. This change poses unique challenges for the patient, caregivers, providers, and the health care system.[5] A notable challenge is ensuring that the patient is supported to adhere to taking their OAC because this can have a significant impact on treatment efficacy and toxicities.[6] The OAC represent a changing paradigm in cancer treatment and are seen as a response to patient preference, new treatment options, and the changing economics of health care.[3,4]

The increased use of oral anticancer agents has been associated with fewer patient visits and can foster a sense of independence for the patient. A significant drawback to this form of chemotherapy, however, includes the failure to take medication as prescribed.[6,7] Adherence to medications across all disease sites is estimated at approximately 50%.[8] Adherence to cancer therapy is documented at less than 80%, including up to 10% of patients not refiling their anticancer prescriptions.[9-11] The therapeutic outcome of treatment of patients taking OAC depends largely on adherence to the regimen. Nonadherence has also been linked to other patient outcomes, including additional inpatient stays, increased health care spending, disease progression, and diminished survival.[12-15]

Moving from Adherence to a Patient-Centered Approach

Adherence to oral medications requires collaboration between the health care team and the patient and caregiver. As such, the term adherence may not be the best to describe the relationship necessary for optimal patient outcomes and may be viewed as a paternalistic term. Recent efforts have focused on patient-centered approaches to medication management.[16,17] Patient-centered care is defined as care that is respectful of and responsive to individual patient preferences, needs, values and that ensures patient values guide clinical decisions.[18] Two strategies that depict the collaborative relationship between providers and patients are shared decision-making and a personal systems approach; both have the potential to improve medication adherence and patient outcomes.

The personal systems approach has grown out of the movement that redirects blame for patient safety errors from individuals to breakdowns within hospital systems and makes the desired behavior more likely to occur by removing environmental barriers.[19] Personal systems interventions focus on shaping routines, involving supportive others in routines, and using medication self-monitoring to change and maintain behavior.[20] Personal systems interventions have been successful in reducing stress, lowering asthma attacks, increasing exercise, improving care for patients with hypertension, and improving medication adherence.[21]

A 4-pronged approach is used for personal systems interventions that target medication adherence. The first step involves assessing individual and key support systems and their impact on medication adherence. The patient and provider work together to look beyond personal motivation to the patient's life routines and their environment. The nurse and patient explore the patient's daily, weekly, and monthly routines and tailor solutions that support optimal medication-taking. This is an important step for patients taking anticancer agents. Motivation is high but environmental or lifestyle routines may prevent patients from taking their oral treatments as prescribed.[22]

Forgetfulness is often noted as a primary reason for not taking oral treatments.[23] The second step in a personal systems intervention involves implementing the proposed solutions to improve adherence. Working with the individual's health care provider, the proposed solutions identified in the first step are implemented and assessed for effectiveness. Changes are incorporated into the patient's life routines and medication-taking becomes linked to these routines. Linking medication-taking to other routines may be useful in helping patients to remember to take their medications.

The third step involves tracking medication adherence data either electronically or by pill counts at office visits. Evaluating these data and reassessing changes that were made and that were effective is the fourth and final step in this personal systems approach.[21,22] For patients taking OAC, each step in this process should occur at each office or clinic visit, and if patients are found to have missed doses routines should be modified to optimize adherence.

Shared decision-making is another aspect of a patient-centered approach that holds promise for improving medication adherence by engaging the patient in prescribing decisions. Evidence-based practice includes making decisions based on the best evidence available and taking into account the unique characteristics and values of each patient.[17] Placing patients at the center of decisions about their treatment ensures that medication adherence is focused on delivering care that incorporates patient beliefs, preferences, goals, practical realities, and concerns into decisions and practices that lead to improved patient outcomes.[16,24]

Emerging research on shared decision-making models to improve adherence suggests that treatment nonadherence may be a result of failure to identify and address individual circumstances and patient goals regarding their medication treatment regimen.[25] In a shared decision-making model, both the patient and the provider share relevant information, express treatment preferences, deliberate options, and agree on the treatment to implement.[26,27] In shared decision-making, the health care professional elicits the patient's goals for treatment and their priorities for care. For example, a patient who is concerned about certain side effects or who is concerned about the cost of OAC, may prefer a regimen of convenience. Treatment options should be discussed along with pros and cons of the recommended treatment. The patient and the provider can then agree on a treatment that best accommodates the patient's goals and the provider's plan of care. Although there may be less flexibility for patient choice with cancer treatments than with other chronic diseases, these discussions are important and highlight barriers or facilitators to treatment that can be managed by both the patient and the provider.

Factors Affecting Patients in Taking Their Medications

Oral treatments for cancer can be effective if adherence is optimized. There are many factors influencing the likelihood that patients will take the right medication, at the right time, in the right amount (dose). Nurses are challenged to determine the strategies that will help their patients achieve this goal. Understanding what works for a specific patient starts with what the nurse knows about the patient and their treatment plan.

Case study

Patient SM is 68-years-old and was recently diagnosed with a chronic lymphocytic leukemia. He is referred to a medical oncologist and, during that visit, his physician recommends that, based on his risk profile, he should begin treatment with imatinib, an oral cancer agent that he will take daily to treat his cancer.

The nurse comes into the examination room and performs patient teaching, using the Multinational Association of Supportive Care in Cancer (MASCC) Oral Agent Teaching Tool (MOATT) for patients receiving OAC. From this assessment, she determines that he is able to take pills, read, and open the medicine bottles. She talks with SM about his routine and support at home. He does not eat breakfast but never misses dinner. The nurse talks with him about taking the imatinib after dinner with a large glass of water. They discuss the potential side effects and SM states he understands them. He also makes a comment that he is not sure a pill is enough to treat his cancer because his friends who have received treatment of other cancers have all had IV treatment. The nurse takes time to talk with SM about the treatment and how oral treatments are very effective for his cancer. She lets him know that he can always ask her or his medical oncologist if he has any questions about his treatment.

As they continue talking, he states that he lives alone but is near his son. The nurse and SM discuss that his son should come to the next appointment and SM agrees. He also states he will review the treatment schedule and materials with his son. SM takes his prescription to the hospital pharmacy. When the pharmacist attempts to fill the prescription, she is notified that prior authorization is required.

The pharmacist then calls SM's nurse and asks her to initiate prior authorization.

The nurse calls SM's insurance company and asks to carry out the prior authorization on the telephone. After filling out the questionnaire with the representative from the insurance company, the nurse is informed that a response will be available within 72 hours and that the office will be contacted via fax once a decision is rendered. The nurse calls the pharmacy and explains that SM will not be able to fill his prescription that day and the patient goes home.

Three days later, the office receives a fax notifying them that prior authorization for SM is granted. The nurse calls SM to let him know his medication is approved and asks the pharmacist to process the imatinib prescription. However, when the pharmacist attempts to fill the medication, it turns out that SM is required by his insurance company to use a mail order pharmacy. The nurse speaks to SM and faxes his prescription to the specialty department of a mail order pharmacy he uses for other medications.

The nurse follows up with SM to let him know that the prescription is with the mail order pharmacy. She reinforces the teaching about the effectiveness of imatinib and some of the common side effects he may see. She also asks him to call her when his prescription arrives so that they can review what he has received together. She reviews his follow-up appointment with him and reminds him to bring his son to the appointment. She ends the call by reinforcing with SM that he can always reach out to her or his physician with any questions or concerns.

The interacting factors of medication adherence are described by the World Health Organization[7] (2003) and include factors related to the patient's social and economic situation, condition, therapy, and physical and psychological, state as well as the patient's interaction with the health care system. Each of these factors is further described by the American Society of Consultant Pharmacists as illustrated in **Box 1.**[28]

Box 1
Factors reported to affect adherence

1. Social and economic dimension
   Limited English language proficiency
   Low health literacy
   Lack of family or social support network
   Unstable living conditions; homelessness
   Burdensome schedule
   Limited access to health care facilities
   Lack of health care insurance
   Inability or difficulty accessing pharmacy
   Medication cost
   Cultural and lay beliefs about illness and treatment
   Elder abuse

2. Health care system dimension
   Provider-patient relationship
   Provider communication skills (contributing to lack of patient knowledge or understanding of the treatment regimen)
   Disparity between the health beliefs of the health care provider and those of the patient
   Lack of positive reinforcement from the health care provider
   Weak capacity of the system to educate patients and provide follow-up
   Lack of knowledge on adherence and of effective interventions for improving it
   Patient information materials written at too high literacy level
   Restricted formularies; changing medications covered on formularies
   High drug costs, copayments, or both
   Poor access or missed appointments
   Long wait times
   Lack of continuity of care

3. Condition-related dimension
   Chronic conditions
   Lack of symptoms
   Severity of symptoms
   Depression
   Psychotic disorders
   Mental retardation or developmental disability

4. Therapy-related dimension
   Complexity of medication regimen (number of daily doses; number of concurrent medications)
   Treatment requires mastery of certain techniques (injections, inhalers)
   Duration of therapy
   Frequent changes in medication regimen
   Lack of immediate benefit of therapy
   Medications with social stigma attached to use
   Actual or perceived unpleasant side effects
   Treatment interferes with lifestyle or requires significant behavioral changes

5. Patient-related dimension
   Physical factors
      Visual impairment
      Hearing impairment
      Cognitive impairment
      Impaired mobility or dexterity
      Swallowing problems
   Psychological or behavioral factors
      Knowledge about disease
      Perceived risk or susceptibility to disease
      Understanding reason medication is needed
      Expectations or attitudes toward treatment

Perceived benefit of treatment
Confidence in ability to follow treatment regimen
Motivation
Fear of possible adverse effects
Fear of dependence
Feeling stigmatized by the disease
Frustration with health care providers
Psychosocial stress, anxiety, anger
Alcohol or substance abuse

Data from American Society of Consultant Pharmacists. Adult Medication. Improving medication adherence in older adults. Available at: http://www.adultmeducation.com/downloads/Adult_Meducation.pdf. Accessed March 15, 2016; with permission.

Additional factors influencing oral adherence described by Johnson[29] include aspects related to beliefs, preferences about health and medication, medication-related experiences, personal factors, treatment factors, health care delivery systems, overall health and disease burden, and patient knowledge and support. Factors identified as having a positive influence on medication adherence include the patient's belief in the necessity of the medication, the patient's knowledge about the medication and management of side effects, the support the patient received during treatment from family and friends and the providers, and the ease of fitting medication administration within the patient's lifestyle. Factors with negative influences on medication adherence included side effects, forgetfulness, and difficulty incorporating medication-taking into lifestyle and the cost or lack of insurance coverage.

Additional factors leading to OAC nonadherence include patient confusion or forgetfulness, chemotherapy-induced and organic cognitive changes, polypharmacy syndrome, side effects, and competing priorities.[30,31] Adherence with oral cancer agents can also be influenced by patient comprehension of the treatment, the patient-provider relationship, and pre-existing attitudes toward health and treatment.[32,33]

Difficult Adherence with Oral Cancer Treatment

Barriers to successful OAC medication adherence can be characterized as an intersection of several factors. It is important that the nurse understands the impact that these factors have on the patient's ability to take medication prescribed for any condition.[33]

Belief about effectiveness of medication

Cancer as a chronic disease is a relatively new concept. The long-term nature of oral cancer therapies may be difficult for patients to fully comprehend. Patients may be accustomed to family or friends having had surgery, radiation, or IV chemotherapy over periods of time and who were then considered cured or in remission. Understanding that cancer is a chronic disease that must be managed like other chronic illnesses, such as hypertension or diabetes, may be a difficult transition for many patients with cancer. This is relevant since a systematic review of 159 qualitative and quantitative studies revealed that "the belief in the necessity of taking medication was the most frequent factor associated with improved adherence." (p.22)[29]

Complexity of oral chemotherapy regimen

The targeted biological and molecular nature of OCA creates a complex medication regimen that may be difficult for patients to follow or keep organized. In addition, many regimens require multiple daily doses, changes in dose depending on the week in a given month, or complicated drug sequencing. An example of a complex regimen is the combination treatment of bleomycin, etoposide, doxorubicin hydrochloride (Adriamycin), cyclophosphamide, vincristine sulfate (Oncovin), procarbazine hydrochloride, and prednisone (BEACOPP) for the treatment of Hodgkin disease. This regimen includes 3 IV agents given on day 1, 1 agent given IV or oral on days 2 and 3, 1 oral agent taken days 1 to 7, a second oral agent taken days 1 to 14, 2 IV agents given on day 8, and a combined oral and IV antiemetic regimen. The cycle is repeated every 21 days. A successful approach to helping patients treated with this regimen might include the oncology nurse preparing a detailed calendar for the patient for the complete 21 day cycle and subsequent treatment cycles identifying specifically which drugs are taken each day.

Side effects

Oncology nurses often tell patients who are receiving IV chemotherapy that these medications will make them sick before they make them better and that the team will help manage their side effects during treatment. Nurses assess patients for medication-related side effects while assisting them to manage the impact of these effects on quality of life. With many OAC, however, there is no foreseeable endpoint for treatment and side effects must be managed on a chronic basis. Patients must be able to manage the side effects from OAC over time and know when to notify the provider with new or uncontrolled symptoms. Plus, the side effects for the OAC are different from the usual side effects of cancer treatments, such as skin reactions that often accompany certain tyrosine kinase inhibitors, making side effect management challenging over a longer period of time.

Relationship with provider

IV chemotherapy infusions are delivered over several hours for extended periods of time. Patients spend significant time with oncology nurses and other cancer care providers establishing relationships that facilitate education and exploration of coping strategies and other concerns that the patient may be experiencing, including fatigue, sleep disturbances, or interference with sexual function. The shift to OAC has changed the nature of this relationship, with patients spending less time in direct contact with their providers. Nurses who spend less direct time with patients may fail to grasp the multiple factors affecting the patient's ability to take their medication as prescribed.

Cost

Financial toxicity is a side effect not addressed in chemotherapy drug handbooks. The payment structure in which costs for therapy are covered by insurance as part of a bundle under inpatient or outpatient care is a sharp contrast to direct medication costs and coinsurance payments incurred by patients treated with OAC. The high cost of anticancer drugs has received considerable attention in the past few years. Kantarjian and colleagues[34] note that "with typical out-of-pocket expenses of 20% to 30%, the financial burden of cancer treatment would be $20,000 to $30,000 a year." (p.e208) Howard and colleagues[35] examined 58 anticancer drugs approved in the United States and noted that the average launch price of anticancer drugs increased approximately $8500 per year from 1995 to 2013. Spending on new oral cancer agents is a driver of these costs and raises serious concerns about the financial hardship imposed by high-cost treatment and its impact on overall cancer survivorship.[36,37]

ASSESSMENT
Nurses Assess, Predict, and Evaluate Medication Adherence

Medication adherence rates are difficult to measure; predicting which patients are likely to be nonadherent to their treatment plan is even more complicated. Spoelstra and Rittenberg[38] distinguish assessment and measurement as 2 related by different concepts. Healthcare providers assess or collect information about self-reporting of medication adherence to make a judgement. Measurement of medication adherence is generally reported as a rate (like an 80% rate of medication adherence) (p.48). Medication adherence assessment methods include direct observation, drug assays, or measurement of prognostic markers. Indirect methods may include self-report, pill counts, electronic measuring systems, and pharmacy records or claims data.

Oncology nurses consider the patient's level of motivation and capacity to assume responsibility for an OAC regimen. Nurses should consider asking the patient and/or caregiver the following questions identified by Moody and Jackowski[39] to facilitate this process:

- Is the patient a highly motivated person who can assume the increased responsibility that comes with self-administration of oral chemotherapy medications?
- Does the patient want to actively participate in his or her treatment?
- Is the patient mentally and cognitively able to be in control of his or her own oral chemotherapy regimen?

Adherence is often in the eye of the beholder. Patients may not what to share information with their providers for fear of disappointing them. Patients may worry about repercussions or consequences if they do not follow doctor's orders. The trust relationship between patient and provider is a strong predictor of successful medication adherence. Supportive provider relations have a positive influence on oral adherence in nearly 20% of the studies reviewed by Irwin and Johnson.[29] These studies included a variety of chronic diseases including human immunodeficiency virus (HIV), osteoporosis, hypertension, coronary artery disease, and stroke. Assessment tools have been developed to determine whether a patient is effectively self-managing their medications and may help providers predict risk of nonadherence. Four of these assessment tools are described in **Table 1**.[38]

MASCC developed a patient assessment and patient education OAC tool kit for health care providers.[40] The tool was used to measure patients' adherence to OAC in a study with subjects with non-small cell lung cancer.[41,42] However, a systematic review of medication adherence to OAC noted that a validated scale to assess adherence is still lacking and that current scales focus on medication-taking behaviors more than on barriers to adherence.[43]

Accurate self-report is the cornerstone of adherence measurement. Encouraging the patient to record each dose of oral chemotherapy in a patient diary provides an opportunity for the oncology nurse, pharmacist, or oncologist to review medication-taking patterns. Kawakami and colleagues[44] used a retrospective cohort analysis of 212 patients with colon cancer to describe adherence to capecitabine during capecitabine plus oxaliplatin (XELOX) treatment using a patient-reported treatment diary in an outpatient clinic in Japan. Nonadherence was identified in approximately 49% of the cases, with the greatest number of missed doses occurring in patients older than 80 years.

Older patients may be at particular risk for nonadherence due to diminished capacity for problem-solving and judgments required to manage complex regimens.[45] A qualitative study of adolescents and young adults (ages 15–31 years) noted that daily adherence decision-making processes used by this population were consistent with the mechanisms used by adults with other chronic medical conditions.[46] A study comparing medication management between older and younger adults living with HIV noted that cognitive ability and depressive symptoms were predictors of

Table 1
Adherence assessment tools

Adherence Tool	Description	Screens for	Advantages	Disadvantages
Adherence Estimator	3-item tool Available: http://www. adherenceestimator.com	Likelihood of nonadherence 3 categories: low, medium, high	May accurately predict risk of nonadherence May be useful in clinical settings	Does not assess adherence rates
ASK-12	12-question tool Asks patients about behaviors that have occurred over time Available: http://www. avoidreadmissions.com/ wwwroot/userfiles/documents/ 204/ask-12-survey-overview.pdf	Inconvenience or forgetfulness and treatment beliefs evaluated on a 5-point Likert scale Behaviors related to taking medications (skipped, stopped, took more or less) evaluated over time (last week, last month, last 3 mo, more than 3 mo, never)	Easy to administer; may help to start a conversation about adherence	Tool is not scored; rate of adherence is not noted
Morisky Medication Adherence Scale	Available in 4- or 8-question formats Questions are asked in Yes/No format Available: http://dmorisky.bol. ucla.edu/MMAS_scale.html	High, medium, low adherence based on: Forgetfulness Carelessness Stop taking medications when feeling worse or better	May be helpful to predict the risk of nonadherence	May not be a reliable tool to measure actual medication adherence
Brief Adherence Rating Scale	3 questions and a visual analog scale (VAS) Available: http://www. psychcongress.com/saundras- corner/scales-screen ersadherence/brief-adherence- rating-scale-bars	Number of prescribed doses taken per day Number of days over past month patient did not take medications Number of days over past month, patient took less than prescribed medications VAS displays proportion of doses taken in the past month	Valid, reliable, sensitive, and specific tool	Limited use compared to other scales

Adapted from Spoelstra SL, Rittenberg CN. Assessment and measurement of medication adherence: oral agents for cancer. Clin J Oncol Nurs 2015;19(3 Suppl):47–52.

medication management. The "predictive value was much stronger in older adults, where cognitive ability alone accounted for 31% of the variability in medication management." (p. 423)[47] However, there may be differences in impact of these factors in different disease states. Younger age was identified as a personal characteristic associated with nonadherence to oral medications in patients with cancer, along with being single, unemployed, and female.[48] The way patients incorporate complex medications regimens into busy lifestyles may be a predictor of nonadherence. In a study of patients with non-small cell lung cancer, a tendency for lower adherence was noted for educated patients with an irregular and active lifestyle.[49]

INTERVENTIONS
Interventions that May Enhance Adherence with Oral Cancer Agents

Oncology nurses are concerned about their patients' ability to take OAC. Spoelstra and Sansoucie[50] note that "nurses should be aware of evidence-based interventions, or lack thereof, when caring for patients prescribed OACs, and use that information to guide decision making in clinical practice" (p.67). Strategies to improve adherence should be multifaceted and practical. Given limited time and resources, strategies and associated interventions should focus on demonstrated drivers of adherence that affect patient behavior and influence positive outcomes.

Several systematic reviews attempt to answer the question about what works to enhance medication adherence to oral cancer agents.[1,51–53] Effective approaches to medication adherence include multiple strategies focused on patient education, convenient care, and patient monitoring and follow-up.

Patient education

Patient education about OAC should include the drug name, dose, how the medication works, when to take it, what to do if a dose is missed, how to manage side effects, and how to get support with taking medications.[54] In a mixed-methods study using a self-report questionnaire with subjects with multiple myeloma who were prescribed cyclophosphamide, thalidomide, and dexamethasone, results indicate that, although 68.8% of the patients indicated that they understood how their medication worked, only 57.8% of the patients reported that they took their medication correctly. Approximately 7 in 10 patients knew what actions to take if they forgot to take their medications.[55]

The American Society of Clinical Oncology (ASCO) and the Oncology Nursing Society (ONS) updated their joint chemotherapy administration safety standards in 2013 to include standards for the safe administration and management of oral chemotherapy.[56] These standards provide guidance for nurses and oncology practices regarding appropriate staffing, documentation, chemotherapy orders or prescription standards, drug preparation, monitoring and assessment, and patient education. Patient education regarding oral cancer agents should include[56]:

- Storage, handling, preparation, administration, and medication disposal
- Supportive care measures, including side effect management
- Possible drug-drug and/or drug-food interactions
- A plan for missed doses
- Contact information and when to notify providers with side effects.

Patient education includes a family member or caregiver whenever possible. Instruction should include patient education materials that are written at an appropriate reading level. The teach-back method allows for opportunities to verify understanding.[54] The patient and/or caregiver's understanding should be documented in the medical record.[56] However, education alone may be insufficient to support medication adherence. Spoelstra and Sansoucie[50] concluded that the effectiveness of education and counseling has not been established and should be supplemented with other patient feedback and monitoring interventions.

Convenient care
The OAC provide patients and caregivers with greater convenience, resulting in fewer office or clinic visits for treatment. The timing of these medications may present problems for some patients. For example, medications that must be taken within specific timeframes, such as before or after food, may present challenges for patients who are trying to fit a new routine into life. Obtaining timely medication refills becomes critical in helping the patient achieve adequate drug levels and relative dose intensity. Specialty pharmacies can assist patients by offering guidance about out-of-pocket costs for medications and linking the patient with pharmaceutical patient assistance programs that may cover a percentage of the costs for these medications. These services should be coordinated with the patient's regular pharmacy to ensure appropriate medication reconciliation and review of potential drug-drug interactions with other medications.

Simplicity of drug regimen may increase the likelihood that patients will take OAC as prescribed by the health care provider or medical oncologist. Johnson[29] noted that the complexity of timing, dose, and complexity related to food interactions is likely to have a negative effect on medication adherence.

It is important to remember that patients may be prescribed medications for other chronic illnesses and OAC may add additional pills. Pill burden refers to the number of pills patients take on a regular basis. An increase in the number of pills is likely to have a negative effect on medication adherence.[29] Nurses should work closely with patient's providers to minimize pill burden when possible.

Monitoring and follow-up
Forgetting to take medication is nearly a universal experience for anyone who has taken a prescription medication. Reminder tools can be as simple as a calendar or patient diary or inexpensive pill box. Sophisticated microelectromechanical medication caps note the date and time that a medication container cap has been opened. Smartphone applications may provide automated text or voice reminders. Keeping medication in a visible location while incorporating taking medication into a daily routine is likely to be an effective strategy. Saying out loud, "I'm taking my medication" or asking family or friends to help with reminders may also be effective.[57]

Providing the patient with feedback about adherence is recommended for practice and may include frequent telephone contact from the nurse in the oncology practice, case manager, and/or pharmacist associated with a specialty pharmacy.[50] Molecular monitoring may be an effective measure of patient adherence with some treatment. For example, the National Comprehensive Cancer Network (NCCN) guidelines for treatment of chronic myelogenous leukemia note that adherence with tyrosine kinase inhibitors is associated with better clinical outcomes and recommend frequent monitoring of drug levels in patients who are nonadherent.[58]

SUMMARY AND IMPLICATIONS FOR THE FUTURE

Increasingly, cancer is treated as a chronic illness managed over time with novel and targeted therapies that hold great promise for cancer control. The OAC have changed the delivery of cancer care by shifting administration of treatment from the provider and oncology nurse to patients and their caregivers. The shift to oral therapies challenges oncology nurses to be informed about best practices for assessing patients regarding barriers to OAC adherence and using strategies that assist patients to

Table 2
Medication adherence resources

Title	Description	URL
Medication Adherence Time Tool: Improving Health Outcomes (American College of Preventive Medicine)	A comprehensive clinical reference for up-to-date information for clinicians and patients regarding medication adherence	http://www.acpm.org/?Adherence
Multinational Association of Supportive Care in Cancer (MASCC) Oral Agent Teaching Tool (MOATT)	Helps minimize the risk of adverse events from oral therapies and increases adherence by ensuring both patients and providers are properly educated Available free of charge in 12 languages	http://www.mascc.org/MOATT
Oncology Nursing Society Oral Chemotherapy Guide for Patients	Video guide to help patients learn about oral cancer drugs and get the most out of their treatment, including safe handling, managing side effects, etc	https://www.onsoralchemoguide.com/
Oncology Nursing Society ONS/ONCC Chemotherapy Biotherapy Certification Course	15 contact hours to equip nurses with the tools needed to safely administer chemotherapy and biotherapy agents to patients	https://www.ons.org/education/courses-articles
NCCN Task Force Report: Oral Chemotherapy	For health care professionals who treat and manage patients with cancer	http://www.nccn.org/JNCCN/PDF/JNSU3_combined_Oral_Chemo_2008.pdf
The American Society of Clinical Oncology and the Oncology Nursing Society Oral Chemotherapy Guidelines	Consensus-based process to develop standards for safe administration of chemotherapy Current ASCO-ONS standards address safety of all routes of chemotherapy administration to adult patients in the outpatient setting and inpatient setting Chemotherapy safety standards are intended to reduce the risk of errors when providing adult patients with chemotherapy and provide a framework for best practices in cancer care; informing practice policies and procedures, internal quality assessment, and external quality monitoring	https://www.ons.org/practice-resources/clinical-practice/ascoons-chemotherapy-administration-safety-standards

Script Your Future	Campaign and website led by the National Consumers League with partners from every sector of the health care system, designed for consumers with chronic illness to help them take medication as directed Includes patient tools for keeping track of medications, how-to videos about taking medications, and tips for talking with their doctor or health care professional.	http://www.scriptyourfuture.org/
National Council on Patient Information and Education (NCPIE)	The is a nonprofit coalition working to stimulate and improve communication of information on the appropriate use of medicines to consumers and health care professionals. Develops and provides patient educational programs and educational resources that promote the latest advances in communication research and practice.	http://www.talkaboutrx.org/index.jsp
Prescriptions for a Healthy America: A Partnership for Advancing Medication Adherence	Raises awareness on the challenges posed by medication nonadherence, as well as advances public policy solutions to help address it	http://adhereforhealth.org/

adhere to their treatment plan. Nurses assess the patient's competence and ability to achieve optimal adherence. Patients and their caregivers with their providers, oncologist, oncology nurse, pharmacist, and other health care team members, engage in shared decision activities conducted in a manner consistent with achieving the patient's treatment goals. Quality care for patients prescribed OAC includes strategies focused on patient education, convenient care, patient monitoring, and follow-up. A list of resources to help nurses learn more about medication adherence is provided in **Table 2**. Research is needed to develop assessment tools that predict or suggest patients who are at risk for nonadherence and standardized approaches to help patients take their medications as prescribed.

REFERENCES

1. Givens BA, Spoelstra SL, Grant M. The challenges of oral agents as antineoplastic treatments. Semin Oncol Nurs 2011;27(2):93–103.
2. O'Neill VJ, Twelves CJ. Oral cancer treatment: developments in chemotherapy and beyond. Br J Cancer 2002;87:933–7.
3. Bedell CH. A changing paradigm for cancer treatment: the advent of new oral chemotherapy agents. Clin J Oncol Nurs 2003;7(6 Suppl):5–9.
4. Moore S. Facilitating oral chemotherapy treatment and compliance through patient/family-focused education. Cancer Nurs 2007;30(2):112–22.
5. Weingart SN, Brown E, Bach PB, et al. NCCN task force report: oral chemotherapy. J Natl Compr Canc Netw 2008;6(Suppl 3):S1–14. Available at: http://www.nccn. org/JNCCN/PDF/JNSU3_combined_Oral_Chemo_2008.pdf. Accessed March 22, 2016.
6. Banna GL, Collova E, Gebbia V, et al. Anticancer oral therapy: emerging related issues. Cancer Treat Rev 2010;36:595–605.
7. Osterberg L, Blaschke T. Adherence to medication. N Engl J Med 2005;353: 487–97.
8. World Health Organization. Adherence to long-term therapies: evidence for action. 2003. Available at: http://apps.who.int/iris/bitstream/10665/42682/1/9241545992. pdf?ua=1. Accessed March 4, 2016.
9. Puts MT, Tu HA, Tourangeau A, et al. Factors influencing adherence to cancer treatment in older adults with cancer: a systematic review. Ann Oncol 2014;25:564–77.
10. Spoelstra SL, Given CW. Assessment and measurement of adherence to oral antineoplastic agents. Semin Oncol Nurs 2011;27:116–32.
11. Streeter SB, Schwartzberg L, Husain N, et al. Patient and plan characteristics affecting abandonment of oral oncolytic prescriptions. J Oncol Pract 2011;7: 46s–51s.
12. Makubate B, Donnan PT, Dewar JA, et al. Cohort study of adherence to adjuvant endocrine therapy, breast cancer recurrence and mortality. Br J Cancer 2013; 108:1515–24.
13. Wu EQ, Johnson S, Beaulieu N, et al. Health-care resource utilization and costs associated with non-adherence to imatinib treatment in chronic myeloid leukemia patients. Curr Med Res Opin 2010;26:61–9.
14. Ganesan P, Sagar TG, Dubashi B, et al. Non-adherence to imatinib adversely affects event free survival in chronic phase chronic myeloid leukemia. Am J Hematol 2011;86:471–4.
15. Hershman DL, Shao T, Kushi LH, et al. Early discontinuation and non-adherence to adjuvant hormonal therapy are associated with increased mortality in women with breast cancer. Breast Cancer Res Treat 2011;126:529–37.

16. McMullen CK, Safford MM, Bosworth HB, et al. Patient-centered priorities for improving medication management and adherence. Patient Educ Couns 2015; 98:102–10.
17. Kuntz JL, Safford MM, Singh JA, et al. Patient-centered interventions to improve medication management and adherence: a qualitative review of research findings. Patient Educ Couns 2014;97:310–26.
18. Committee on Quality of Health Care in America Institute of Medicine. Crossing the quality chasm: a new health system for the 21st century. Washington, DC: The National Academy Press; 2001.
19. Kohn KT, Corrigan JM, Donaldson MS. To err is human: building a safer health system. Washington, DC: National Academy Press; 1999.
20. Alemi F, Neuhauser D, Ardito S, et al. Continuous self-improvement: systems thinking in a personal context. Jt Comm J Qual Improv 2000;26(2):74–86.
21. Russell CL, Ruppar TM, Matteson M. Improving medication adherence: moving from intention and motivation to a personal systems approach. Nurs Clin North Am 2011;46:271–81.
22. Russell CL. A clinical nurse specialist-led intervention to enhance medication adherence using the plan-do-check-act cycle for continuous self-improvement. Clin Nurse Spec 2010;24:69–75.
23. DiBonventura M, Copher R, Basurto E, et al. Patient preferences and treatment adherence among women diagnosed with metastatic breast cancer. Am Health Drug Benefits 2014;7(7):386–96.
24. Lambert BL, Levy NA, Winer J. Keeping the balance and monitoring the self-system towards a more comprehensive model of medication management in psychiatry. In: Brashers DE, Goldsmith DJ, editors. Communicating to manage health and illness. New York: Routledge/Taylor and Francis Group; 2009. p. 179–211.
25. Wilson SR, Strub P, Buist AS, et al. Shared treatment decision making improves adherence and outcomes in poorly controlled asthma. Am J Respir Crit Care Med 2010;181:566–77.
26. Charles C, Gafni A, Whelen T. Shared decision-making in the medical encounter: what does it mean? (or it takes at least two to tango). Soc Sci Med 1997;44: 681–92.
27. Charles C, Gafni A, Whelen T. Decision-making in the physician-patient encounter: revisiting the shared-treatment decision making model. Soc Sci Med 1999;49:651–61.
28. American Society of Consultant Pharmacists. Adult medication: improving medication adherence in older adults. Available at: http://www.adultmeducation.com/. Accessed March 15, 2016.
29. Irwin M, Johnson LA. Factors influencing oral adherence: qualitative metasummary and triangulations with quantitative evidence. Clin J Oncol Nurs 2015; 19(3 Suppl):6–30.
30. Halfdanarson TR, Jatoi A. Oral cancer chemotherapy: the critical interplay between patient education and patient safety. Curr Oncol Rep 2010;12(4):247–52.
31. Ruddy K, Mayer E, Partridge A. Patient adherence and persistence with oral anticancer treatment. CA Cancer J Clin 2009;59(1):56–66.
32. Hollywood E, Semple D. Nursing strategies for patients on oral chemotherapy. Oncology (Williston Park) 2001;15(1 Suppl 2):37–9.
33. Moore S. Adherence to oral therapies for cancer: barriers and models for change. J Adv Pract Oncol 2010;1(3):155–64.
34. Kantarjian H, Steensma D, Rius JR, et al. High cancer drug prices in the United States: reason and proposed solutions. J Oncol Pract 2014;10(4):e208–11.

35. Howard DH, Bach PB, Berndt ER, et al. Pricing in the market for anticancer drugs. J Econ Perspect 2015;29(1):139–62.
36. Conti RM, Fein AJ, Bhatta SS. National trends in spending on and use of oral oncologics, first quarter 2006 through third quarter 2011. Health Aff 2014;33(10): 1721–7.
37. Yabroff KR, Dowling EC, Guy GP Jr, et al. Financial hardship associated with cancer in the United States: findings from a population-based sample of adult cancer survivors. J Clin Oncol 2015;34(3):259–67.
38. Spoelstra SL, Rittenberg CN. Assessment and measurement of medication adherence: oral agents for cancer. Clin J Oncol Nurs 2015;19(3 Suppl):47–52.
39. Moody M, Jackowski J. Are patients on oral chemotherapy in your practice setting safe? Clin J Oncol Nurs 2010;14(3):339–46.
40. Kav S, Schulmeister L, Nirenberg A, et al. Development of the MASCC teaching tool for patients receiving oral agents for cancer. Support Care Cancer 2010;18: 583–90.
41. Boucher J, Lucca J, Hooper C, et al. A structured nursing intervention to address oral chemotherapy adherence in patients with non-small cell lung cancer. Oncol Nurs Forum 2015;42(4):383–9.
42. Ribed A, Escudero-Vilaplana V, Romero-Jiménezm RM. Guiding pharmacist clinical interviews: a safety tool to support the education of patients treated with oral antineoplastic agents. Expert Opin Drug Saf 2016. Published online: Mar 9, 2016.
43. Huang WC, Chen CY, Lin SJ, et al. Medication adherence to oral anticancer drugs: Systematic Review. Expert Rev Anticancer Ther 2016.
44. Kawakami K, Nakamoto E, Yokokawa T, et al. Patients' self-reported adherence to capecitabine on XELOX treatment in metastatic colorectal cancer: findings from a retrospective cohort analysis. Patient Prefer Adherence 2015;9:561–7.
45. Maloney KW, Kagan SH. Adherence and oral agents with older patients. Semin Oncol Nurs 2011;27(2):154–60.
46. McGrady ME, Brown GA, Pai AL. Medication adherence decision-making among adolescents and young adults with cancer. Eur J Oncol Nurs 2016;10:207–14.
47. Frain J, Barton-Burke M, Bachman J, et al. A comparison of medication management between older and younger adults living with HIV. J Assoc Nurses AIDS Care 2014;25(5):414–26.
48. Berry DL, Blonquist TM, Halpenny B, et al. Self-reported adherence to oral cancer therapy: relationships with symptom distress, depression, and personal characteristics. Patient Prefer Adherence 2015;9:1587–92.
49. Bourmand A, Henin E, Tinquaut F, et al. Adherence to oral anticancer chemotherapy: what influences patients' over or non-adherence? Analysis of the OCTO study through quantitative–qualitative methods. BMC Res Notes 2015;8:291.
50. Spoelstra SL, Sansoucie H. Putting evidence into practice: evidence-based interventions for oral agents for cancer. Clin J Oncol Nurs 2015;19(3 Suppl):60–72.
51. Verbrugghe M, Verhaeghe S, Lauwaert K, et al. Determinants and associated factors in influencing medication adherence and persistence to oral anticancer drugs: a systematic review. Cancer Treat Rev 2013;39:610–21.
52. Mathes T, Antoine SL, Pieper D, et al. Adherence enhancing interventions for oral anticancer agents. Cancer Treat Rev 2013;40:102–8.
53. Bassan F, Peter F, Houbre B, et al. Adherence to oral antineoplastic agents by cancer patients: definition and literature review. Eur J Cancer Care (Engl) 2014; 23:22–35.
54. McCue DA, Lohr LK, Pick AM. Improving adherence to oral cancer therapy in clinical practice. Pharmacotherapy 2014;34(5):48–494.

55. Arber A, Odelius A, Williams P, et al. Do patients on oral chemotherapy have sufficient knowledge for optimal adherence? A mixed methods study. Eur J Cancer Care (Engl) 2015. [Epub ahead of print].
56. Neuss MN, Polovich M, McNiff K, et al. 2013 updated American Society of Clinical Oncology/Oncology Nursing Society chemotherapy administration safety standards including standards for the safe administration and management of oral chemotherapy. Oncol Nurs Forum 2013;40(3):225–33. Available at: https://www. ons.org/sites/default/files/2013chemostandards.pdf. Accessed March 13, 2016.
57. Burhenn PS, Smudde J. Using tools and technology to promote education and adherence to oral agents for cancer. Clin J Oncol Nurs 2015;19(3):53–9.
58. National Comprehensive Cancer Network. National Comprehensive Cancer Network NCCN guidelines® chronic myelogenous leukemia. Available at: http://www.nccn.org/professionals/physician_gls/f_guidelines.asp. Accessed March 12, 2016.

Clinical Trials and the Role of the Oncology Clinical Trials Nurse

Elizabeth A. Ness, MS, BSN, RN[a],*, Cheryl Royce, MS, RN, CRNP[b]

KEYWORDS

- Clinical trials • Oncology trial design • Clinical trials nurse
- Research nurse competencies • Research nursing office

KEY POINTS

- Genomic profiling and the development of molecularly targeted agents have led to novel designs for oncology clinical trials.
- Ensuring human subject protections and quality data are responsibilities for all individuals involved in clinical trials; however, the principal investigator is ultimately accountable for the overall conduct of the trial.
- Oncology clinical trials nurses (CTNs) are critical to the implementation of oncology clinical trials.
- Competencies developed by the Oncology Nursing Society help define the specialized role of the oncology CTN.

INTRODUCTION

Today's standard of care was yesterday's clinical trial. Oncology clinical trials have been and will continue to be the cornerstone for improving outcomes for individuals at risk for and living with cancer. A clinical trial is a type of patient-oriented clinical research study that prospectively assigns participants, also known as human subjects, to one or more biomedical or behavioral interventions to evaluate health-related outcomes.[1] Discovering these new interventions and developing, implementing, and monitoring a clinical trial involves many groups and individuals (**Box 1**). Collectively their responsibility is to ensure that the rights and well-being of the research participants are protected and to advance scientific knowledge by ensuring

Disclosures: None.
[a] Office of Education and Compliance, Center for Cancer Research, National Cancer Institute, 10 Center Drive, Room 3-2571, MSC 1206, Bethesda, MD 20892, USA; [b] Office of Research Nursing, Center for Cancer Research, National Cancer Institute, 10 Center Drive, Room 3-2571, MSC 1206, Bethesda, MD 20892, USA
* Corresponding author.
E-mail address: nesse@mail.nih.gov

Box 1
Key groups and individuals responsible for ensuring good clinical practice

Clinical trial sponsors including:
  Pharmaceutical companies
  Government agencies (eg, National Cancer Institute)

Research teams
  Principal investigator
  Subinvestigators
  Research participant
  Study coordinator (nurse or non-nurse)
  Clinical data manager
  Statistician

Research site collaborators
  Staff/infusion nurses
  Basic science and clinical laboratory staff
  Radiology staff
  Pharmacists
  Contract and billing staff

Federal agencies
  Office for Human Research Protections
  US Food and Drug Administration (FDA)

---

that data generated by the trial are accurate, verifiable, and reproducible.[2,3] A key role in successful implementation of a clinical trial is the study coordinator.[4]

Clinical trials nursing is a specialty practice that includes a variety of roles (eg, study coordinator, direct care nurse, nurse manager, nurse educator), settings (eg, academic medical center, private practice, research unit), and clinical specialties (eg, oncology, cardiology, infectious disease). The clinical trials nurse (CTN) serves as a study coordinator but may have different job titles (eg, Research Nurse Coordinator, Clinical Research Nurse, Clinical Research Coordinator) and may be supervised by a physician, investigator, or a non-nurse research manager.[5–9] This article provides an overview of clinical trials, highlights the role of the oncology CTN (ie, the nurse in the role of study coordinator), and shares one organization's process to unite all CTNs under one nursing office.

OVERVIEW OF CLINICAL TRIALS

Good Clinical Practice (GCP) is an international ethical and scientific set of standards for the design and conduct of research involving humans, including protocol design, conduct, performance, monitoring, auditing, recording, analyses, and reporting.[10] It includes both regulations, which are binding, and guidelines or guidances, which are not binding but recommended to be followed. In response to historical events, regulations and guidelines have been developed (**Box 2**).[2,3]

Several groups with regulatory authority are involved in the conduct of clinical trials in the United States. In the Code of Federal Regulations (CFR), the 2 main titles related to clinical trials are Title 45 (Public Welfare) and Title 21 (Food and Drugs). Guidance documents describe an agency's interpretation of or policy on a regulatory issue. Title 45 Part 46 is interpreted by the Office for Human Research Protections. The US Food and Drug Administration (FDA) interprets Title 21 and its subparts.[11,12]

There are 5 types of clinical trials (**Table 1**).[13,14] Treatment clinical trials can further be characterized by phases (**Table 2**).[14–16] Advancements in cancer biology, genomic

Box 2
United States regulations related to clinical trials
Title 45 Part 46
Subpart A: Protection of Human Subjects (1974, revised in 1981, 1991, 2005); also referred to as the Common Rule (1991)
Subpart B: Pregnant Women, Human Fetuses and Neonates in Research (1975, revised 2001)
Subpart C: Biomedical and Behavioral Research Involving Prisoners as Subjects (1978)
Subpart D: Children Involved as Subjects in Research (1983)
Subpart E: Registration of IRBs (2009)
Title 21
Part 11: Electronic Records; Electronic Signatures
Part 50: Protection of Human Subjects
Part 54: Financial Disclosure by Clinical Investigators
Part 56: Institutional Review Boards
Part 312: Investigational New Drug Application
Part 600: Biologic Products
Part 812: Investigational Drug Exemptions

Table 1		
Types of clinical trials		
Trial Type	**Purposes**	**Examples**
Prevention	Evaluate better ways to prevent a disease[a] from developing or returning	Vaccine (eg, HPV vaccine) Exercise
Screening	Discover the best ways to detect a disease[a] in the general population, or, for individuals who have a higher than normal risk of developing a disease, before symptoms start	Laboratory test (eg, BRCA1) Imaging (eg, mammogram) Health history (eg, pedigree)
Diagnostic	Evaluate better ways to identify a particular disease[a]	Genetic tests (eg, VHL syndrome) Imaging tests (eg, PET scan)
Quality of life/supportive care	Explore ways to improve the comfort and the quality of life for individuals with a chronic illness	Antiemetic Support group
Treatment	Develop better interventions for disease[a]	Drug Vaccine Device Surgery Radiation Psychotherapy Combination modalities

Abbreviations: BRCA1, breast cancer genes 1; HPV, human papillomavirus; VHL, von Hippel Lindau.
[a] Disease includes a disorder or health condition.

Table 2
Phases of clinical trials

Phase	Goals	Traditional Design
I	Determine dosing in humans - known as the MTD; conducted in adults before children Assess safety Evaluate pharmacokinetics and pharmacodynamics May also be used to evaluate new treatment schedule, new drug combination strategy, and new multimodality regimen	Open label, nonrandomized, dose escalation with cohorts of 3–6 research participants; known as a 3 + 3 design Increase dose gradually, most commonly using a modified Fibonacci schema Low starting dose based on the animal models to avoid serious toxicity
II	Provide initial assessment of efficacy or clinical activity Further define safety and toxicity	Open label, 1 dose level based on the MTD; also known as the recommended phase 2 dose Most commonly a 2-stage design with an early stopping rule Increasing use of randomized designs
III	Efficacy compared with standard therapy Further evaluation of safety	Randomization with or without blinding May include stratification based on disease-specific prognostic factors (eg, hormone receptor status in breast cancer) or other factors (eg, age, gender)

Abbreviation: MTD, maximum tolerated dose.

profiling, and the development of molecularly targeted agents (MTAs) have led trialists to rethink traditional trial designs. Basket, umbrella, and adaptive trials are examples of novel designs now being used in oncology clinical trials (**Table 3**).[17,18]

PROTOCOL DEVELOPMENT AND REVIEW PROCESS

A protocol is the written detailed action plan that provides background about the clinical trial, specifies trial objectives, describes the trial's design and organization, and

Table 3
Trials designs for targeted therapies

Trial Type	Description	Example
Basket trial	Test an MTA on the same genomic mutation regardless of tumor histology	NCI-MATCH (ClinicalTrials.gov identifier: NCT02465060)
Umbrella trial	Test an MTA on a single tumor type/histology with different genomic mutations	Lung-MAP (ClinicalTrials.gov identifier: NCT02154490)
Adaptive designs	Use accumulating data to decide how to modify aspects of the trial on an ongoing basis without undermining the validity and integrity of the trial	I-SPY 2 (ClinicalTrials.gov identifier: NCT01042379)

Abbreviations: I-SPY 2, Investigation of Serial Studies to Predict Your Therapeutic Response With Imaging And Molecular Analysis 2; Lung-MAP, Lung Cancer Master Protocol; MATCH, Molecular Analysis for Therapy Choice; MTA, molecular target agent; NCI, National Cancer Institute.

ensures that trial procedures are performed consistently, protecting the research participants and providing appropriate data to answer the trial objectives. **Box 3** outlines the various sections of a protocol. Protocols undergo various reviews before participant enrollment. Some protocols undergo a scientific review (eg, National Cancer Institute [NCI]–designated cancer centers) and some need to have additional safety reviews:

- Radiation safety review if ionizing radiation is used at a frequency greater than standard of care
- Institutional Biosafety Committee and Office of Biotechnology Activities if human gene transfer is a component of the trial
- Sponsor review if the protocol was written by an investigator and not the sponsor (eg, NCI-sponsored trials)[19]

All clinical trial protocols including the informed consent (IC) document undergo an ethical review by an institutional review board (IRB) before their implementation. The IRB is a committee charged with the review of human subject research. Its primary mandate is to protect and safeguard the rights and welfare of human subjects. Internationally, the IRB may be known by other names, such as ethical review board or research ethics committee.[19,20] Note that a clinical trial cannot begin to enroll participants until it has been approved by the IRB.

Box 3
Content of a protocol: section titles vary based on the clinical trial sponsor or Institutional Review Board

Title page

Précis/synopsis

Table of contents, including subsections and accurate pagination

Objectives: primary and secondary

Background information

Study design and methods

Inclusion and exclusion criteria

Clinical and laboratory methods

Collection and storage of human specimens or data

Statistical analysis

Human subject protection

Privacy and confidentiality

Pharmaceutical interventions

Event reporting requirements

Data and safety monitoring plan

Data/record management

Compensation

References

Appendices

INFORMED CONSENT

IC is a legal and ethical requirement for most health care matters and when conducting clinical research. IC involves subjects having the capacity to agree for themselves to participate in a given situation (eg, clinical research). Informed consent is an important process in the clinical research.[21] The IC document is a written tool used by the investigator and/or other research team members to guide and reinforce the discussion with each patient about a research study. The IC document includes 8 required and 6 additional elements depending on the type of study and IRB policy (**Box 4**).[11,22] Each IRB has an IC document template that needs to be used. When working on industry-sponsored trials or trials that are conducted at multiple sites (ie, multisite

---

Box 4
Elements of an informed consent document (21 Code of Federal Regulations Part 50 and 45 Code of Federal Regulations Part 46)

Eight essential elements

A statement disclosing that the study involves research, including
  Explanation of the purpose of the research
  Invitation to participate
  Expected duration of participation
  Description of procedures to be followed
  Identification of any procedures that are experimental (eg, MRI that would not be done as part of standard of care, but for research only)

Description of any foreseeable risks/discomforts

Description of any benefits to patient or others

Disclosure of any appropriate alternatives to study participation (eg, standard comfort measures)

How patient's confidentiality will be maintained

For research that involves more than minimal risk, an explanation regarding compensation if injury occurs, what that compensation is, and how to obtain further information

Contact persons for questions related to research and research subjects' rights

A statement regarding the voluntary nature of participation, including that refusal to participate does not involve any penalty or loss of benefit to the patient

For applicable clinical trials under the FDA Amendment Act (sections 505 or 351), the statement, "A description of this clinical trial will be available on (www.clinicaltrials.gov). This Web site will not include information that can identify you. At most, the Web site will include a summary of results. You can search this Web site at any time."

Six additional elements

The intervention or procedure may cause unforeseeable risks (eg, risk to fetus if patient should become pregnant)

Circumstance for termination of participation by the investigator (eg, noncompliance with protocol's safety assessments, sponsor terminates an Investigational New Drug application)

Additional costs to the patient from participation

Consequences of the patient's decision to discontinue research participation

Statement that the patient will be notified of significant new findings that may affect their decision to continue participation

Approximate number of subjects

trials), a sample IC document is provided to each investigator for reformatting per the reviewing IRB's template.

Individuals' voluntary agreement to participate in a clinical trial is shown by their signatures on the IC document; this is referred to as obtaining consent. However, IC is an ongoing process of communication and mutual understanding between individuals and investigators. The research participants need to be provided with additional pertinent new information (eg, new risks, new procedures) throughout their participation on a clinical trial in order to make a decision to remain on the clinical trial.

The advancements in genomic profiling affect not only trial design but the IC document and process as well. The National Human Genome Research Institute recommends that the following be considered when addressing IC:

- Broad versus specific consent
- Considerations for families
- Considerations for identifiable populations
- Studies involving children
- Studies involving participants who cannot give consent
- Data and sample sharing through data repositories and biobanks
- Return of results to participants[23]

THE RESEARCH TEAM

Once the IC document is signed, protocol-specific procedures for eligibility screening begin. If eligible, the intervention begins, data are collected, monitoring and quality control activities occur, participants are removed from the protocol based on prespecified criteria, and data are analyzed. The results may be published and, if applicable, the results are reported in ClinicalTrials.gov, a registry for publicly and privately supported clinical studies. It is the research team that orchestrates these activities. It is essential for all individuals involved in clinical research to have knowledge and understanding of research-related laws and regulations to ensure GCP.[24–26]

Every clinical trial has a principal investigator (PI) who is accountable for the overall conduct of the trial and enrolls research participants. Other team members may include subinvestigators, study coordinator (nurse or non-nurse), clinical data manager, and statistician. The types of individuals and responsibilities vary based on the clinical setting. **Table 4** outlines the general responsibilities of the PI, study coordinator, and research participant.[24–29] Note that US regulations only outline the role of the investigator, not other research team members.

ONCOLOGY CLINICAL TRIALS NURSE

In the 1960s, early chemotherapy clinical trials provided new roles for nurses. Oncology nurses needed to develop new skills and new partnerships with physician investigators while caring for patients on clinical trials. This requirement not only included administering investigational agents but also coordinating the clinical trial.[30] As nurses, oncology CTNs must adhere to the American Nursing Association Scope and Standards of Practice and Code of Ethics along with their state's Practice Act. In addition to the responsibilities of the study coordinator listed in **Table 4**, oncology CTNs:

- Provide and coordinate the care of the research participant
- Know the diseases being studied
- Understand the basics of genomics and molecularly targeted therapies, including implications for participant education and IC

| Table 4 |
| Responsibilities of the principal investigator, study coordinator, and research participant |

Role	General Responsibilities
PI	Comply with all applicable federal regulations and state laws affecting the protection of human subjects Comply with all applicable IRB policies, procedures, decisions, conditions, and requirements Conduct study in accordance with the current IRB-approved protocol Design the clinical trial and/or provide study oversight Personally conduct and supervise the clinical trial
Study coordinator	Recruit and retain research participant Schedule protocol-specific procedures Secure and reinforce IC Prepare for and participate in monitoring visits and audits Ensure integrity of protocol is maintained by enforcing timelines for study visits and other procedures Maintain regulatory files Assist PI in submitting protocol and consent for initial review, continuing review and amendments Report serious adverse events and unanticipated problems Participate in data management and data quality assurance
Research participants	Respect research staff and other participants Read the consent form and other documents Ask questions if they do not understand something about the study, their rights and responsibilities Know when the study begins and ends Follow directions for all protocol-related procedures Show up at scheduled appointments on time or inform research staff within a reasonable time if they need to reschedule Report symptoms and other problems they experience during the study Provide truthful answers to questions asked throughout the study Inform staff if they decide to withdraw from the study

- Assess adverse events using the Common Terminology Criteria for Adverse Events
- Manage toxicities within the scope of license and protocol
- Educate research staff and collaborators on an ongoing basis
- Educate research participants and their significant others about:
  ○ Underlying disease processes
  ○ The clinical trial (eg, objectives, schema, adverse events) and their roles
  ○ Expectations for cure, control, palliation, or no benefit
- Facilitate the ongoing IC process
- Advocate for the patients (ie, research participants) and protocol[26]

Based on the wide variation of how the oncology CTN role was implemented across various practice settings and with feedback from the Oncology Nursing Society (ONS) CTN Special Interest Group, the ONS developed competencies for oncology CTNs. A complete set of the competencies can be found at https://www.ons.org/sites/default/files/ctncompetencies.pdf.[31] Initially published in January 2010, the ONS CTN competencies are undergoing a revision that will:

- Include new functional areas (eg, data management) incorporating some previous categorizations
- Separate required knowledge from skills and behaviors

- Add recommended resources to aid in knowledge and competency achievement
- Add a more advanced level of competencies for those with more experience or who are functioning at a higher level than novice CTNs

THE REORGANIZATION OF CLINICAL TRIALS NURSES: ONE INSTITUTION'S EXPERIENCE

Necessity is the mother of taking chances.
—From Roughing It by Mark Twain, American author and humorist

The Center for Cancer Research (CCR) is the basic and clinical intramural research program of the NCI. Within the CCR is the Office of the Clinical Director, which supports CCR's clinical research program by providing biostatistical expertise, education and training, data management, auditing and monitoring activities, regulatory support and expertise, and informatics for data collection and storage.

The growth of CCR clinical research programs requiring support of the CTN has increased over the years. Historically the management of CTNs was within the specific programs including CTN recruitment, supervision, training, personnel actions, and performance evaluations. The programs were silos in which the team functioned. By 2011, there were 74 CTNs across 13 programs, supporting 68 PIs. As the workload of one program grew there was little to no flexibility to have CTNs cross-cover from another program. The scope and volume of work were discrepant across programs. When programs expanded their research portfolios, necessitating more CTN staff, the request was forwarded to the Office of the Clinical Director for evaluation and approval. There were no standard performance evaluation metrics. Work practices for leave and attendance and telecommuting were different across programs. Communication practices were not efficient or timely. There were a multitude of reasons that supported the CCR leadership to consider centralizing the CTNs.

In 2011 the CCR leadership recognized that the organization would benefit from an integrated infrastructure for CTNs. The primary purpose was to allow nurses to report to nurses in the hopes of:

- Establishing a career path for CTNs
- Establishing core CTN competencies
- Increasing training
- Developing standard policies for time and attendance
- Allowing for the cross-training required to respond to variances in workload
- Establishing an esprit de corps
- Efficiently recruiting and hiring CTNs
- Implementing human resource actions consistently
- Establishing efficient mechanisms for communication
- Ensuring collaboration with the PIs

OFFICE OF RESEARCH NURSING

The new office would be called the Office of Research Nursing (ORN) and would become part of the Office of the Clinical Director. The Deputy Director for the CCR was aware that this was a major cultural shift for CTNs and the PIs. Several town hall meetings for CTNs and PIs were held in the fall of 2012 to present the idea for a new model and to elicit feedback from these stakeholders.

Building the infrastructure for this office took place between September 2012 and March 2013. The ORN was given a budget to include salaries, travel, training, and supplies. A director needed to be recruited for the office and 3 team leaders needed to be hired into the ORN. The director was an experienced leader in nursing within the CCR with background as a CTN and nurse practitioner. The team leaders selected had strong backgrounds in research nursing and leadership, and strong institutional knowledge. A leadership team was formed and an administrative assistant hired with responsibilities for travel, supplies, management of timecards, and facilitation of the recruitment and hiring processes. Performance evaluations were created using the ONS competencies. The ORN director thought that the consolidation of nursing under nursing leadership had the potential to develop quality CTNs to support clinical research within the organization.

LEADING CHANGE THROUGH ENGAGEMENT

In order for the new model to be successful, the chief needed to lead change by engaging clinical research staff in a mutually supported vision of the future while being sensitive to the cultural change experienced by the CTNs and the PIs. In *Getting Change Right*, Seth Kahan[32] shares tips for successful change:

> *So what's a change leader to do? Create ways for people to get together and converse. Get them participating, engaged, and involved. This is the road to personal investment, enthusiastic support, and genuine buy-in. This is how you move people across the line from "I have to do this" to "I want to do this." And that makes all the difference in the world.*[32]

The challenge with the reorganization was getting engagement across the research team.

On the first day in office, the director made appointments with each of the 74 CTNs and interviewed them to understand their background (**Box 5**), motivations, and career aspirations. CTNs were asked:

- How long they had been in their jobs
- What kept them in their jobs
- What obstacles they faced that prevented them from getting their jobs done
- What was on their wish list

Overwhelmingly, the CTNs said that what kept them in their jobs were the relationships with their colleagues, including investigators and other physicians. They were intellectually challenged by the research protocols and science, autonomous in their positions, and driven to help patients. The overriding impediment related to performing their jobs better was a lack of communication about policies and procedures. They wanted to know best practices and what other nurses were doing that improved their efficiency. Much of the information gained from these interviews was congruent with the reasons for the reorganization of the CTNs. The director was comfortable knowing that the needs of the CCR and the CTNs were in alignment.

Establishing Structure

The ORN leadership team met and developed the ORN draft mission and vision statement, which was presented to the CTNs for their input and feedback. This draft was a key first step to engaging staff in decision making for what was to be a long-term meaningful partnership between leadership and staff.

> *To provide a unique, cohesive team of superior research nurse specialists to carry out the mission of the CCR through a culture that supports continuing education, mentorship, professional development, and collaboration while balancing*

Box 5
Research nurses demographics
Educational background
Master's degree in nursing: 14
Master's degree in other (in addition to the nursing degree): 7
Bachelor of Science in nursing: 52
Associate degree: 8
Years in nursing
Less than 5: 3
From 5 to 10: 12
From 11 to 15: 8
Greater than 15: 51
Certification in nursing
Oncology certified nurse: 20
Bone marrow transplant certified nurse: 2
Advanced practice nurse in genetics: 2
Certification in clinical research
Certified clinical research coordinator: 1
Certified clinical research professional: 2

comprehensive patient coordination and quality clinical and translational research.

—Vision statement for the ORN, 2013

The leadership team participated in a 12-week supervisory course on self-development, program development, and leading though change. Training included the legalities of supervision, conflict resolution, leadership development, forming and leading teams, and handling human resource issues. In addition, the director and team leads were afforded the opportunity to have 3 months of individual executive coaching, which has proved to be invaluable for the development of the ORN.

The ORN established 4 teams, each with a team lead (**Fig. 1**). The ORN leadership took the following into account while creating teams:

- CTN experience
- Existing research team dynamics
- Research team workload (eg, types of protocols, phases of clinical trials, number of protocols)
- Support staff (eg, data manager, scheduling support staff, midlevel providers)

The aim was to provide manageable teams for each team leader to supervise while supporting the vision statement of the ORN.

Communication and Transparency

An immediate response to the needs of both the CCR and the CTN was to initiate a communication plan. The ORN developed a monthly newsletter that includes staff recognition, educational opportunities, new policies/procedures, staff departures,

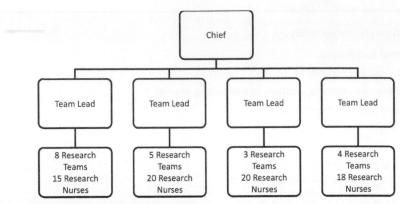

Fig. 1. Organizational chart for the ORN.

staff hires, and regulatory updates. The newsletter is distributed via e-mail and posted on a dedicated Web site. Informal staff meetings called Coffee and Chats began and are held monthly on 3 different days of the week so that all staff have an opportunity to attend. The purpose of these meetings is for staff to network, share best practices, and receive up-to-date information from the leadership team. The CTNs are invited to join the meetings but not required to attend the meetings. Part of the communication plan includes the development of the ORN Wiki page. The site is maintained by the ORN chief and contains newsletters, listing of the nurses, their contact information, and procedures for promotion. An e-mail distribution list with all research nurses, ORN leadership, and additional staff from the Office of the Clinical Director (eg, deputy clinical director, nurse educator, protocol support office director, and quality management coordinator) allows rapid, thorough communication to all CTNs.

All team leaders developed relationships with their CTNs, the teams in which the team leaders worked, and the respective PIs. It was imperative to know what each individual on the research team valued and find ways to help them achieve that as quickly as possible. The team leaders attended research team and data management meetings as well as clinic when needed. The team leaders continue to meet regularly with PIs.

Quickly work groups began to emerge composed of staff who identified a need or a problem and developed a team to address solutions. One work group emerged to address documentation needs in the electronic medical record. Other work groups developed, including:

- Wellness Committee with a goal of helping CTNs strike work-life balance
- Journal Club to provide CTNs with a forum to discuss peer-reviewed literature related to oncology, nursing, or clinical trials
- Model for cross-coverage and what it meant to cover for a CTN who was out of the office

Making Changes

From its inception the ORN leadership made a strategic decision that changes in practice would be small with a likelihood of being successful, and that we would build from there. It was about building trust and respecting staff input. A decision was made that all changes would be presented to the staff with rationale for the change, they would have input, and leadership would listen. The PIs and other stakeholders were included in the communications. We would use champions to advocate for new ideas and change that needed to be addressed. We would communicate to the staff the final proposal and then roll out the changes and fully communicate to all involved. The first change that was presented was standard operating procedures for time, attendance, and telework. This process was successful, because the staff trusted the process, allowing for subsequent changes. We established ground rules for conducting business, including work schedule options, performance evaluations, and promotion procedures. All changes were approached in the manner of our change management philosophy.

NOW THAT THERE IS ENGAGEMENT, TIME TO GET DOWN TO BUSINESS

A priority of the CCR was to improve cross-coverage and flexibility to cover workload. There were 4 programs that included only 1 CTN. We paired these single CTN teams with other CTNs to cover workload in times of absences. We also identified the need to have a senior resource CTN who could be deployed to teams for various reasons (eg, cover for CTNs out on extended leave, audit assistance, or coverage because of a temporary increase in workload). This resource CTN was available to precept new staff. In addition, all team leaders ensured that they had a working knowledge of their team's protocols so that they could back up a CTN if necessary.

There had been a promotion process in place at the CCR for CTNs who want to be considered for promotion. The process was evaluated by leadership and senior staff who had previously gone through the process. Feedback was elicited from staff and the process was finalized. Five nurses have been promoted using the new promotion process incorporating a leadership initiative as part of their senior CTN status.

New CTN orientation has been redesigned. Each new CTN is assigned a preceptor. New CTN orientation procedures and standardized checklists have been developed to guide the new CTNs and their preceptors. An integral piece of the orientation is the formalized clinical trial training provided by the nurse educator.

COMPETENCY ASSESSMENT AND VALIDATION

Once the basic infrastructure of the ORN was created and engagement started, the next initiative was competency assessment and validation. Working with the CCR nurse educator, the ORN embarked on developing behavioral indicators for 2 of the 9 ONS competencies (ie, professional development and documentation) using working groups that included CTNs and leadership. A validation tool was created (**Table 5**) and the nurse educator developed a facilitator's guide (**Table 6**) with input from ORN leadership.

The nurse educator validated the competency for the ORN director and each of the team leaders using the facilitator's guide. Time was spent discussing how the team leaders would use the guide to validate the research nurses' competency. In January 2015 CTNs were notified that competency sign-off was to be performed in March. Between January and March 2015 educational sessions were offered to staff and by the end of March all CTNs were signed off on their professional development competency by their team leader. Additional competency validation is ongoing.

ASSESSMENT OF THE OFFICE OF RESEARCH NURSING AND FUTURE PLANS

Three years following the inception of the ORN, consolidating the CTNs under 1 office has been viewed as success by the CTNs and the research teams. This new infrastructure was supported by an organizational commitment to optimize this key resource for the clinical program. Future strategic direction includes completion of competency assessment and validation using the ONS competencies, development of a workload

Table 5
Professional development competency validation sign-off log

Behavioral Indicators	Assessment Method	Rating Self	Rating Validator	Comments
1. Participate in at least 4 h annually of research educational activities and document in the Professional Development log	DR			
2. Participate in at least 4 h annually of oncology nursing educational activities and document in the Professional Development log.	DR			
3. Maintain curriculum vitae	DR			
4. Identify professional organizations related to clinical trials and oncology nursing	V			
5. Use resources related to clinical trials, oncology, and nursing practice on an ongoing basis	V			

Rating indicators: 1, requires assistance and supervision; 2, requires supervision; 3, independent; 4, assists and instructs others.

Note: see facilitator's guide for specific criteria for each indicator and rating.

Assessment method used for validation: D, demonstration; DR, document review; V, verbalization; O, other (specify).

Table 6
Sample of professional development competency facilitator's guide

Indicator #2: Participate in at least 4 h annually of oncology nursing educational activities
    Oncology nursing or professional development activities include any of the following:
        ONS Congress, Chapter meetings, and clinical webinars
        Other disease specialty conferences/meetings
        Nursing grand rounds (offered 3–4 times per year)
        Brown bag lunch (offered monthly September–June)
        Clinical Center genetics and genomics courses (basic or intermediate)
        Professional development series (offered 3–4 times per year)
        Other CE activities (ie, reading a journal article that offers CE units)
    Oncology nursing or professional development activities do not include:
        CPR/ACLS/PALS

Instructions: using the research nurse's professional development log for the previous 12 mo, evaluate the indicator using the criteria below:

1	Requires assistance and supervision	0–3.5 h listed in the last quarter
2	Requires supervision	0.5–3.5 h listed to reflect ongoing learning (ie, not just in the last quarter)
3	Independent	≥4 h listed to reflect ongoing learning (ie, not just in the last quarter)
4	Assists and instructs others	NA

Abbreviations: ACLS, advanced cardiac life support; CE, continuing education; CPR, cardiopulmonary resuscitation; NA, not applicable; PALS, pediatric advanced life support.

assessment tool, development of a training and resource manual, and continued commitment to improve communication.

SUMMARY

Clinical research is the foundation for improving human health. Clinical trials, a type of clinical research, explore ways to prevent, screen, diagnose, treat, and improve quality of life for individuals with a chronic illness. Protecting research participants and ensuring quality data are the responsibility of many individuals and groups. Participant protection includes the ethical review of protocols and the IC of the participants. The protocol serves as a written, detailed action plan that supports the scientific rationale for conducting the trial and outlines all trial procedures to be conducted all to ensure the participants' safety and the quality of the data. A key member of the oncology research team is the oncology CTN, who may or may not be supervised by a nurse. Using the process of engagement, one organization has been able to restructure the CTNs into a nurse-supervisor model with direct benefits to the CTNs.

REFERENCES

1. National Institutes of Health. NIH definition of clinical trial. Available at: https://auth.osp.od.nih.gov/sites/default/files/NIH%20Definition%20of%20Clinical%20Trial%2010-23-2014-UPDATED_0.pdf. Accessed March 11, 2016.
2. Woltz PC, Moore AC. Good clinical practice. In: Klimaszewski A, Bacon MA, Ness EA, et al, editors. Manual for clinical trials nursing. 3rd edition. Pittsburgh (PA): Oncology Nursing Society; 2016. p. 67–76.
3. Brown S, Markus S, Bales CA. Legal, regulatory, and legislative issues. I. In: Klimaszewski A, Bacon MA, Ness EA, et al, editors. Manual for clinical trials nursing. 3rd edition. Pittsburgh (PA): Oncology Nursing Society; 2016. p. 51–66.
4. Fisher J, Kalbaugh C. Altruism in clinical research: coordinators' orientation to their professional roles. Nurs Outlook 2012;60(3):143–8.e1.
5. International Association of Clinical Trials Nurses Scope and Standards of Practice Committee report. Enhancing Clinical research quality and safety through specialized nursing practice. Available at: http://iaCTN.memberlodge.org/aboutus. Accessed March 11, 2016.
6. Jones CT, Hastings C, Wilson LL. Research nurse manager perceptions about research activities performed by non-nurse clinical research coordinator. Nurs Outlook 2015;63(4):474–83.
7. Castro K, Bevans M, Miller-Davis C, et al. Validating the clinical research nursing domain of practice. Oncol Nurs Forum 2011;38(2):E72–80.
8. Hastings CE, Fisher CA, McCabe MA. Clinical research nursing: a critical resource in the national research enterprise. Nurs Outlook 2012;60(3):149–56.
9. Hastings C. Clinical research nursing: a new domain of practice. In: Gallin JI, Ognibene FP, editors. Principles and practice of clinical research. 3rd edition. Boston: Elsevier; 2012. p. 649–63.
10. International Conference on Harmonisation of Technical Requirements for Registrations of Pharmaceuticals for Human Use. ICH harmonised tripartite guideline: guidelines for good clinical practice. Available at: http://www.ich.org/fileadmin/Public_Web_Site/ICH_Products/Guidelines/Efficacy/E6/E6_R1_Guideline.pdf. Accessed March 11, 2016.
11. Office for Human Research Protections. Title 45 Part 46-Protection of human research subjects. Available at: http://www.hhs.gov/ohrp/humansubjects/guidance/45cfr46.html. Accessed March 11, 2016.

12. US Food and Drug Administration. Title 21, Food and Drug Administration. Available at: https://www.accessdata.fda.gov/scripts/cdrh/cfdocs/cfcfr/cfrsearch.cfm. Accessed March 11, 2016.

13. National Cancer Institute. Types of clinical trials. Available at: http://www.cancer.gov/about-cancer/treatment/clinical-trials/what-are-trials/types. Accessed March 11, 2016.

14. Ness E, Parreco LK, Galassi A, et al. Clinical trials 101. Am Nurse Today 2012;7(4). Available at: https://www.americannursetoday.com/clinical-trials-101/.

15. Ness E, Cusack G. Types of clinical research: experimental. In: Klimaszewski A, Bacon MA, Ness EA, et al, editors. Manual for clinical trials nursing. 3rd edition. Pittsburgh (PA): Oncology Nursing Society; 2016. p. 23–34.

16. Stoney C, Johnson LL. Design of clinical studies and trials. In: Gallin JI, Ognibene FP, editors. Principles and practice of clinical research. 3rd edition. Boston: Elsevier; 2012. p. 225–42.

17. Redig A, Janne P. Basket trials and the evolution of clinical trial design in an era of genomic medicine. J Clin Oncol 2015;33(9):975–7.

18. Mandrekar S, Dahlberg S, Simon R. Improving clinical trial efficiency: thinking outside the box. Am Soc Clin Oncol Educ Book 2015;35:e141–7.

19. Filchner K. Protocol review and approval process. In: Klimaszewski A, Bacon MA, Ness EA, et al, editors. Manual for clinical trials nursing. 3rd edition. Pittsburgh (PA): Oncology Nursing Society; 2016. p. 141–54.

20. Grady C. Institutional review boards. Chest 2015;148(5):1148–55.

21. The Belmont report: Ethical principles and guidelines for the protection of human subject of research. 1979. Available at: http://www.hhs.gov/ohrp/humansubjects/guidance/belmont.html. Accessed March 4, 2016.

22. US Food and Drug Administration. Title 21 Part 50-Protection of human subjects. Available at: https://www.accessdata.fda.gov/scripts/cdrh/cfdocs/cfcfr/CFRSearch.cfm?CFRPart=50. Accessed March 11, 2016.

23. National Human Genome Research Institute. Informed consent elements: considerations for genomics research and sample language. Available at: http://www.genome.gov/27559024#_Return_of_results. Accessed March 11, 2016.

24. Baer AR, Devine S, Beardmore CD, et al. Clinical investigator responsibilities. J Oncol Pract 2011;7(2):124–8.

25. Baer A, Zon R, Devine S, et al. The clinical research team. J Oncol Pract 2011;7(3):188–92.

26. Schmotzer GL, Ness E. The research team. In: Klimaszewski A, Bacon MA, Ness EA, et al, editors. Manual for clinical trials nursing. 3rd edition. Pittsburgh (PA): Oncology Nursing Society; 2016. p. 77–88.

27. Office for Human Research Protection. Investigator responsibilities—FAQs. Available at: http://www.hhs.gov/ohrp/policy/faq/investigator-responsibilities/index.html. Accessed March 7, 2016.

28. US Food and Drug Administration. Responsibilities of sponsors and investigators. Available at: http://www.accessdata.fda.gov/scripts/cdrh/cfdocs/cfcfr/CFRSearch.cfm?CFRPart=312&showFR=1&subpartNode=21:5.0.1.1.3.4. Accessed March 7, 2016.

29. Resnik D, Ness E. Participants' responsibilities in clinical research. J Med Ethics 2012;38(12):746–50.

30. Hubbard SM, DeVita V. Chemotherapy research nurse. Am J Nurs 1976;76:560–6.

31. Lubejko B, Good M, Weiss P, et al. Oncology clinical trials nursing. Clin J Oncol Nurs 2011;15(6):637–43.

32. Kahan S. Getting change right. San Francisco (CA): Jossey-Bass; 2010.

Organizational Strategies for Building Capacity in Evidence-Based Oncology Nursing Practice

A Case Report of an Australian Tertiary Cancer Center

Raymond Javan Chan, RN, BN, MAppSc (Research), PhD, FACN[a,*],
Alison Bowers, RN, BN (Child), MClin Res[b,c],
Margaret Barton-Burke, PhD, RN, FAAN[d]

KEYWORDS

- Evidence-based practice • Oncology nursing • Cancer nursing research
- Embedded-scholar model • Cancer nursing professorial precinct
- Knowledge translation

KEY POINTS

- Despite the many efforts to promote evidence-based practice in the clinical setting, barriers remain.
- The literature is clear that a supportive infrastructure and environment for evidence generation and use is necessary to inform safe, effective and quality nursing care.
- There are 4 successful organizational strategies in the Embedded Scholar: Enabler, Enactor and Engagement (4 Es) Model.
- The 4Es model includes a 12-week evidence-based practice program that prioritizes clinically relevant research proposed by clinical staff.
- The 4Es model endorses high-quality, evidence-based point-of-care resources such as the Cochrane Database of Systematic Reviews and the Oncology Nursing Society Putting Evidence into Practice.

Dr Barton-Burke acknowledges funding support from MSK Cancer Center Support Grant/Core Grant (P30 CA008748).

[a] Cancer Nursing Professorial Precinct, Royal Brisbane and Women's Hospital and Queensland University of Technology, Level 2, Building 34, Butterfield Street, Herston, Brisbane, Queensland 4029, Australia; [b] West Moreton Hospital and Health Service, Queensland 4305, Australia; [c] School of Nursing, Queensland University of Technology, Level 3, N Block, Victoria Park Road, Kelvin Grove, Brisbane, Queensland 4059, Australia; [d] Nursing Research, Memorial Sloan Kettering Cancer Center, Room 251, Concourse Level, 205 East 64th Street, New York, NY 10065, USA
* Corresponding author.
E-mail address: Raymond.Chan@qut.edu.au

INTRODUCTION

The demand for cancer care is growing exponentially owing to the increasing cancer incidence and the improved efficacy of cancer treatments. According to the World Health Organization International Agency for Research on Cancer, the number of new cancer cases is projected to increase from 14.1 million in 2012 to 21.4 million in 2030.[1] In response to this growing demand and the stringent health economic climate, oncology nurses are expected to deliver more care activities with finite resources. Developing and implementing evidence-based, innovative, and cost-effective interventions is key to sustainable cancer care. At the organizational level, demonstrating exemplary integration of evidence-based practice (EBP) and research into care in the clinical setting is one of the key assessment criteria for institutions that seek the Magnet recognition.[2]

Obstructions to the Timely Translation of Research Findings into Real-World Practice Settings

Although there have been reports of tremendous efforts to promote EBP in oncology nursing,[3–7] a number of barriers that impede timely translation of evidence into practice remain.[8,9] These persisting barriers include lack of required EBP knowledge, skills, and training; lack of support from support from managers; and lack of opportunity or time to be involved in EBP activities.[8,9] A recent study of 276 American Chief Nurse Executives revealed that, although they believe strongly in EBP, up to 44% felt they cannot implement it in a time-efficient manner.[10] For EBP to sustain, cultures and environments that include EBP resources, mentors, and easy-to-access tools for EBP must be developed.[11] To facilitate this, we discuss 4 successful organizational strategies for building EBP capacity in this paper using a case report of an Australian tertiary cancer center. For each strategy discussed, at least 1 example of clinical application is provided. The clinical setting of this case report is a cancer center of a tertiary referral hospital in Queensland, Australia. Each day, the center serves approximately 68 inpatients, 200 radiation therapy outpatients, 200 patients attending specialized cancer care clinics, and 90 patients attending the day therapy unit. In total, approximately 270 full-time registered nurses provide nursing services to the departments of hematology, bone marrow transplantation, medical oncology, radiation oncology, and the hemophilia center.

Embedded Scholar: Enabler, Enactor, and Engagement Model

In 2008, the inaugural nurse researcher was appointed using an Embedded Scholar Model,[12] and was responsible for supporting and facilitating EBP for a team of approximately 270 oncology nurses. The role of the nurse researcher and the role evaluation was reported elsewhere.[12] Over the past 8 years (2008–2016), the model has evolved from the original Embedded Scholar Model into the Embedded Scholar: Enabler, Enactor and Engagement (4 Es) Model, where there is a full appreciation of the importance of the whole system approach at the organizational level.

Cancer Nursing Professorial Precinct In this paper, the Royal Brisbane and Women's Hospital (RBWH) and Queensland University of Technology Cancer Nursing Professorial Precinct is used as an exemplar to illustrate the 4 Es Model (**Fig. 1**).[13] The success of the 4 Es Model requires the commitment of hospital executives, experienced senior researchers, and a number of engagement strategies that aim to overcome the barriers commonly reported to impede EBP. In the 4Es Model, the nursing executives, nursing leadership committee, and university academics act as the enablers. The nurse researchers are responsible for directly enacting the research strategy. The

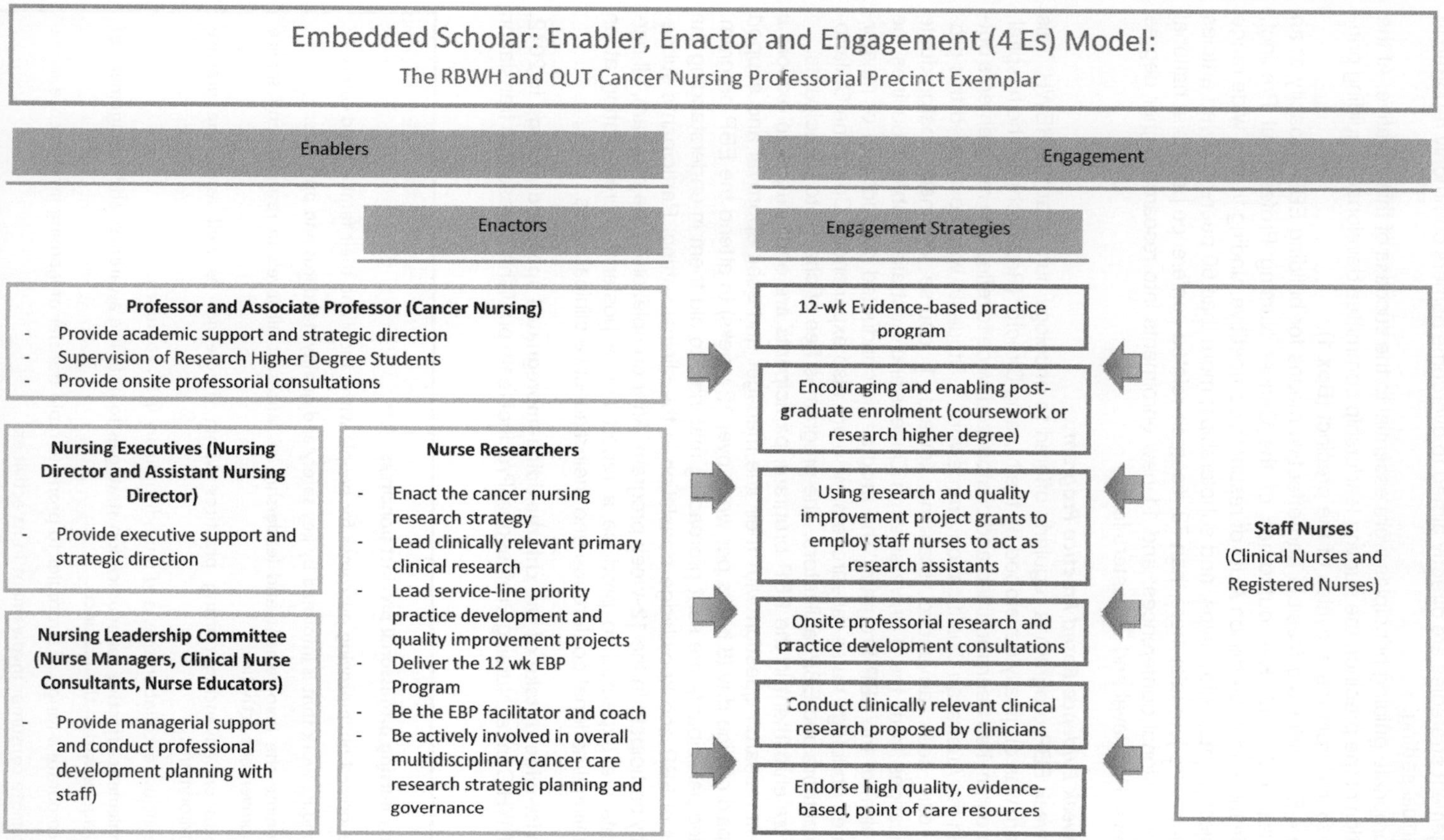
Embedded Scholar: Enabler, Enactor and Engagement (4 Es) Model:
The RBWH and QUT Cancer Nursing Professorial Precinct Exemplar
Enablers
Engagement
Enactors
Engagement Strategies
Professor and Associate Professor (Cancer Nursing)
- Provide academic support and strategic direction
- Supervision of Research Higher Degree Students
- Provide onsite professorial consultations
Nursing Executives (Nursing Director and Assistant Nursing Director)
- Provide executive support and strategic direction
Nursing Leadership Committee (Nurse Managers, Clinical Nurse Consultants, Nurse Educators)
- Provide managerial support and conduct professional development planning with staff)
Nurse Researchers
- Enact the cancer nursing research strategy
- Lead clinically relevant primary clinical research
- Lead service-line priority practice development and quality improvement projects
- Deliver the 12 wk EBP Program
- Be the EBP facilitator and coach
- Be actively involved in overall multidisciplinary cancer care research strategic planning and governance
12-wk Evidence-based practice program
Encouraging and enabling post-graduate enrolment (coursework or research higher degree)
Using research and quality improvement project grants to employ staff nurses to act as research assistants
Onsite professorial research and practice development consultations
Conduct clinically relevant clinical research proposed by clinicians
Endorse high quality, evidence-based, point of care resources
Staff Nurses
(Clinical Nurses and Registered Nurses)

Fig. 1. Embedded scholar: enabler, enactor and engagement (4 Es) model for achieving excellence in evidence-based oncology nursing practice. EBP, evidence-based practice; QUT, Queensland University of Technology; RBWH, Royal Brisbane and Women's Hospital.

engagement strategies are directly aimed to overcome barriers commonly reported in the clinical setting.

Appropriate guiding principles were essential to the success of this initiative. At the inception of the precinct, the nursing leadership committee developed 8 guiding principles to underpin the activities of the precinct (**Box 1**).

The 4 Es model is a feasible and effective means for building EBP capacity at an organizational level. Key outcomes of the Cancer Nursing Professorial Precinct, include more than $4 million AUD of research competitive funding from a wide range of project grants, fellowships, and scholarships; more than 60 peer-reviewed articles in cancer care journals; more than 70 research-related conference papers at national and international conferences; and 11 new enrolments into research higher degree studies (4 PhD level and 7 masters level).

A 12-week Evidence-Based Practice Program

A 12-week EBP program is regularly offered to oncology nurses at the RBWH. This program was originally developed by the Nursing Director (Research) for the hospital. This program has been modified and customized twice to reflect the requirements outlined in the Australian Qualification Framework.[14] Students who completed this program can seek advanced standing toward 1 course of their postgraduate qualifications from the 3 universities in Queensland Australia. **Table 1** outlines the curriculum of the EBP Program. The program is conducted by doctoral- or master-prepared oncology nurse researchers, who are also experienced Cochrane Collaboration authors and EBP facilitators. The program is free of charge to participants.

Before enrollment in the EBP program, participants are encouraged to explore a relevant research question with their line manager and seek approval and support for 1 paid off-line day (8 hours per week over 12 weeks) to attend the EBP program. Enrolled participants are sent prereading materials to aid them in understanding the basics of EBP and knowledge translation in the clinical setting. Participants subsequently participate in the 12-week program. After completion of the program, all participants are expected to produce a report and a poster for presentation at an international/national conference and their respective clinical areas.

A service-wide uptake of the chlorhexidine-impregnated sponge dressings In 2012, the RBWH Cancer Nursing Professorial Precinct team published a research translation

---

Box 1
Cancer nursing professorial precinct principles

- Be focused on improving outcomes for people with cancer and their families and carers.
- Conduct work that is informed by key safety and quality standards and priorities.
- Promote the involvement and leadership of nurses at all levels in research and service improvement activities.
- Focus on advancing nursing practices within the service as well as in the practice environment.
- Be inclusive, collaborative, and multidisciplinary in its approach.
- Implement effective communication strategies to optimize awareness and engagement of all nurses within the precinct.
- Incorporate a range of strategies to promote rapid transfer of learning into practice.
- Promote consumer involvement in its activities.

Table 1		
The current Royal Brisbane and Women's Hospital 12-week evidence-based practice program		
Week	Content	Number of hours
Preworkshop	Prereadings	22
Week 1	Introduction to evidence-based practice Workshop discussion: Exploring and developing clinical questions using the PICO format Online tutorials • Cochrane tutorial • PubMed tutorial • Medline tutorial • CINAHL tutorial Practical demonstration on literature searching Begin literature search	8

Week 2	Literature searching
	Title and abstracts screening, and decide which full
	    articles to retrieve
	• Do they provide an answer to your question or are
	    they just interesting? (Do they include the right
	    population, the intervention of interest, and results
	    about the outcomes of interest?)
	• Are they the correct study design to answer your
	    question?
		8

Weeks 3–4	Terminology used in evidence-based health care:
	    understanding the basics
	Statistics: understanding the basics
	Literature searching and critical appraisal
	• Randomized controlled trials
	If relevant to the research questions, below types of
	    research can be included, critically appraised and
	    synthesized
	• Qualitative studies
	• Diagnostic studies
	• Systematic reviews
	• Clinical guidelines
		8 per week

Weeks 5–10	Data extraction, data entry, and data synthesis • Using standard Cochrane data extraction form and Review Manager[a] • Interpret Forest plots and the results table[a] • Narrative synthesis of data	8 per week

Weeks 11–12	Prepare a report and recommendations for practice
	• Formulation of implications for practice and future
	    research
	• Preparation of an A0 poster for conference and local
	    presentations
		8 per week

		Total: 96

Abbreviation: PICO, population/disease, intervention, comparison, outcome.
    This curriculum was developed by Professor Joan Webster, Nursing Director Research, Royal Brisbane and Women's Hospital.
    [a] If applicable.

paper illustrating how a staff nurse who worked at the outpatient therapy unit changed practice based on the findings of a meta-analysis, as an outcome of the 12-week EBP program.[15] The research question was: Is the routine use of chlorhexidine-impregnated sponge dressings effective for reducing catheter-related blood stream infections in cancer patients with central venous access devices? As part of the 12-week EBP program, the clinical nurse conducted a systematic review and metaanalysis including data of 5295 participants from 5 randomized controlled trials. The results strongly favored the routine use of chlorhexidine-impregnated sponge dressings on central catheter entry sites for reducing catheter-related blood stream infections (odd ratio [OR], 0.43; 95% confidence interval [CI], 0.29–0.64). After presenting the results to the nursing executives, nurse managers and nurse clinicians in all clinical areas, the clinical nurse received support to implement the routine use of chlorhexidine-impregnated sponge dressings throughout the entire cancer care center.

Prioritizing clinically relevant research proposed by clinical staff
A range of engagement strategies within the 4 Es model allow opportunities for clinicians to propose research that is directly relevant to clinical care. The EBP program is limited in that relevant research questions can only be answered sufficiently where there is strong evidence in the literature to inform practice. Where there is insufficient evidence available to answer a specific clinical question, it creates an opportunity for a primary research project to be conducted. The progression from an EBP project to a primary research project is advantageous, because the participant can use the existing data from the EBP program to inform a research grant application, and potentially be employed as the research assistant responsible for collecting to project data. Such involvement allows the participant to further gain experience in the conduct of clinical research.

Management of treatment-related skin toxicity Between 2012 and 2014, the Cancer Nursing Professorial Precinct research team conducted 2 EBP projects[16,17] that investigated the best intervention for preventing and reducing skin toxicities related to radiation therapy and/or targeted therapies. Despite the number of clinical trials conducted in this area, it is clear that there is no evidence suggesting any topical preparation being superior in comparison with any other topical preparation. In 2012, the Nurse Unit Manager (Radiation Oncology) noticed a rapid uptake of a specific skin preparation in patients receiving radiation therapy across Australia. Anecdotal evidence from radiation oncologists, nurses, and patients strongly suggested the efficacy of this skin preparation for preventing and reducing skin toxicities. This particular new preparation began to gain popularity in Australia and some Asian countries, and was considerably more expensive than the other basic moisturizers used in usual care, such as the aqueous cream or sorbolene.[18]

At the request of the nurse manager and staff nurses at the department of radiation oncology, the precinct research team undertook a double-blind randomized controlled trial comparing the effects of the new preparation versus aqueous cream (usual care).[18] This trial included 174 patients receiving radiation therapy without and without concurrent systemic therapy (n = 89 in intervention group; n = 85 in the control group), with results indicating that patients receiving the new topical preparation had significantly more severe skin toxicities at week 7, 8, and 9 of radiation treatment.[18] Considering the undesirable outcomes and significantly higher cost compared with usual care, all patients are now advised to avoid using this particular preparation. This exemplar not only demonstrates the process that led to the conduct of a clinically relevant research project, but also the active involvement of management and clinical staff, and a rapid translation of knowledge into practice.

Endorsing high-quality, evidence-based point-of-care resources
Given lack of time is a well-reported barrier that impedes EBP, it is important organizational leaders endorse high-quality, evidence-based, point-of-care resources for

busy clinicians. Below are some examples of high-quality evidence-based resources that can be used at the point of care by oncology nurses.

The Cochrane Database of Systematic Reviews The Cochrane Collaboration is a not-for-profit organization established in 1993.[19] When celebrating the 20th anniversary of the Cochrane Collaboration in 2013, the Cancer Nursing Professorial Precinct research team published an editorial to explain why the Cochrane Database of Systematic Reviews should be the place of choice to obtain evidence in informing care.[20] Systematic reviews are considered the highest level of evidence and the standard approach in summarizing health research and influencing health care decisions.[21] Cochrane systematic reviews, are required to be of a set standard, to include having a clearly stated set of objectives with predefined eligibility criteria for studies; an explicit reproducible methodology; a systematic search that attempts to identify all studies that would meet the eligibility criteria; an assessment of the validity of the findings of the included studies, for example, through the assessment of risk of bias; and a systematic presentation and synthesis of the characteristics of findings of the included study.[22] At the end of 2015, more than 9143 systematic reviews or protocols have been published online in the Cochrane Database of Systematic Reviews.[19]

It is important to inform oncology nurses that the quality of non-Cochrane systematic reviews varies largely.[23,24] In contrast, the Cochrane Collaboration has credibility because its reviews consistently adhere to the strict standards listed. In addition to the high-quality systematic reviews, the Cochrane Collaboration has also developed a number of resources to increase the accessibility of the evidence generated by the collaboration. The collaboration creatively has used strategies to reach busy clinicians such as the Evidently Cochrane blog, social media such as Facebook and Twitter, and a number of Cochrane Review Summaries (published in specialty journals such as *Cancer Nursing: An International Journal for Cancer Care*). All these additional greatly enhanced the accessibility of Cochrane systematic reviews at the point of care.

The Oncology Nursing Society's Putting Evidence into Practice Institutionalizing EBP requires oncology nurses to be knowledgeable about the available evidence and its usefulness at the bedside or chairside. This should not be difficult given the resources developed by and available to oncology nurses. The Oncology Nursing Society 'Putting Evidence into Practice' (ONS PEP) resources are available in a ready to use format designed to provide evidence-based interventions for oncology patient care.

During the development process, professional librarians assist in the literature search. Panels of advanced practice nurses, staff nurses, and doctorally prepared nurse researchers, also called ONS PEP topic teams, review the relevant literature and summarize and synthesize the available evidence in various PEP topic areas. Based on the analysis, the panel formulates a judgment about the body of evidence related to the intervention under consideration. The panel classifies the evidence into one of 6 weight of evidence categories based on the quality of the data, with more weight assigned to levels of evidence higher in the Partnership for Research Integrity in Science & Medicine (PRISM) categorization (eg, randomized trials, meta-analyses), the magnitude of the outcome (eg, effect size, minimal clinically important difference), and the concurrence among the evidence (based on the premise that an investigator has less confidence in findings in which the lines of evidence contradict one another; **Box 2**). The classification schema does not guide the decision about using a particular intervention for an individual patient. Those decisions should be made by the interdisciplinary team based on key components of EBP (ie, individual patient

Box 2
The Oncology Nursing Society Putting Evidence into Practice

Recommended for Practice

Interventions for which effectiveness has been demonstrated by strong evidence from rigorously designed studies, metaanalysis, or systematic reviews and for which expectation of harm is small compared with the benefits.

Likely to Be Effective

Interventions for which effectiveness has been demonstrated from a single rigorously conducted controlled trial, consistent supportive evidence from well-designed controlled trials using small samples, or guidelines developed from evidence and supported by expert opinion

Benefits Balanced with Harm

Interventions for which clinicians and patients should weigh the beneficial and harmful effects according to individual circumstances and priorities

Effectiveness Not Established

Interventions for which insufficient or conflicting data or data of inadequate quality currently exist, with no clear indication of harm

Effectiveness Unlikely

Interventions for which lack of effectiveness has been demonstrated by negative evidence from a single rigorously conducted controlled trial, consistent negative evidence from well-designed controlled trials using small samples, or guidelines developed from evidence and supported by expert opinion

Not Recommended for Practice

Interventions for which lack of effectiveness or harmfulness has been demonstrated by strong evidence from rigorously conducted studies, metaanalyses, or systematic reviews, or interventions where the costs, burden, or harm associated with the intervention exceed anticipated benefit

Expert Opinion

Low-risk interventions that are consistent with sound clinical practice, suggested by an expert in a peer reviewed publication, and for which limited evidence exists (an expert is an individual who has published peer-reviewed material in the domain of interest)

From PEP Rating System Overview. Reused courtesy of the Oncology Nursing Society (ONS). Available at https://www.ons.org/practice-resources/pep. Accessed April 1, 2016. Copyright © 2016 by ONS. All rights reserved.

characteristics, values, and preferences; consideration of potential benefit and harm; and an assessment of the feasibility of implementing the intervention) within a specific care setting.

The ONS PEP topics focus on patient-centered outcomes, such as symptoms, selected by a survey of ONS members combined with the best available evidence in the topic. The ONS PEP evidence synthesis provides interventions that are effective in preventing or treating the outcome of interest. The ONS PEP resources can be used to plan patient care, patient education, nursing education, quality improvement, and research. The ONS PEP resources can be embedded into cancer care interventions or incorporated into telephone triage protocols. They could be included in oncology policies and procedures, quality/performance improvement activities, standards of care, and physician order sets. The ONS PEP information can be integrated into orientation, educational programs, nursing grand rounds, and journal clubs.

SUMMARY

This paper demonstrates the feasibility and effectiveness of several organizational strategies. The 12-week EBP program aims to develop EBP skills among oncology nurses. It can be integrated easily to any cancer center where a masters/doctorally prepared nurse researcher with advanced EBP skills can deliver the program. Prioritizing clinically relevant research through involving departmental nurse managers and staff nurses is a key strategy that can enable rapid translation of research evidence into care. Another strategy is endorsing high-quality EBP resources that can inform oncology nurses of best available evidence at the point of care. For the full potential of these strategies to be realized, it is critical that they be implemented in a systematized approach at an organizational level. In this paper, we illustrate the feasibility and effectiveness the 4 Es Model for facilitating EBP at an organizational level. A supportive infrastructure and environment for evidence generation and use is necessary to inform safe, effective, and quality nursing care. The authors acknowledged the limitation that this paper uses a single center's experience to depict a feasible model for facilitating EBP, various components of the model can be adapted by other cancer centers according to their context.

REFERENCES

1. International Agency for Research on Cancer (IARC). GLOBOCAN 2012: Estimated Cancer Incidence, Mortality and Prevalence Worldwide in 2012. Available at: http://www.globocan.iarc.fr/Pages/fact_sheets cancer.aspx. Accessed March 1, 2016.
2. American Nurses Credentialing Center (ANCC). Getting started: an overview of the ANCC magnet recognition program and pathway to excellence program. Silver Spring (MD): American Nurses Credentialing Center; 2013.
3. Harvey G, Kitson A. PARIHS revisited: from heuristic to integrated framework for the successful implementation of knowledge into practice. Implement Sci 2016; 11(1):33.
4. Rycroft-Malone J, Seers K, Chandler J, et al. The role of evidence, context, and facilitation in an implementation trial: implications for the development of the PARIHS framework. Implement Sci 2013;8:28.
5. Damschroder LJ, Aron DC, Keith RE, et al. Fostering implementation of health services research findings into practice: a consolidated framework for advancing implementation science. Implement Sci 2009;4:50.
6. Melnyk BM, Gallagher-Ford L, Long LE, et al. The establishment of evidence-based practice competencies for practicing registered nurses and advanced practice nurses in real-world clinical settings: proficiencies to improve healthcare quality, reliability, patient outcomes, and costs. Worldviews Evid Based Nurs 2014;11(1):5–15.
7. Flodgren G, Rojas-Reyes MX, Cole N, et al. Effectiveness of organisational infrastructures to promote evidence-based nursing practice. Cochrane Database Syst Rev 2012;(2):CD002212.
8. Caldwell B, Coltart K, Hutchison C, et al. Research awareness, attitudes and barriers among clinical staff in a regional cancer centre. Part 1: a quantitative analysis. Eur J Cancer Care (Engl) 2016. [Epub ahead of print].
9. Johnson C, Lizama C, Harrison M, et al. Cancer health professionals need funding, time, research knowledge and skills to be involved in health services research. J Cancer Educ 2014;29(2):389–94.

10. Melnyk B, Gallagher-Ford L, Thomas B, et al. A study of chief nurse executives indicates low prioritization of evidence-based practice and shortcomings in hospital performance metrics across the United States. Worldviews Evid Based Nurs 2016;13(1):6–14.

11. Melnyk B. An urgent call to action for nurse leaders to establish sustainable evidence-based practice cultures and implement evidence-based interventions to improve healthcare quality. Worldviews Evid Based Nurs 2016;13(1):3–5.

12. Chan R, Gardner G, Webster J, et al. Building research capacity: the design and evaluation of the nurse researcher model. Aust J Adv Nurs 2010;27(4):62–9.

13. Chan R, Geary A, Yates P, et al. Building capacity for cancer nursing research and evidence-based practice: the cancer nursing professorial precinct initiative. Asia Pac J Oncol Nurs 2016;3(1):28–9.

14. Australian Qualifications Framework Council. Australian qualifications framework. In: A council of the ministers responsible for tertiary education SAE, South Australia. 2nd edition. (South Australia): National Library of Australia; 2013. p. 1–119.

15. Chan R, Northfield S, Alexander A, et al. Using the collaborative evidence-based practice model: a systematic review and uptake of chlorhexidine impregnated sponge dressings on central venous access devices in a tertiary cancer care centre. Aust J Cancer Nurs 2012;13(2):10–5.

16. Chan RJ, Webster J, Chung B, et al. Prevention and treatment of acute radiation-induced skin reactions: a systematic review and meta-analysis of randomized controlled trials. BMC Cancer 2014;14:53.

17. Chan RJ, Larsen E, Chan P. Re-examining the evidence in radiation dermatitis management literature: an overview and a critical appraisal of systematic reviews. Int J Radiat Oncol Biol Phys 2012;84(3):e357–62.

18. Chan RJ, Mann J, Tripcony L, et al. Natural oil-based emulsion containing allantoin versus aqueous cream for managing radiation-induced skin reactions in patients with cancer: a phase 3, double-blind, randomized, controlled trial. Int J Radiat Oncol Biol Phys 2014;90(4):756–64.

19. Cochrane Collaboration. Cochrane collaboration home page- about us 2012. Available at: http://www.cochrane.org/about-us. Accessed March 1, 2016.

20. Chan RJ, Wong A. Two decades of exceptional achievements: does the evidence support nurses to favour Cochrane systematic reviews over other systematic reviews? Int J Nurs Stud 2012;49(7):773–4.

21. Grimshaw JM, Russell IT. Effect of clinical guidelines on medical practice: a systematic review of rigorous evaluations. Lancet 1993;342(8883):1317–22.

22. Higgins J, Green S, editors. Cochrane handbook for systematic reviews of interventions. Chichester (England): John Wiley & Sons Ltd; 2008.

23. Choi PT, Halpern SH, Malik N, et al. Examining the evidence in anesthesia literature: a critical appraisal of systematic reviews. Anesth Analg 2001;92(3):700–9.

24. Hoving JL, Gross AR, Gasner D, et al. A critical appraisal of review articles on the effectiveness of conservative treatment for neck pain. Spine (Phila Pa 1976) 2001;26(2):196–205.

The Hidden Morbidity of Cancer

Burden in Caregivers of Patients with Brain Metastases

Marlon Garzo Saria, PhD, RN, AOCNS[a],*, Adeline Nyamathi, PhD, ANP[b],
Linda R. Phillips, PhD, RN[b], Annette L. Stanton, PhD[c],
Lorraine Evangelista, PhD, RN[d], Santosh Kesari, MD, PhD[e],
Sally Maliski, PhD, RN[b,f]

KEYWORDS

- Cancer • Caregivers • Brain metastases • Caregiver burden • Neuro-oncology

KEY POINTS

- The cancer caregiving experience can be distinguished from caregiving for other chronic conditions by the rapid and unpredictable deterioration of the health of patients with cancer.
- Caregivers of persons with brain metastases find themselves in an overwhelming and unpredictable role that is primarily influenced by the patient's cognitive and functional decline and aggravated by household, occupational, or societal demands.
- Although many studies have established the negative effects associated with caregiving, it is equally important to consider the reported positive effects of caregiving, as well as effects not directly related to caregivers.

Disclosures: American Cancer Society Doctoral Degree Scholarships in Cancer Nursing, Oncology Nursing Society Doctoral Scholarship, The DAISY Foundation Research Grant (JPB-2013-45-A).
[a] Clinical Trials and Research, John Wayne Cancer Institute, Providence Saint John's Health Center, University of California, Los Angeles, School of Nursing, 2200 Santa Monica Boulevard, Santa Monica, CA 90404, USA; [b] University of California, Los Angeles, School of Nursing, 700 Tiverton Avenue, Los Angeles, CA 90095, USA; [c] Department of Psychology, University of California, Los Angeles, 1285 Franz Hall, Box 951563, Los Angeles, CA 90095-1563, USA; [d] Nursing Science, University of California, Irvine, 106 Berk Hall, Irvine, CA 92697-3959, USA; [e] Department of Translational Neuro-Oncology and Neurotherapeutics, John Wayne Cancer Institute, Providence Saint John's Health Center, 2200 Santa Monica Boulevard, Santa Monica, CA 90404, USA; [f] University of Kansas Medical Center, University of Kansas School of Nursing, Mail Stop 2029, 3901 Rainbow Boulevard, Kansas City, KS 66160, USA
* Corresponding author.
E-mail address: sariam@jwci.org

INTRODUCTION

Despite remarkable progress in cancer prevention, early detection, and treatment, many people still encounter the catastrophic experience of a cancer diagnosis. After diagnosis, patients and caregivers begin a journey on which they encounter the cognitive, psychosocial, emotional, physical, and practical consequences of the disease and its treatment. Although the diagnosis of cancer, in itself, can lead to significant changes in all aspects of patients' and caregivers' lives, the subsequent diagnosis of brain metastases can be even more devastating. Brain metastasis has an annual incidence estimated between 98,000 and 170,000.[1–3] It can elicit rapid deterioration in quality of life brought on by progressive neurologic deficits, which can be daunting challenges for family caregivers.[4] In addition, median survival between 2 and 25 months despite treatment suggests that brain metastases indicate poor prognosis and are associated with increased mortality and morbidity.[5] Recently, novel therapeutic discoveries have been shown to improve survival in a subset of patients; however, for most patients with brain metastases, palliation of symptoms, preservation of function, and maintenance of quality of life (QOL) are still considered to be the primary goals of treatment.[4]

Although there is a wealth of literature on the caregiving challenges associated with cancer, less is written about the caregiving challenges associated with brain metastases. This article describes some of these challenges and identifies implications of these challenges for health care professionals. Given the paucity of caregiving research in brain metastases, the discussion relies heavily on research about caregiving in general, with a particular focus on caregiving for individuals who have diagnoses associated with similar progressive neurologic deficits (eg, dementia).

CAREGIVING BURDEN AND THE EXPERIENCE OF CARING FOR PERSONS WITH BRAIN METASTASIS

The cancer caregiving experience can be distinguished from caregiving for other chronic conditions by the rapid and unpredictable deterioration of the health of patients with cancer. Cancer is unique in that it can be marked by active disease, followed by prolonged remission that may be abruptly interrupted by recurrence, metastases, or a new primary site. In addition, cancer caregivers report spending more time in caregiving, providing higher acuity care in a shorter time frame, and being predisposed to higher financial burden than caregivers of persons with other diseases.[6]

From the first publications introducing the concept to the current state of the science, caregiver burden remains one of the most commonly studied variables in caregiving research.[7–18] Caregiver burden is defined as the cognitive appraisal of the multidimensional response to demands and their consequences within the context of an evolving caregiving experience.[19,20] The critical attributes of caregiver burden include subjective perception, multidimensional phenomena, dynamic change, and overload.

Subjective Perception

Consistent with reports that the degree and kind of reaction to the stress produced by environmental demands vary among individuals,[21] studies show that, after controlling for patient characteristics and the type of stressors, perception of caregiver burden varies among individuals.[13,22–25] These findings can be linked to the varied sensitivity and vulnerability of individual caregivers to certain types of experiences and to differences in caregivers' interpretations and reactions.[21]

Research suggests that the dynamics of caregiving may differ by diagnosis but study results are equivocal.[26–28] Studies comparing caregiver burden present divergent findings, including higher caregiver burden in psychiatric illness compared with other chronic medical illness and no differences in caregiver burden for caregivers of older adults with different diagnoses.[29,30] Meanwhile, 2 other studies report few differences in caregiver burden by diagnosis and conclude that caregiver resources, not patient diagnosis or illness severity, are primary correlates of caregiver burden.[31,32]

These studies are relevant to caregiving for persons with brain metastases, suggesting that findings from research on the general caregiving population apply to caregivers of patients with brain metastases. They underscore the importance of individual difference. As Ankri and colleagues[33] noted, even when using valid and reliable measures, a score may not provide complete and accurate assessment because caregivers may be affected by different aspects of burden; although one caregiver may be overwhelmed with the physical demands of caregiving, another may experience emotional stress or feel socially marginalized because of the situation.

Multidimensional Phenomena

Chou[19] describes multidimensional characteristics of burden in terms of outcomes; that is, caregiver burden can affect the physical, psychological, social, and spiritual domains of the caregiver. In addition, the multidimensional nature of the antecedents of burden have been explored. In cancer, variables that have been shown to affect caregiver burden include caregiver age, gender, relationship to the care recipient, length of time providing care, and care recipient tumor type.[34,35] In community-based caregivers (N = 92), the strongest predictors of caregiver burden were the health-related needs of the care receivers, including their behavioral and mental health problems ($P = .01$). Also, 2 personal resources of caregivers (ie, having less resilience and using negative emotion-focused coping) were significantly, but less strongly, correlated with caregiver burden.[36]

The relationships of variables in caregiving situations to caregiver burden are described in the literature[37,38] for many conditions. These studies provide insight into the complexity of caregiver burden for caregivers of persons with brain metastases, a diagnosis that often implies significant physical and psychosocial burden.

Dynamic Change

From the time of initial cancer diagnosis throughout the illness trajectory, caregivers face challenges.[39] Caregivers are subject to multiple transitions as they adapt to new demands brought on by disease progression, changes in physical and cognitive function, or acquisition of new debilities. Situations that may contribute significantly to caregiver burden may no longer be as stressful as the caregiver adapts and copes, but stress may increase as new problems or crisis situations arise.[19]

Among caregivers of persons with cancer, Kim and Given[40] reported that QOL varied along the illness trajectory. Caregivers of women with advanced breast cancer were more depressed (30% vs 9%; $P = .02$) and experienced higher levels of burden (mean score, 26.2 vs 19.4; $P = .02$) at the start of the terminal period (n = 84) than at the start of the palliative period (n = 15).[10] However, caregivers of patients with dementia reported fewer differences, with 98.9% reporting problems in the initial stage of dementia, 99.1% within 1 to 4 years, and 98% beyond 4 years (χ^2test, $P>.01$),[41] although the types of problems varied based on stage. In later stages, 49.1% experienced more problems in their social networks compared with initial stage (25.6%). Likewise, no significant differences in mental health and health-related QOL, a concept associated with caregiver burden, were found in caregivers of patients with cancer (N = 167) in the palliative and the curative phases, respectively.[42] In caregivers of persons with a guarded prognosis such as brain metastases, usually identified after a sudden unexpected event (eg, severe headaches, focal weakness, gait disturbances, seizures, nausea and vomiting),[4] the impact of dynamic changes can be profound.

Overload

Caregivers' responses to the caregiving experience range from low to high stress and result from an imbalance of care demand relative to resources; that is, knowledge or training, personal time, social roles, physical and emotional states, financial resources, and formal care resources.[17,43] Demands may come from patients, other family members, employment, or society, whereas resources may be internal or external.[19] The caregiving experience can create physical and psychological strain over extended periods of time and is usually accompanied by high levels of unpredictability and loss of control.[44] These life stressors and demands increase the risk for caregiver burden by exacerbating role conflict and disruption.

Caregivers are responsible for tasks, from managing household chores and finances to assisting with medical and personal care. For persons with brain metastases, caregivers may have been performing the tasks for some time. Caregivers of persons with brain metastases face plural challenges of living their own lives, in addition to providing physical care and extending emotional support while also coping with the anticipated decline of the patient's health.

These critical attributes, subjective perceptions, multidimensional phenomena, dynamic changes, and overload, experienced in combination, can be stressful to caregivers and can be severe enough to result in serious consequences and outcomes.

DEMANDS OF CAREGIVING

The caregiver role is associated with many demands. For many, these demands result in caregiving burden (an incongruity between demands and the caregiver's ability to cope) and negative biopsychosocial effects.[45,46] These effects can be classified into primary and secondary caregiving demands, defined as stressors inherent in the caregiving situation and those that come from other areas in the caregiver's life, respectively.

Primary Demands of Caregiving

Primary demands are dictated by the health-related needs of the care receiver. They include cognitive deficits associated with the diagnosis of brain metastases and the functional impairment observed in patients with cancer (**Box 1**).

Neurocognitive impairment of care receivers
Patients with brain cancers often endure a variety of neurologic, cognitive, and emotional problems that, even with the slightest impairment, can significantly alter QOL.[47] In the past, these problems have not been adequately addressed because of the dismal outcome associated with the diagnosis. However, in the milieu of improved survival with the accompanying neurorehabilitative potential of the patient, recognition of cancer-related and cancer therapy–related neurologic outcomes has recently become an indispensable step that precedes therapy selection.

Assessment and interpretation of neurocognitive function in patients with brain cancer is confounded by multiple variables that include neurotoxic effects of anticancer therapies and supportive care agents and the presence of mood disorders. In clinical trials, neurocognitive function has now been proposed as a secondary end point that

---

Box 1
Primary demands of caregiving

Neurocognitive impairment

- Patients with brain cancers often endure a variety of neurologic, cognitive, and emotional problems.

- Assessment and interpretation of neurocognitive function in patients with brain cancer is confounded by multiple variables.

- Neurocognitive assessment includes measures of general intellectual functioning (ie, intelligence quotient [IQ]), language, memory, attention, information processing speed, motor speed and dexterity, and executive functioning.

- Cognitive dysfunction has been identified as a leading cause of disability and the single greatest cause of burden in patients with primary brain tumors.

- Mechanisms of cognitive dysfunction in brain cancers are diverse and may include direct damage caused by cancer, indirect effects of cancer (paraneoplastic syndrome), and effects of cancer treatment on the brain.

Functional impairment

- Patients with brain cancer may not be able to perform activities of daily living because of neurologic disorders such as paralysis, paresis, sensory loss, blindness, decreased level of consciousness, ataxia, and headaches.

- Care recipients' functional status has been consistently reported as a common predictor of negative caregiver outcomes.

- Functional status was not as strong a predictor of burden as the care recipients' cognitive and neuropsychiatric status.

Data from Refs.[35,47,50–53]

---

can provide significant information otherwise not observed in traditional end points, including overall survival, progression-free survival, and radiographic changes. It is viewed as more than just a surrogate marker of disease response to therapy.[48,49] Neurocognitive assessment includes measures of general intellectual functioning (ie, intelligence quotient [IQ]), language, memory, attention, information processing speed, motor speed and dexterity, and executive functioning. In addition, self-reported measures of mood may be obtained in order to estimate the influence of depression on cognitive performances.[50]

Cognitive deficits create care demands for the caregivers and increase the number of tasks with which the caregiver must render assistance. Cognitive dysfunction was identified as a leading cause of disability and the single greatest cause of burden in patients with primary brain tumors.[35,47] Most patients with brain metastases have some degree of neurocognitive impairment, which may even be more common than functional impairment.[51] Mechanisms of cognitive dysfunction in brain cancers are diverse and may include direct damage caused by cancer, indirect effects of cancer (paraneoplastic syndrome), and effects of cancer treatment on the brain.[51–53] These causes add to preexisting neurologic and psychiatric disorders that alter the patient's cognition and mood.

It is important to highlight findings from studies that distinguish between the characteristics and outcomes of caregivers of individuals who have cognitive symptoms with different causes or whose symptoms occur during different time points during the disease trajectory. One study found that depressive symptoms were more commonly reported by caregivers of patients with dementia compared with caregivers of patients with non–dementia-related cognitive impairment.[54] Another study reported divergence in caregiver burden in patients with amnesic mild cognitive impairment and mild Alzheimer disease, in which burden was more severe in patients with mild Alzheimer disease.[55] These studies highlight the findings that multiple factors contribute to caregiver burden at different stages of the disease.

Many other studies explored the relationship between the patient's cognitive impairment and caregiver burden in a variety of diagnoses. One study reported that caregiver burden is directly associated with an increase in patients' comorbidities, independent of behavioral status, functional status, and cognitive impairment.[56] Compared with functional status, cognitive status is a much stronger predictor of caregiver burden in caregivers of patients with dementia according to a meta-analysis of 228 studies of the relationship between caregiving stressors, caregiver burden, and depression,[57] which was supported by a study in patients with Alzheimer disease.[58]

In a study of burden and depressive symptoms in caregivers of geriatric patients, the care recipients' mental status was almost twice as powerful in predicting caregiver burden as the care recipients' functional status.[59] However, in several studies of the relationship between cognitive abilities of patients with dementia and their caregivers' burden, there were either no or weak relationships between the variables. Findings from one study indicated that cognitive impairment did not contribute significantly to caregiver burden.[60] However, Etters and colleagues[8] postulated that it may be the patients' behavioral disturbances associated with cognitive impairment that predict caregiving burden rather than the cognitive impairment.

Functional impairment of care receivers
Functional status is defined as an individual's ability to perform a task. Patients with brain cancer may not be able to perform activities of daily living because of neurologic disorders such as paralysis, paresis, sensory loss, blindness, decreased level of consciousness, ataxia, and headaches. These problems may be complicated by treatment-related toxicities, comorbidities, and mood disorders.[35]

In caregivers of patients with cancer, care recipients' functional status has been consistently reported as a common predictor of negative caregiver outcomes. However, although caring for someone with functional limitations added to burden, functional status was not as strong a predictor of burden as the care recipients' cognitive and neuropsychiatric status. In 488 family caregivers of patients with diverse diagnoses (eg, cerebrovascular, circulatory, musculoskeletal, or pulmonary disorders; fractures of hip or major limb; and cancer), the care recipient's mental status was almost twice as powerful (standardized path coefficient of −0.37) in predicting caregiver burden as was the care recipient's functional status (standardized path coefficient of −0.23).[59] Similar outcomes were reported in a study involving caregivers of patients with amyotrophic lateral sclerosis (N = 140); behavioral changes had greater impact on caregiver burden (odds ratio of 1.4) than the level and pattern of physical disability.[61]

In oncology caregiving, there is a lack of information on caregiver outcomes when multiple variables (ie, alterations in functional, cognitive, and neuropsychiatric status) are examined together.[62] In a study of 95 caregivers of patients with primary malignant brain tumors, the patient's functional status as measured by activities of daily living (eating, bathing dressing, toileting, walking inside the house, and getting out of bed) and instrumental activities of daily living (transportation, laundry, shopping, housework, meal preparation) affected a subscale of caregiver burden but the patient's cognitive status was not associated with caregiver burden, whereas neuropsychiatric status consistently affected every subscale of caregiver burden. However, the investigators suggested that the lack of a significant relationship between the patient's cognitive status and caregiver burden might have been caused by the lack of an objective measure of cognitive status.[35]

Caregivers are key participants in the care of persons with brain metastases and are compelled to take more important roles compared with many other clinical situations. The additional tasks of managing the functional and cognitive deficits of the patient increase the demands on caregivers who must deal with the changes that accompany a diagnosis that is the most common neurologic complication of cancer.

Secondary Demands of Caregiving

Family, work, and/or society contribute to the secondary demands on caregivers (**Box 2**). These demands come from outside the caregiving relationship between patients with metastatic brain tumors and their caregivers.

Family

Caregiver burden has been reported to be specifically related to multiple roles assumed by the caregiver. Family roles of caregivers directly affect their ability to take on new responsibilities and adjust to living with constant uncertainty.[63] The presence of young children in the household and single-parent families with a female head of household are some of the family structures that have been reported as significant predictors of caregiver burden.[19]

Work

The impact of the caregiver's employment on caregiver burden is not clear. Although it is intuitive that work outside the caregiving relationship is a competing priority for caregivers that adds to perceived caregiver burden, several studies have reported that employment or other roles outside the family may be the key to caregiver well-being.[64] In 205 family caregivers of hospitalized patients with cardiovascular disease who participated in a family intervention trial, time demands (38%) and work adjustments (25%) were among the most commonly reported causes of burden.[65]

In contrast, a cross-sectional household survey conducted among 2458 adult residents having at least 1 close relative with any chronic physical and/or mental illness revealed that employment did not significantly contribute to caregiver burden (67.1% of the 1720 who were employed full time did not perceive burden; $P = .0747$).[66] In another study of caregivers of 7 geographically and institutionally defined cohorts of patients with newly diagnosed colorectal and lung cancer

---

Box 2
Secondary demands of caregiving

Family

- Family roles of caregivers directly affect their ability to take on new responsibilities and adjust to living with constant uncertainty.

Work

- Work outside the caregiving relationship can contribute to either increased caregiver burden or improved caregiver well-being.

Society

- Health and labor policies have been shown to differentially affect caregiver financial burden.

Data from Refs.[63,64,67]

(N = 677), 21% (n = 142) cared for at least 1 other individual, 49% (n = 312) were employed (including two-thirds full time), and 28% (n = 86) of the respondents who were working either full or part time reported having difficulty balancing work and caregiving demands. In the same study, 67% (n = 453) of caregivers faced at least 1, and 19% (n = 131) faced 2 or more, of these additional demands, with 1 in 5 reporting poor to fair health.[17]

Society

Several studies confirmed that many family caregivers experience financial difficulties related to lost wages from reduced work hours.[63] However, another study revealed that very few caregivers reported financial burden and even fewer caregivers had to give up employment to continue to care for a family member.[67] The differences were attributed to differing health policies between the countries where the studies were conducted.

Caregivers of persons with brain metastases find themselves in an overwhelming and unpredictable role that is primarily influenced by the patient's cognitive and functional decline and aggravated by household, occupational, or societal demands. The caregiving experience presents a situation in which multiple concurrent stressful demands compete for the caregiver's attention. It is therefore important that caregivers be supported to meet the escalating demands of the caregiving experience with as little impact on their emotional and physical well-being as possible.

CONSEQUENCES AND OUTCOMES OF CAREGIVER BURDEN

The caregiving experience is commonly perceived as chronically stressful and can lead to negative outcomes. In caregivers of patients with brain metastases, that experience begins with the diagnosis of the primary cancer and is relived on diagnosis of brain metastases.

Although the nature and magnitude of caregiver burden vary in the context of different clinical and medical diagnoses, many studies have established the negative effects associated with caregiving.[13,22,68,69] Although not as well documented, it is equally important to consider the reported positive effects of caregiving,[44,64,70–74] as well as effects not directly related to the caregiver. The indirect effects include clinical outcomes of patients (care recipients), effects on the other members of the household, and impact on the health care system in general (**Box 3**).

Consequences to Caregivers

The high incidence of brain metastases resulting from improved therapy for systemic disease is contributing to the increase in the number of cancer caregivers. Historically, caregiving was considered a stressor that leads to implications, usually negative, for the caregivers' well-being. More recently, research in this tradition has evolved from an emphasis on the role-specific negative outcome of burden (eg, caretaker role fatigue, spousal burnout, and role engulfment) to more general well-being considerations, including positive psychological well-being (eg, improved relationships, and improved self-satisfaction, gratification, self-efficacy, and self-respect), negative psychological well-being (eg, depression, anxiety), and physical health and immune functioning.[20,64,75–79]

Results of a systematic review to identify the types of problems and burdens faced by family caregivers of patients with cancer reported that 97 of the 164 research-based studies described the physical, social, and/or emotional problems related to caregiving.[69] Investigators assessing the caregivers of patients with newly diagnosed colorectal and lung cancer (N = 677) reported that the relationship between objective

---

Box 3
Consequences and outcomes of caregiver burden

Consequences to caregivers

- Caregiving research has evolved from an emphasis on the role-specific negative outcome of burden to more general well-being considerations, including positive psychological well-being, negative psychological well-being, and physical health and immune functioning.

- Caregivers can develop their own health problems from their caregiving responsibilities.

- Caregivers have been reported to be less likely to engage in preventive health activities and are at a high risk of contracting serious illnesses.

- Most common and severe health effects of caregiving are found within the psychological and emotional domains.

- Caregivers have to adjust their work schedules, take leaves of absence, or reduce work hours as a result of care responsibilities.

- Caregivers may have to spend their own money to take care of their sick family members.

Consequences to care receivers

- Caregivers can place their family members at risk if they lack the knowledge and skills to perform their work or if they engage in harmful behaviors, intentional or unintentional, because of their lack of capacity to provide the level of care that is needed.

Consequences to the family

- The stress of caring for a relative with cancer can create new conflicts or can bring long-standing unresolved family issues to the surface.

Consequences to the health care system

- Caregiver burden has been associated with the caregiver's own poor health status, a decrease in health maintenance behaviors, and increase in health-risk behaviors and prescription drug use.

- Family caregiving can also have a positive impact on health care expenditure.

Data from Refs.[19,20,64,75–79,81,91,95]

---

burden and caregiver mental and physical health outcomes varied by caregiver resources. More specifically, caregivers with significant coping, social, and material resources were less likely to have deleterious consequences as a result of caregiving demands, whereas those with few resources were at increased risk.[17] In caregivers of patients with prostate cancer who were to begin radiation therapy (N = 60), 12.2% had clinically meaningful levels of depression, 40.7% anxiety, 15.0% pain, 36.7% sleep disturbance, 33.3% morning fatigue, and 30.0% evening fatigue. In addition, those who were older and who had lower levels of state anxiety and higher levels of depression, morning fatigue, and pain reported significantly poorer functional status (R^2 = 38.7%). Moreover, those who were younger, had more years of education, were working, and had higher levels of depression, morning fatigue, sleep disturbance, and lower levels of evening fatigue reported significantly lower QOL scores (R^2 = 70.1%).[80]

Physical/physiologic/biological implications to caregivers

The increase in the length of time providing care and the corresponding burden perceived by family caregivers of patients with brain cancers have negatively affected the physical well-being of caregivers.[79] Caregivers can develop their own health problems from their caregiving responsibilities (**Table 1**).

Table 1 Most common aspects of caregiver health that have deteriorated as a result of caregiving (n = 528)	
Symptom	Frequency (%)
Energy and sleep	87
Stress and/or panic attacks	70
Pain, aching	60
Depression	52
Headaches	41
Weight gain/loss	38

Data from Evercare in collaboration with National Alliance for Caregiving. Evercare study of caregivers in decline: A close-up look at the health risks of caring for a loved one. Evercare, Minnetonka, MN and NAC, Bethesda, MD; 2006.

Caregivers are less likely to engage in preventive health activities and have a higher risk of contracting serious illnesses.[81] Approximately 50% of caregivers report at least 1 chronic condition, 20% describe their health as fair or poor, and 17% think that their health has deteriorated as a result of caregiving.[81–83] Older spousal caregivers who reported caregiver stress had a 63% higher mortality than noncaregivers of the same age.[84] In addition, data obtained from salivary biomarkers of caregivers of patients with cancer has shown marked changes in neurohormonal and inflammatory processes within the year of the cancer diagnosis[85] whereas a more recent study found higher levels of proinflammatory cytokines in male caregivers with anxiety, in obese caregivers who reported higher burden from disrupted schedules, and in younger caregivers with low self-esteem.[79]

Psychological/emotional implications to caregivers
The confounding problems, including fear, uncertainty, and lack of hope, that accompany the diagnosis of cancer continue to surround patients and caregivers throughout the continuum of care.[39] These psychological responses may be heightened on receiving a diagnosis of brain metastases. On the grounds that cancer caregiving has the features of a chronic stress experience,[44] it can be expected that the most common and severe health effects of caregiving are found within the psychological and emotional domains.

In caregivers of individuals with schizophrenia, the psychological impact of traumatic experiences from the patient's violent behavior was significantly associated with caregiver burden ($P<.05$).[86] A systematic review of 164 research-based studies of family caregivers of patients with cancer identified more than 200 problems and burdens related to caregiving responsibilities, with social and emotional implications as the most frequently studied categories.[69]

The National Alliance for Caregiving[87] reported a link between caregiving and higher rates of insomnia and depression, with rates reported as high as 91% for depression, of which 60% was rated as moderate or severe. In addition, a high prevalence of psychological distress in caregivers has been documented in caregivers of patients with cancer in Italy, where more than half scored positive in screening for mood disorders, more than 10% experienced severe levels of posttraumatic stress disorder, and 37% scored positive for clinically relevant emotional disturbance.[88]

Results from a cross-sectional, descriptive, and correlational study involving 410 caregivers recruited from the community indicate a high level of burden and depression among all caregivers. Significant differences ($P<.001$; F = 26.11) between the 3 caregiving groups (Alzheimer disease, cancer, schizophrenia) were detected in terms of burden, with the highest reported for Alzheimer disease caregivers. One-way analysis of variance showed significant differences ($P = .008$; F = 4.85) between the 3 caregiving groups in terms of depression, with the highest depression levels being for cancer caregivers.[89]

Caregivers of terminally ill patients with cancer in Taiwan showed the dynamic change and multidimensional attributes that can also be observed with the consequences of caregiver burden. In that study, caregivers' depressive symptoms increased as the patients' deaths approached. Adult children or spousal caregivers experienced more depressive symptoms if they self-identified as lacking social support and confidence in offering substantial assistance for younger terminally ill patients with cancer with higher levels of symptom distress. Likewise, the study reported that caregivers were susceptible to higher levels of depressive symptoms if they were heavily burdened by caregiving; that is, experienced more disruptions in schedules, greater health deterioration, stronger sense of family abandonment, and lower caregiver esteem.[90]

Social implications to caregivers
The cancer experience can significantly affect the social well-being of caregivers. For caregivers of patients with brain metastases, the uncertain disease trajectory containing a variety of distressing events presents a unique challenge. Caregivers have trouble balancing their work and family responsibilities and many have to adjust their work schedules, take leaves of absence, or reduce work hours as a result of care responsibilities.[91] Caregivers may have to spend their own money to take care of their sick family members. The average out-of-pocket expense for caregivers in 2007 was $5531, which is approximately 10% of the annual household income for more than 40% of caregivers in the United States. The cost did not include the loss of salary, benefits, and the reduction in retirement savings and social security benefits.[81]

A 2012 study of caregivers of patients with lung cancer (N = 74) reported that close to three-fourths (74%) had 1 or more adverse economic or social changes, such as disengagement from most of their regular social and leisure activities and hours of work lost caused by the illness.[92] The investigators further reported that 16 was the average number of hours of work lost each week because of the illness (standard deviation, 13; range, 1–50). In addition, 28% of the caregivers (n = 21) reported that their families lost their major source of income or made a major change in plans that included delaying medical care for another family member or altering educational plans (22%) because of the high cost of the illness.[92] Nearly one-fifth (18%) of caregivers reported losing most or all of the family savings and another 18% indicated that a family member made a major life change (eg, quit work) to care for the patient.[92]

In a similar study of 70 caregivers of patients in palliative care, Mazanec and colleagues[93] reported that the overall work productivity loss in their sample was 22.9%, which was slightly higher than the number (20.1%) previously reported by Giovannetti and colleagues.[94] This study also found associations between greater work productivity loss and higher levels of depression and anxiety, and greater perceived caregiver burden related to financial problems, disrupted schedule, and health problems.[93]

Consequences to Care Receivers
Although most studies on cancer caregiving focus on either patient or caregiver outcomes, addressing each as separate individuals, a few studies explored caregiver-patient dyads and dyadic outcomes.[6] This focus is of particular importance to

caregivers of patients with brain metastases because of the multiple assaults to the physical and mental health of both the patient and the caregiver. Despite their good intentions and hard work, caregivers can place their family members at risk if they lack the knowledge and skills to perform their work or if they engage in harmful behaviors, intentional or unintentional, because of their lack of capacity to provide the level of care that is needed.[95] Studies in noncancer caregiver–care-receiver dyads have documented that depressed caregivers are more likely to engage in neglect or abusive behaviors.[96] In a systematic review of risk factors for elder abuse among community-dwelling elders, caregiver burden was a risk factor in 3 studies of elders requiring assistance with daily activities and in 4 studies of elders with dementia.[97] Studies have also linked cognitive behavioral problems of care receivers with an increased risk for abusive behaviors by the caregivers.[98,99]

The stressful work associated with caregiving can increase the risk of the caregiver engaging in harmful behaviors toward the care recipients. In addition, caregiver burden can affect patient outcomes. The National Alliance for Caregiving reported that one-half of caregivers thought that the decline in their own health compromised their ability to provide care for the care recipient.[81,82]

Consequences to the Family

Cancer significantly affects the entire family and is not an isolated experience for 1 individual.[100] The stress of caring for a relative with cancer can create new conflicts or can bring long-standing unresolved family issues to the surface. Conflicts arise when patients and caregivers avoid discussion of sensitive issues surrounding the cancer diagnosis and its treatments. Barriers to communication and negotiation of family roles hinder the caregivers' and the patients' abilities to support one another, decrease spousal intimacy, or have a detrimental effect on marital and family relationships.[101]

Family caregivers assume more load when they assume the responsibilities of the sick family member in addition to their own. It has been reported that primary caregivers need not only the assistance of family members but their expressed encouragement and appreciation as well.[8] Family conflicts have also been found to be predictors of caregiver depression but, on a positive note, prior good family dynamics have been associated with significantly less caregiver burden.[8] It may be that positive family support can be an important resource to caregivers in mitigating some of their perceived burden.

Consequences to the Health Care System

Brain metastases are 10 times more common that primary brain tumors and have been reported in as many as 40% of patients with systemic cancer.[4,102,103] With the increase in the number of patients with brain metastases comes a corresponding increase in the number of caregivers. Although the role of caregivers has been well recognized, most health care systems have yet to develop a formal process to integrate caregiver health into their structures. Caregiver burden has been associated with the caregiver's own poor health status, a decrease in health maintenance behaviors, and increase in health-risk behaviors and prescription drug use.[81,95] In terms of use of acute care services, investigators studying caregivers of patients with Alzheimer dementia reported that 24% of the caregivers (N = 153) had at least 1 emergency room visit or hospitalization in the 6 months before study enrollment.[104] In addition, caregivers who reported higher levels of burden had a higher Framingham Stroke Risk and an increased all-cause mortality risk.[81]

Family caregivers constitute the foundation of the long-term care system and although many studies have reported on the negative impact of caregiver burden on the health care system, family caregiving can also have a positive impact on health care expenditure. Family caregiving saves billions of dollars that would otherwise be required for long-term hospitalization and care.[19] The Association of American Retired Persons estimated that the economic value of unpaid contributions of family caregivers was approximately $450 billion in 2009.[105]

Caregiving at the end of life

Although a subset of patients benefit from novel treatments, cure remains an unrealistic expectation for most patients with brain metastases.[4] Multiple prognostic models predicting the overall survival of patients with brain metastases reiteratively report a median survival of 2 to 7 months,[106] and, because of this, the diagnosis of metastatic disease is often considered an eligibility criteria for admission to hospice (University of Texas Health Sciences Center San Antonio, [http://geriatrics.uthscsa.edu/tools/Hospice_elegibility_card__Ross_and_Sanchez_Reilly_2008.pdf], Hospice and Palliative Care of Greensboro [https://www.hospicegso.org/wp-content/uploads/2013/07/AdmissionCriteriaBooklet-8-2013.pdf], Optum [https://campaign.optum.com/hospice/clinical-professionals/hospice-eligibility.html], Hospice of the Valley [https://www.hov.org/hospice-eligibility-guidelines]). In contrast with the traditional health care delivery model, which is centered on patients' individual needs, hospice provides support with the patient and the family as the unit of care.[107] However, referral to hospice typically occurs very late in the dying process and whether patients and caregivers receive hospice support depends on many things, including patients', caregivers', and health care providers' preferences for aggressive treatment.[108] Hence, these individuals often deal with end-of-life issues before hospice care is even offered as an option.

When caregivers of patients with brain metastases transition from usual care provided in hospitals and ambulatory care settings to the specialized end-of-life care, they receive minimal preparation and limited information from health care providers.[109,110] The lack of preparation and limited information are reflected in the themes that emerged from a qualitative study exploring caregivers' perspectives in providing end-of-life care. In the study, caregivers described end-of-life care as unpredictable, intense, and complex, but at the same time profoundly moving and affirming.[110]

IMPLICATIONS FOR PRACTICE

It is worth noting that caregivers have regular interactions with the health care system but may not receive the attention they need.[111] Caregivers who continue to suffer in silence as they juggle the tasks and prioritize the needs of the patients, and those who knowingly suppress their needs so as not to contribute to the guilt or remorse of patients with cancer over being the cause of the burden, can be helped by comprehensive and holistic care provided by those same health care systems. Stakeholders need to develop a plan to integrate the care of caregivers into formal health care systems in cancer care. Clinicians and researchers need to work together to create an infrastructure for more comprehensive caregiver surveillance at national and/or state levels.

Although routine interactions between patients and providers that are focused on an integrated care is the cornerstone of quality comprehensive care, the well-being assessment of family caregivers is currently not considered standard of care. In the age of precision medicine, the care of the caregiver is several years behind the powerful advances in the diagnosis and treatment of cancer. Clinicians need to identify the factors that cause burden, relationship conflicts in the patient-caregiver dyad and among other members of the household, and financial toxicity in caregivers of patients with cancer. More importantly, clinicians need to provide an individualized plan of care for caregivers, including respite for caregivers, supplemental services, and interventions to reduce burden and improve health.[111]

SUMMARY

Caregiving is a highly individualized experience, as seen in caregivers of patients with brain metastases. Whether expressed or implied, the responsibilities they take up on assuming the caregiving role place additional demands that the caregivers must adapt to and cope with. Although some demands of caregiving are more likely to increase caregiver burden, every caregiver has a different threshold and the variation in responses are as diverse as the characteristics of caregivers.

What is unique about the features of caregiving in patients with brain metastases that would warrant the development of a program of research that does not duplicate the work already done with other caregiver populations? As described in previous articles, improving long-term survival of patients has corresponded with an increased incidence of brain metastases. This sequence of events in the trajectory of patients with cancer has extended the length of the caregiving experience. In addition, the universal concerns about disease recurrence or progression that are unique to cancer predispose patients and the caregivers to uncertainty and stress. Likewise, the diagnosis of cancer takes the patients and their caregivers through a journey that winds through unique stages: initial diagnosis, treatment, survivorship, recurrence, progression, and end of life. The route that patients with cancer and their caregivers take can put them on a direct path to remission or end of life, but can also maneuver them on a path that circles through these stages. In addition, developments in cancer research have increased the complexity of cancer treatment because new therapies, devices, and clinical trials are now available to patients when, only a years ago, options for further treatment did not exist. All these contribute to the demands placed on the patients and their caregivers.

This article describes the challenges of caregiving in brain metastases. It reviews the critical attributes of caregiver burden: subjective perception, multidimensional phenomena, dynamic change, and overload. These attributes have been examined in many caregiver studies within a variety of diagnoses and health conditions. It also describes the demands of caregiving, classifying them into primary and secondary demands, with primary demands being dictated by direct health-related needs of the care receiver and secondary demands being determined by factors outside the environment of the caregiver-patient dyad (ie, family, work, and society). In addition, it presents the consequences and outcomes of caregiver burden. Although the article mostly describes the negative consequences of caregiving, it acknowledges the growing body of work highlighting positive outcomes and more general well-being considerations for individuals in the caregiving role.

Caregiver burden is an important component of comprehensive and holistic clinical care. It is a consequence of a process that involves several interrelated conditions within the caregiving experience. As health care providers prepare to care for an aging population, and with advancing age being a known risk factor for cancer, it becomes increasingly important to address the needs of caregivers, in effect the other patients, who are at an increased risk for various psychological, physical, financial, and social problems.

REFERENCES

1. Hutter A, Schwetye KE, Bierhals AJ, et al. Brain neoplasms: epidemiology, diagnosis, and prospects for cost-effective imaging. Neuroimaging Clin North Am 2003;13(2):237–50, x–xi.
2. Levin VA, Leibel SA, Gutin PH. Neoplasms of the central nervous system. In: DeVita VT Jr, Hellman S, Rosenberg SA, editors. Cancer: principles and practice of oncology. 6th edition. Philadelphia: Lippincott Williams & Wilkins; 2001. p. 2100–60.
3. National Cancer Institute. Adult brain tumors treatment (PDQ). 2010. Available at: http://www.cancer.gov/cancertopics/pdq/treatment/adultbrain/Health Professional/page2#Reference2.11. Accessed August 21, 2010.
4. Saria MG, Piccioni D, Carter J, et al. Current perspectives in the management of brain metastases. Clin J Oncol Nurs 2015;19(4):475–9.
5. Leone JP, Leone BA. Breast cancer brain metastases: the last frontier. Exp Hematol Oncol 2015;4:33.
6. Kent EE, Rowland JH, Northouse L, et al. Caring for caregivers and patients: research and clinical priorities for informal cancer caregiving. Cancer 2016; 122(13):1987–95.
7. Dionne-Odom JN, Hull JG, Martin MY, et al. Associations between advanced cancer patients' survival and family caregiver presence and burden. Cancer Med 2016;5:853–62.
8. Etters L, Goodall D, Harrison BE. Caregiver burden among dementia patient caregivers: a review of the literature. J Am Acad Nurse Pract 2008;20(8):423–8.
9. Francis LE, Worthington J, Kypriotakis G, et al. Relationship quality and burden among caregivers for late-stage cancer patients. Support Care Cancer 2010; 18(11):1429–36.
10. Grunfeld E, Coyle D, Whelan T, et al. Family caregiver burden: results of a longitudinal study of breast cancer patients and their principal caregivers. CMAJ 2004;170(12):1795–801.
11. Mausbach BT, Harmell AL, Moore RC, et al. Influence of caregiver burden on the association between daily fluctuations in pleasant activities and mood: a daily diary analysis. Behav Res Ther 2011;49(1):74–9.
12. McLennon SM, Habermann B, Rice M. Finding meaning as a mediator of burden on the health of caregivers of spouses with dementia. Aging Ment Health 2011; 15(4):522–30.
13. Moller-Leimkuhler AM, Wiesheu A. Caregiver burden in chronic mental illness: the role of patient and caregiver characteristics. Eur Arch Psychiatry Clin Neurosci 2011;262:157–66.
14. Poulshock SW, Deimling GT. Families caring for elders in residence: issues in the measurement of burden. J Gerontol 1984;39(2):230–9.
15. Rafiyah I, Sutharangsee W. Review: burden on family caregivers caring for patients with schizophrenia and its related factors. Nurse Media Journal of Nursing 2011;1(1):29–41.
16. Rha SY, Park Y, Song SK, et al. Caregiving burden and the quality of life of family caregivers of cancer patients: the relationship and correlates. Eur J Oncol Nurs 2015;19(4):376–82.
17. van Ryn M, Sanders S, Kahn K, et al. Objective burden, resources, and other stressors among informal cancer caregivers: a hidden quality issue? Psychooncology 2011;20(1):44–52.
18. Zarit SH, Reever KE, Bach-Peterson J. Relatives of the impaired elderly: correlates of feelings of burden. Gerontologist 1980;20(6):649–55.

19. Chou KR. Caregiver burden: a concept analysis. J Pediatr Nurs 2000;15(6): 398–407.
20. Hoffmann RL, Mitchell AM. Caregiver burden: historical development. Nurs Forum 1998;33(4):5–11.
21. Lazarus RS, Folkman S. Stress, appraisal, and coping. New York: Springer; 1984.
22. Connell CM, Janevic MR, Gallant MP. The costs of caring: impact of dementia on family caregivers. J Geriatr Psychiatry Neurol 2001;14(4):179–87.
23. Luchetti L, Uhunmwangho E, Dordoni G, et al. The subjective feeling of burden in caregivers of elderly with dementia: how to intervene? Arch Gerontol Geriatr 2009;49(Suppl 1):153–61.
24. Nguyen M. Nurse's assessment of caregiver burden. Medsurg Nurs 2009;18(3): 147–51 [quiz: 152].
25. Stinson JM, Collins RL, Maestas KL, et al. Dependency aspect of caregiver burden is uniquely related to cognitive impairment in veterans. J Rehabil Res Dev 2014;51(8):1177–88.
26. Harding R, Gao W, Jackson D, et al. Comparative analysis of informal caregiver burden in advanced cancer, dementia, and acquired brain injury. J Pain Symptom Manage 2015;50(4):445–52.
27. Kim Y, Schulz R. Family caregivers' strains: comparative analysis of cancer caregiving with dementia, diabetes, and frail elderly caregiving. J Aging Health 2008;20(5):483–503.
28. Whisenant M. Informal caregiving in patients with brain tumors. Oncol Nurs Forum 2011;38(5):E373–81.
29. Ampalam P, Gunturu S, Padma V. A comparative study of caregiver burden in psychiatric illness and chronic medical illness. Indian J Psychiatry 2012;54(3): 239–43.
30. Garlo K, O'Leary JR, Van Ness PH, et al. Burden in caregivers of older adults with advanced illness. J Am Geriatr Soc 2010;58(12):2315–22.
31. Burton AM, Sautter JM, Tulsky JA, et al. Burden and well-being among a diverse sample of cancer, congestive heart failure, and chronic obstructive pulmonary disease caregivers. J Pain Symptom Manage 2012;44(3):410–20.
32. Sautter JM, Tulsky JA, Johnson KS, et al. Caregiver experience during advanced chronic illness and last year of life. J Am Geriatr Soc 2014;62(6): 1082–90.
33. Ankri J, Andrieu S, Beaufils B, et al. Beyond the global score of the Zarit Burden Interview: useful dimensions for clinicians. Int J Geriatr Psychiatry 2005;20(3):254–60.
34. Jeong YG, Jeong YJ, Kim WC, et al. The mediating effect of caregiver burden on the caregivers' quality of life. J Phys Ther Sci 2015;27(5):1543–7.
35. Sherwood PR, Given BA, Given CW, et al. Predictors of distress in caregivers of persons with a primary malignant brain tumor. Res Nurs Health 2006;29(2): 105–20.
36. Chappell NL, Dujela C. Caregiving: predicting at-risk status. Can J Aging 2008; 27(2):169–79.
37. Lou Q, Liu S, Huo YR, et al. Comprehensive analysis of patient and caregiver predictors for caregiver burden, anxiety and depression in Alzheimer's disease. J Clin Nurs 2015;24(17–18):2668–78.
38. Sherwood PR, Donovan HS, Given CW, et al. Predictors of employment and lost hours from work in cancer caregivers. Psychooncology 2008;17(6):598–605.
39. Khalili Y. Ongoing transitions: the impact of a malignant brain tumour on patient and family. Axone 2007;28(3):5–13.

40. Kim Y, Given BA. Quality of life of family caregivers of cancer survivors: across the trajectory of the illness. Cancer 2008;112(11 Suppl):2556–68.
41. Zwaanswijk M, Peeters JM, van Beek AP, et al. Informal caregivers of people with dementia: problems, needs and support in the initial stage and in subsequent stages of dementia: a questionnaire survey. Open Nurs J 2013;7:6–13.
42. Grov EK, Valeberg BT. Does the cancer patient's disease stage matter? A comparative study of caregivers' mental health and health related quality of life. Palliat Support Care 2012;10(3):189–96.
43. Sherwood PR, Given B, Given C, et al. Caregivers of persons with a brain tumor: a conceptual model. Nurs Inq 2004;11(1):43–53.
44. Schulz R, Sherwood PR. Physical and mental health effects of family caregiving. Am J Nurs 2008;108(9 Suppl):23–7 [quiz: 27].
45. Hunt CK. Concepts in caregiver research. J Nurs Scholarsh 2003;35(1):27–32.
46. Kruithof WJ, Post MW, Visser-Meily JM. Measuring negative and positive caregiving experiences: a psychometric analysis of the Caregiver Strain Index Expanded. Clin Rehabil 2015;29(12):1224–33.
47. Davis ME, Stoiber AM. Glioblastoma multiforme: enhancing survival and quality of life. Clin J Oncol Nurs 2011;15(3):291–7.
48. Wefel JS, Cloughesy T, Zazzali JL, et al. Neurocognitive function in patients with recurrent glioblastoma treated with bevacizumab. Neuro Oncol 2011;13(6):660–8.
49. Weller M. Neurocognitive function: an emerging surrogate endpoint for neuro-oncology trials. Neuro Oncol 2011;13(6):565.
50. Witgert ME, Meyers CA. Neurocognitive and quality of life measures in patients with metastatic brain disease. Neurosurg Clin North Am 2011;22(1):79–85, vii.
51. Khuntia D, Mathew BS, Meyers CA, et al. Brain metastases. In: Meyers CA, Perry JR, editors. Cognition and cancer. New York: Cambridge University Press; 2008. p. 170–86.
52. Schagen SB, Klein M, Reijneveld JC, et al. Monitoring and optimising cognitive function in cancer patients: present knowledge and future directions. EJC Suppl 2014;12(1):29–40.
53. Shen C, Bao WM, Yang BJ, et al. Cognitive deficits in patients with brain tumor. Chin Med J (Engl) 2012;125(14):2610–7.
54. Fisher GG, Franks MM, Plassman BL, et al. Caring for individuals with dementia and cognitive impairment, not dementia: findings from the aging, demographics, and memory study. J Am Geriatr Soc 2011;59(3):488–94.
55. Ikeda C, Terada S, Oshima E, et al. Difference in determinants of caregiver burden between amnestic mild cognitive impairment and mild Alzheimer's disease. Psychiatry Res 2015;226(1):242–6.
56. Dauphinot V, Ravier A, Novais T, et al. Relationship between comorbidities in patients with cognitive complaint and caregiver burden: a cross-sectional study. J Am Med Dir Assoc 2016;17(3):232–7.
57. Pinquart M, Sorensen S. Associations of stressors and uplifts of caregiving with caregiver burden and depressive mood: a meta-analysis. J Gerontol B Psychol Sci Soc Sci 2003;58(2):P112–28.
58. Germain S, Adam S, Olivier C, et al. Does cognitive impairment influence burden in caregivers of patients with Alzheimer's disease? J Alzheimers Dis 2009;17(1):105–14.
59. Sherwood PR, Given CW, Given BA, et al. Caregiver burden and depressive symptoms: analysis of common outcomes in caregivers of elderly patients. J Aging Health 2005;17(2):125–47.

60. Rosdinom R, Zarina MZ, Zanariah MS, et al. Behavioural and psychological symptoms of dementia, cognitive impairment and caregiver burden in patients with dementia. Prev Med 2013;57(Suppl):S67–9.

61. Lillo P, Mioshi E, Hodges JR. Caregiver burden in amyotrophic lateral sclerosis is more dependent on patients' behavioral changes than physical disability: a comparative study. BMC Neurol 2012;12:156.

62. Russell B, Collins A, Dally M, et al. Living longer with adult high-grade glioma: setting a research agenda for patients and their caregivers. J Neurooncol 2014;120(1):1–10.

63. Northfield S, Nebauer M. The caregiving journey for family members of relatives with cancer: how do they cope? Clin J Oncol Nurs 2010;14(5):567–77.

64. Given BA, Given CW. Family caregiving for the elderly. In: Fitzpatrick JJ, Taunton RL, Jacox AK, editors. Annual review of nursing research, vol. 9. New York: Springer; 1991. p. 77–101.

65. Mochari-Greenberger H, Mosca L. Caregiver burden and nonachievement of healthy lifestyle behaviors among family caregivers of cardiovascular disease patients. Am J Health Promot 2012;27(2):84–9.

66. Vaingankar JA, Subramaniam M, Abdin E, et al. "How much can I take?": predictors of perceived burden for relatives of people with chronic illness. Ann Acad Med Singap 2012;41(5):212–20.

67. Abernethy A, Burns C, Wheeler J, et al. Defining distinct caregiver subpopulations by intensity of end-of-life care provided. Palliat Med 2009;23(1):66–79.

68. Rodriguez-Sanchez E, Perez-Penaranda A, Losada-Baltar A, et al. Relationships between quality of life and family function in caregiver. BMC Fam Pract 2011;12:19.

69. Stenberg U, Ruland CM, Miaskowski C. Review of the literature on the effects of caring for a patient with cancer. Psychooncology 2010;19(10):1013–25.

70. Beattie S, Lebel S. The experience of caregivers of hematological cancer patients undergoing a hematopoietic stem cell transplant: a comprehensive literature review. Psychooncology 2011;20(11):1137–50.

71. Guetin S, Portet F, Picot MC, et al. Impact of music therapy on anxiety and depression for patients with Alzheimer's disease and on the burden felt by the main caregiver (feasibility study). Encephale 2009;35(1):57–65 [in French].

72. Picot S. Choice and social exchange theory and the rewards of African American caregivers. J Natl Black Nurses Assoc 1995;7(2):29–40.

73. Picot SJ. The relationship between the rewards, costs, and coping strategies of black family caregivers [Doctoral dissertation - research]. Baltimore (MD): University of Maryland; 1991.

74. Picot SJ, Youngblut J, Zeller R. Development and testing of a measure of perceived caregiver rewards in adults. J Nurs Meas 1997;5(1):33–52.

75. Dias R, Santos RL, Sousa MF, et al. Resilience of caregivers of people with dementia: a systematic review of biological and psychosocial determinants. Trends Psychiatry Psychother 2015;37(1):12–9.

76. Li Q, Loke AY. The positive aspects of caregiving for cancer patients: a critical review of the literature and directions for future research. Psychooncology 2013; 22(11):2399–407.

77. Marks NF, Lambert JD. Family caregiving: contemporary trends and issues. Madison (WI): University of Wisconsin; 1997.

78. Sherwood PR, Cwiklik M, Donovan HS. Neuro-oncology family caregiving: review and directions for future research. CNS Oncol 2016;5(1):41–8.

79. Sherwood PR, Price TJ, Weimer J, et al. Neuro-oncology family caregivers are at risk for systemic inflammation. J Neurooncol 2016;128:109–18.
80. Fletcher BS, Paul SM, Dodd MJ, et al. Prevalence, severity, and impact of symptoms on female family caregivers of patients at the initiation of radiation therapy for prostate cancer. J Clin Oncol 2008;26(4):599–605.
81. Collins LG, Swartz K. Caregiver care. Am Fam Physician 2011;83(11):1309–17.
82. Aldrich N. CDC seeks to protect health of family caregivers. 2009.
83. Family Caregiver Alliance. Family caregiving: state of the art, future trends. Report from a national conference. San Francisco (CA): 2007.
84. Schulz R, Beach SR. Caregiving as a risk factor for mortality: the Caregiver Health Effects Study. JAMA 1999;282(23):2215–9.
85. Rohleder N, Marin TJ, Ma R, et al. Biologic cost of caring for a cancer patient: dysregulation of pro- and anti-inflammatory signaling pathways. J Clin Oncol 2009;27(18):2909–15.
86. Hanzawa S, Bae JK, Bae YJ, et al. Psychological impact on caregivers traumatized by the violent behavior of a family member with schizophrenia. Asian J Psychiatr 2013;6(1):46–51.
87. National Alliance for Caregiving. Evercare study of caregivers in decline: a close-up look at the health risks of caring for a loved one. 2006.
88. Mazzotti E, Sebastiani C, Antonini Cappellini GC, et al. Predictors of mood disorders in cancer patients' caregivers. Support Care Cancer 2013;21(2):643–7.
89. Papastavrou E, Charalambous A, Tsangari H, et al. The burdensome and depressive experience of caring: what cancer, schizophrenia, and Alzheimer's disease caregivers have in common. Cancer Nurs 2012;35(3):187–94.
90. Tang ST, Chang WC, Chen JS, et al. Course and predictors of depressive symptoms among family caregivers of terminally ill cancer patients until their death. Psychooncology 2012;22(6):1312–8.
91. Family Caregiver Alliance. Caregiving. San Francisco. 2009.
92. Mosher CE, Champion VL, Azzoli CG, et al. Economic and social changes among distressed family caregivers of lung cancer patients. Support Care Cancer 2013;21(3):819–26.
93. Mazanec SR, Daly BJ, Douglas SL, et al. Work productivity and health of informal caregivers of persons with advanced cancer. Res Nurs Health 2011;34(6):483–95.
94. Giovannetti ER, Wolff JL, Frick KD, et al. Construct validity of the work productivity and activity impairment questionnaire across informal caregivers of chronically ill older patients. Value Health 2009;12(6):1011–7.
95. Reinhard S, Given B, Petlick N, et al. Supporting family caregivers in providing care. In: Hughes R, editor. Patient safety and quality: an evidence-based handbook for nurses. Rockville (MD): Agency for Healthcare Research and Quality; 2008. p. 341–404.
96. Beach SR, Schulz R, Williamson GM, et al. Risk factors for potentially harmful informal caregiver behavior. J Am Geriatr Soc 2005;53(2):255–61.
97. Johannesen M, Logiudice D. Elder abuse: a systematic review of risk factors in community-dwelling elders. Age Ageing 2013;42:292–8.
98. Fulmer T, Paveza G, VandeWeerd C, et al. Dyadic vulnerability and risk profiling for elder neglect. Gerontologist 2005;45(4):525–34.
99. Heath JM, Kobylarz FA, Brown M, et al. Interventions from home-based geriatric assessments of adult protective service clients suffering elder mistreatment. J Am Geriatr Soc 2005;53(9):1538–42.

100. Otis-Green S, Juarez G. Enhancing the social well-being of family caregivers. Semin Oncol Nurs 2012;28(4):246–55.
101. Northouse LL, Katapodi MC, Song L, et al. Interventions with family caregivers of cancer patients: meta-analysis of randomized trials. CA Cancer J Clin 2010; 60(5):317–39.
102. Chamberlain MC. Brain metastases: a medical neuro-oncology perspective. Expert Rev Neurother 2010;10(4):563–73.
103. Lorger M, Felding-Habermann B. Capturing changes in the brain microenvironment during initial steps of breast cancer brain metastasis. Am J Pathol 2010; 176(6):2958–71.
104. Schubert CC, Boustani M, Callahan CM, et al. Acute care utilization by dementia caregivers within urban primary care practices. J Gen Intern Med 2008;23(11): 1736–40.
105. Feinberg L, Reinhard SC, Houser A, et al. Valuing the invaluable: 2011 update the growing contributions and costs of family caregiving. Washington, DC: AARP Public Policy Institute; 2011.
106. Stavas M, Arneson K, Friedman J, et al. From whole brain to hospice: patterns of care in radiation oncology. J Palliat Med 2014;17(6):662–6.
107. Oliver DP, Demiris G, Washington KT, et al. Challenges and strategies for hospice caregivers: a qualitative analysis. Gerontologist 2016. [Epub ahead of print].
108. Wright AA, Keating NL, Ayanian JZ, et al. Family perspectives on aggressive cancer care near the end of life. JAMA 2016;315(3):284–92.
109. Guo G, Phillips LR, Reed PG. End-of-life caregiver interactions with health care providers: learning from the bad. J Nurs Care Qual 2010;25(4):334–43.
110. Phillips LR, Reed PG. End-of-life caregiver's perspectives on their role: generative caregiving. Gerontologist 2010;50(2):204–14.
111. Adelman RD, Tmanova LL, Delgado D, et al. Caregiver burden: a clinical review. JAMA 2014;311(10):1052–60.

Symptom Management and Palliative Care for Patients with Cancer

Patsy Yates, PhD, RN

KEYWORDS

• Advanced cancer • Palliative care • Symptom management

KEY POINTS

- Advanced cancer is often characterized by multiple physical and psychological symptoms that can be chronic in nature.
- Contemporary models of symptom management emphasize the importance of understanding the multifactorial causes of symptoms and diversity of individual responses to these symptoms.
- Optimal symptom management for patients with advanced cancer includes eliminating the cause of the problem where possible while responding to individual experience and impacts of the symptoms.
- Effective communication and continuity and coordination of care are required to ensure high-quality person-centered palliative care.

INTRODUCTION

Palliative care services have evolved considerably over the past few decades. Originally pioneered in the United Kingdom by Dame Cicely Saunders as a reformist movement to address deficiencies in oncology care, palliative care today is considered an integral component of quality cancer care. Palliative care today is delivered via many modes and in many different care settings. It has become synonymous with the physical, social, psychological, and spiritual support of patients with life-limiting illness, delivered by a multidisciplinary team.[1] There is also a growing evidence base to underpin palliative interventions, in particular the management of physical and psychological symptoms. Professional guidelines thus recommend combined standard oncology care and palliative care early in the course of illness for any patient with metastatic cancer.[2,3] This article explores scientific advances in palliative care and the way in which these advances can be integrated into cancer nursing practice.

School of Nursing, Queensland University of Technology, Victoria Park Road, Kelvin Grove, QLD 4059, Australia
E-mail address: p.yates@qut.edu.au

Nurs Clin N Am 52 (2017) 179–191
http://dx.doi.org/10.1016/j.cnur.2016.10.006
0029-6465/17/© 2017 Elsevier Inc. All rights reserved.

THE CLINICAL CONTEXT FOR MODERN PALLIATIVE SYMPTOM MANAGEMENT
Extended Survival

The cancer trajectory has changed significantly in recent years as treatment advances and increased survival rates mean that cancer has been transformed as a chronic disease. These extended survival rates are seen for the majority of cancers and for people with both early-stage and advanced-stage disease. For example, median survival after a metastatic breast cancer diagnosis today is 3 years, up from 18 months in 1970.[4] As a result, many patients whose disease is considered incurable are living for extended periods of time with cumulative morbidity from their disease and treatment, requiring health care professionals to develop new approaches to optimize quality of life.[5]

More Diverse Cancer Trajectories

Advanced cancer trajectories vary according to many disease and treatment-related factors and require different health care responses. For example, one study of the last 90 days of life of patients with prostate, lung, or hematological cancer identified varying symptomatology, which, in turn, influenced clinical management, use of palliative care services, the site of care, and the site of death.[6] A summary of the key features of the trajectories for this study sample is presented in **Box 1**.

The diverse nature of these disease trajectories, coupled with increasing and prolonged use of many anticancer therapies to gain control and/or palliation of advancing disease, means that determining when a person can benefit from palliative care referral is not always clear. Ongoing and thorough assessment of need is important to ensure the appropriate services are provided according to individual clinical and psychosocial circumstances.

Box 1
Disease trajectories for patients with prostate, lung, and hematological malignancies in the last 90 days of life

Prostate cancer patients
- Deteriorated over many months
- Rarely required aggressive medical inpatient management
- Increasing dependency
- Often frail/elderly spouses
- Most died after a hospice admission of at least 1 month

Lung cancer patients
- Developed significant acute symptoms, in particular dyspnea and moderate-to-severe delirium
- Palliative care services were generally involved late or not at all

Hematological cancer patients
- Long course from diagnosis but generally a rapid rate of decline
- Palliative care referrals frequently belated

Data from William L, Jackson K, Bostanci A, et al. Diagnosis matters: the differing clinical trajectories for terminal prostate, lung and haematological cancers. Aust Fam Physician 2015;44(7):479–84.

Complex Symptom Profiles

Patients with advanced cancer often experience multiple physical and psychological symptoms as a result of progressing disease or anticancer treatment. **Table 1** presents data from a systematic review of symptom prevalence for patients with advanced cancer.[7] Symptoms where the pooled prevalence was greater than 30% are included in the table. Data indicate that the top 5 most common symptoms, all experienced by more than 50% of patients, include fatigue, pain, lack of energy, weakness, and appetite loss.

In addition, many patients experience multiple co-occurring symptoms. One recent systematic review involving 33 articles identified 4 common groupings of symptoms that were present across the disease trajectory: anxiety-depression, nausea-vomiting, nausea–appetite loss, and fatigue-dyspnea-drowsiness-pain. In most cases, these symptom clusters were not stable longitudinally.[8] The existence of such symptom clusters has important implications for practice, because they suggest potential causes that can be targeted, possible predictors of quality of life, and management strategies that might have greater impact.

Developing Evidence Base for Integrated Models

Given the changing trajectories associated with advanced cancer, more recent therapeutic models describe incorporation of gradual or phased transitions, which emphasize palliative input and quality-of-life considerations during the active phase of treatment.[9] Such models emphasize that the simultaneous palliative care approach

Table 1
Symptom prevalence in advanced cancer

	Symptom Prevalence		
	Number of Studies	Number of Patients	Pooled Prevalence (%)	95% CI (%)
N	40	25,074	—	—
Fatigue	17	6727	74	(63, 83)
Pain	37	21,917	71	(67, 74)
Lack of energy	6	1827	69	(57, 79)
Weakness	18	14,910	60	(51, 68)
Appetite loss	37	23,112	53	(48, 59)
Nervousness	5	727	48	(39, 57)
Weight loss	17	13,167	46	(34, 59)
Dry mouth	20	6359	40	(29, 52)
Depressed mood	19	8678	39	(33, 45)
Constipation	34	22,437	37	(33, 40)
Worrying	6	1378	36	(21, 55)
Insomnia	28	18,597	36	(30, 43)
Dyspnea	40	24,490	35	(30, 39)
Nausea	39	24,263	31	(27, 35)
Anxiety	12	7270	30	(17, 46)
Irritability	6	1009	30	(22, 40)

Adapted from Teunissen SC, Wesker W, Kruitwagen C, et al. Symptom prevalence in patients with incurable cancer: a systematic review. J Pain Symptom Manage 2007;34:94–104; with permission.

allows for treatment goals to evolve while concurrent curative and palliative care are provided.[10] **Fig. 1** illustrates how such models can be conceptualized.

Several recent landmark studies confirm the benefit of this type of early referral and integrated model of palliative care.[11,12] Temel and colleagues[12] randomized patients with newly diagnosed metastatic non–small cell lung cancer to receive early palliative care integrated with standard oncological care or standard oncological care alone. Results confirmed that compared with the standard care group, the intervention group had better quality of life, lower rates of depression, and a 2.7-month survival benefit. Other studies have also confirmed that early access to palliative care leads to cost reductions of up to 24%, with the intervention reducing both the length and intensity of hospital stay for patients.[13]

THEORETIC PERSPECTIVES ON CANCER SYMPTOM MANAGEMENT

Nurse scientists have led the way in developing comprehensive theoretic and conceptual models to inform investigations of cancer-related symptoms. One of the first of these models, the theory of symptom management,[14] has underpinned numerous research studies over the past 2 decades. The theory specifies 3 concepts as core dimensions to consider in research and practice: symptom experience, symptom management strategies, and symptom outcomes. The strengths of this theory are its comprehensive approach, recognition of contextual variables, acknowledgment of individual perception and evaluation of the symptom, and specification of a wide range of symptom outcomes.[15] Similarly, the more recent theory of unpleasant symptoms focuses on explanation of the physiologic, psychological, and situational factors

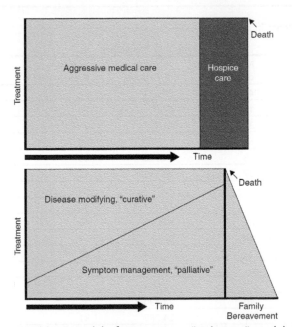

Fig. 1. The older "transition" model of care versus a "trajectory" model. (*Reprinted from* Lynn J, Adamson D. Living well at the end of life: adapting health care to serious chronic illness in old age. Santa Monica (CA): RAND Corporation; 2003. Available at: http://www. rand.org/pubs/white_papers/WP137.html; with permission expressly granted by the RAND Corporation, Santa Monica, CA. Also available in print form.)

that influence the symptom experience.[16] These categories are broad and the model has less of a focus on an intervention component.[15]

This pioneering work has enabled researchers to make significant advances in the field and has provided practitioners with a better understanding of the various dimensions of cancer-related symptoms that need to be considered in practice. Although the relationships between the various dimensions, the interactions between symptoms, and the temporal aspects of symptoms are acknowledged, these aspects of the models require further development.[15] The symptom experience of patients with advanced cancer in particular is, by nature, complex and constantly changing. This is because the basis for these symptoms is often the multisystem effects of progressive disease, physiologic changes associated with advancing disease, and psychological and existential challenges associated with an uncertain future.

Current symptom management theories are being reconceptualized to reflect new directions and scientific discoveries in nursing and other disciplines. One recent review identified specific evaluation components and criteria for determining the utility of symptom management models in contemporary research and practice (**Box 2**).[15]

PRINCIPLES OF PALLIATIVE SYMPTOM MANAGEMENT
Mechanistic Approaches

Theoretic models and empirical research highlight the multidimensional nature of cancer-related symptoms, the constantly changing patterns of such symptoms, and the multifactorial etiologic mechanisms and interactions between symptoms. The complex nature of advanced cancer-related symptoms thus requires that nurses implement regular screening to identify the occurrence of symptoms. When symptoms occur, comprehensive focused assessment to identify the broad range of factors contributing to the symptoms as well as the impact and meaning of the symptoms is then required. Because symptom experiences typically change over time, ongoing assessment is essential. Key components of symptom assessment in advanced cancer are listed in **Box 3**.

Patient-reported measures

Table 2 provides examples of patient-reported screening and assessment tools in palliative symptom management

The Edmonton Symptom Assessment Scale (ESAS) is a commonly used screening tool in clinical practice because it is simple and easy for both patients and clinicians to

---

Box 2
Evaluation components for model or theory for symptom management research

- Antecedents or precipitating factors
- Symptom appraisal
- Symptom pair and cluster components
- Outcomes or consequences
- Temporal components
- Intervention components

Reproduced from Brant JM, Beck S and Miaskowski C. Building dynamic models and theories to advance the science of symptom management research. J Adv Nurs 2010;66:228–40; with permission.

Box 3
Essential components of symptom assessment in advanced cancer

Patient reports of symptom

- Frequency
- Severity
- Impact
- Meaning

Clinical history and investigations to identify contributing factors, including

- Multisystem effects of disease progression and treatment
- Comorbidities

---

use. The Memorial Symptom Assessment Scale (MSAS) is more comprehensive, assessing dimensions of distress and frequency in addition to severity. The length of the MSAS means it is not as useful for screening in clinical practice; however, it is a useful instrument to investigate patient experience in research.

More recently, the Patient-Reported Outcomes Version of the Common Terminology Criteria for Adverse Events (PRO-CTCAE)[19] has been developed as a patient-reported outcome measure to evaluate symptomatic toxicity in patients on cancer clinical trials. The PRO-CTCAE comprises 124 items representing 78 symptomatic toxicities drawn from the CTCA. These items incorporate various rating scales of severity, frequency, and interference. The simplicity of these items means that they have potential use in screening for symptom experiences in patients with advanced cancer; however, the instrument was developed for use in assessing toxicity in clinical trials situations and has not been validated in the advanced cancer population.

Clinical history and investigations

Patient-reported assessment needs to be accompanied by a comprehensive clinical assessment to ascertain likely causes of the symptoms and to guide intervention. For example, nausea in advanced cancer can have many different causes. Each cause can be associated with different underlying mechanisms, which can have unique clinical manifestations. Depending on the underlying mechanisms, specific treatment approaches may be required. For some symptoms, structured tools have been used to assist with the assessment of underlying cause of the problem. For example, the Brief Pain Inventory[20] has been developed to provide detailed information about a person's pain experience to help diagnose pain type and thus guide intervention. As with other symptom tools, the 20-item Brief Pain Inventory assesses pain severity and

---

Table 2
Instruments for assessing multiple symptoms in advanced cancer

Instrument	Scope	Measurement
ESAS – Revised[17]	9 Symptoms plus 1 "other"	Symptoms rated on an 11-point scale ranging from no symptom to worst possible symptom
MSAS[18]	32 Physical and psychological symptoms	Each symptom rated on three dimensions (frequency, severity, and distress) using 4-point rating scale

interference, but, in addition, items are included to assess pain history, location, and quality, to enable identification of underlying mechanisms.

Similar structured tools have not been developed for other symptoms, requiring nurses to draw on their knowledge of the pathophysiology of symptoms to guide clinical assessment and identify etiologic mechanisms. **Table 3** provides a summary of potential causes of nausea in advanced cancer and the key manifestations of each potential cause in patients experiencing this symptom.

Targeted, Tailored, and Integrated Approaches

Targeted approaches

Palliative symptom management models highlight the need to ensure symptom management interventions are targeted to the cause. Selected examples of evidence/etiology-based approaches to managing common symptoms in palliative care are summarized in **Table 4**.

In practice, determining a cause may be difficult in many cases, and often causes of a symptom are multifactorial. Care, therefore, needs to be taken to consider the interactions between various symptoms, their cases, and any treatments implemented to address the symptoms.

Tailored approaches

Consistent with contemporary symptom management models, an individual's response to symptoms can be influenced by a range of social, cultural demographic, and environmental circumstances. For example, there are some differences between older and younger people in symptom experiences. One study that identified symptom clusters in older patients typically included a larger and more diverse range of physical and psychological symptoms than were found in the clusters for younger patients. This was attributed to the multiple risk factors and organ systems that are often involved in how older patients present in clinical practice as well as factors such as differences in reporting.[23]

A person's ability to adapt to circumstances is also dependent on personal and social circumstances. Health literacy has been defined as "an individuals' ability to obtain, understand, and use health information and services in order to make appropriate health decisions within a healthcare system."[24] In palliative care, limited health literacy limits patients' and caregivers' ability to navigate the health care system, creates additional barriers to communication, and hinders patient self-care and caregiver support.[24] Assessment of health literacy, therefore, enables nurses to identify additional action that may be needed to ensure effective symptom management.

For patients with advanced disease, symptoms can be a reminder of progressive disease and be associated with existential threats. Management of symptoms requires an understanding of the perceptions and meanings attributed to the symptom by the individual, because these meanings influence how management strategies are approached. To explore personal meanings and concerns, nurses can ask questions, such as "What is your biggest concern about your pain? and "Some people find these symptoms to be very frightening. How does your breathing problem make you feel?" Patient's responses to such questions can inform the focus of supportive interventions.

Integrated approaches

The multidimensional nature of symptoms means that both pharmacologic and non-pharmacologic approaches to symptom management are required. This is especially important in palliative care, where attention to psychological, social, and spiritual

Table 3
Potential causes of nausea in advanced cancer

Syndrome	Causes	Key Features
Chemically induced nausea	• Drugs: opioids, digoxin, anticonvulsants, antibiotics, cytotoxics • Toxins: food poisoning; ischemic bowel, for example, gut obstruction • Metabolic: organ failure, hypercalcaemia, ketoacidosis	Of drug toxicity or of underlying disease plus constant nausea, variable vomiting
Gastric stasis	• Anticholinergic drugs, opioids • Ascites • Hepatomegaly • Peptic ulcer • Gastritis • Stress • Drugs • Radiotherapy • Autonomic failure	Epigastric pain, fullness, nausea, early satiety, flatulence, acid reflux, hiccup, large volume vomits (possibly projectile) gastric regurgitation, other features of autonomic failure
Stretch/distortion of gastrointestinal tract	• Constipation • Intestinal obstruction • Mesenteric metastases	Altered bowel habit, nausea, vomiting, may be feculent, colic
Serosal stretch/irritation	• Liver metastases • Ureteric obstruction • Retroperitoneal cancer	Of underlying condition, nausea, occasional vomiting
Irritation of gastrointestinal tract	• Cryptospordiosis	Profuse diarrhea, nausea, occasional vomiting
Raised intracranial pressure/meningism	• Cerebral edema • Intracranial tumor • Intracranial bleeding • Meningeal infiltration by tumor • Skull metastases • Cerebral infections (AIDS)	Headache (diurnal); papilledema, photophobia may be absent. Nausea may be diurnal; neurologic signs may be absent.
Movement-associated emesis	• Opioids (more common in ambulant patients) • Gut distortion • Gastroparesis → passive regurgitation	Nausea and/or sudden vomits on movement/turning in bed

Anxiety-induced emesis	• Anxiety
	  ○ About self
	  ○ About others
	  ○ About disease
	  ○ About symptoms
	• Anticipatory emesis with cytotoxics
		Waves of nausea ± vomiting, reminders trigger nausea; may be relieved by distraction

Adapted from Hardy J, Glare P, Yates P, et al. Palliation of nausea and vomiting. In: Cherny N, Fallon N, Kaasa S, et al, Editors. Oxford textbook of palliative medicine 5th Edition, Oxford: Oxford University Press; 2015. p. 1661–74; with permission.

Table 4
Selected Etiology-based approaches to palliative symptom management

Symptom	Potential Causes	Etiology-Based Management Approaches
Nausea[21]	Chemotherapy induced	Serotonin antagonists; neurokinin-1 antagonists
	Raised intracranial pressure	Corticosteriods
Pain[22]	Nerve compression or inflammation	Corticosteriods
	Neuropathic pain	Antidepressants, anticonvulsants
	Bone pain without oncological emergency	Non-opioid analgesia; bisphosphonates
Dyspnea	Fluid overload	Low-dose diuretics
	Pleural effusion	Therapeutic procedures, for example, pleurodesis
	Airway obstruction	Low-dose opioids Bronchodilators
	Compression	Radiotherapy, chemotherapy

Table 5
Selected nonpharmacologic strategies for symptom management

Therapy	Potential Uses
Cognitive-behavioral therapies	Address knowledge, beliefs, and behaviors Can assist individuals to reframe misconceptions and disruptive thoughts Promote a sense of control
Mindfulness and relaxation-based therapies	Assist to reduce anxiety and fear
Physical therapy	Optimizes function
Counseling approaches, for example, acceptance commitment therapy and expressive therapies	Promote control Promote expression of feelings

Table 6
Evidence-based principles for communication in palliative care

P	Prepare for the Discussion, Where Possible.
R	Relate to the person.
E	Elicit patient and caregiver preferences.
P	Provide information tailored to the individual needs of both patients and their families.
A	Acknowledge emotions and concerns.
R	(Foster) realistic hope (eg, peaceful death, support).
E	Encourage questions and further discussions.
D	Document.

Adapted from Clayton J, Hancock K, Butow P, et al. Clinical practice guidelines for communicating prognosis and end-of-life issues with adults in the advanced stages of a life-limiting illness, and their caregivers. Med J Aust 2007;186(12):S77–108; with permission.

Box 4
Recommendations for establishing an advance care plan

Ask patient if he/she has a living will, medical power of attorney, health care proxy or patient surrogate for health care; if not, encourage patient to prepare one.

Explore fears about dying and anxiety.

Assess decision-making capacity and need for surrogate decision maker.

Initiate discussions of personal values and preferences for end-of-life care.

If patient values and goals lead to a clear recommendation regarding future treatment in light of disease status, physician should make a recommendation about future care.

Document patient values and preferences in an accessible site in the medical record.

Encourage the patient to discuss wishes with family/proxy.

Initiate discussions of palliative care options including hospice, if appropriate.

Introduce palliative care team if appropriate.

Refer to state and institutional guidelines for additional guidance.

Adapted with permission from the NCCN Clinical Practice Guidelines in Oncology (NCCN Guidelines®) for Palliative Care V.1.2016. © 2016 National Comprehensive Cancer Network, Inc. All rights reserved. The NCCN Guidelines® and illustrations herein may not be reproduced in any form for any purpose without the express written permission of the NCCN. To view the most recent and complete version of the NCCN Guidelines, go online to NCCN.org. NATIONAL COMPREHENSIVE CANCER NETWORK®, NCCN®, NCCN GUIDELINES®, and all other NCCN Content are trademarks owned by the National Comprehensive Cancer Network, Inc.

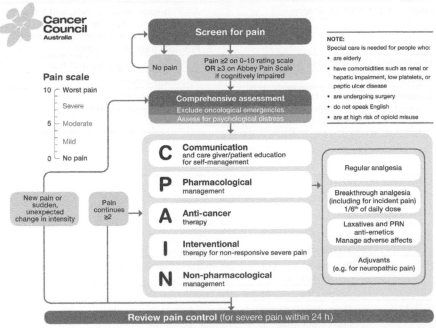

Fig. 2. Putting it all together: a pathway for cancer pain management. (*Reproduced from* Australian Cancer Pain Management Guideline Working Party, Australian Clinical Pathway for Screening, Assessment and Management of Cancer Pain in Adults, Sydney: Cancer Council Australia. Available at: http://wiki.cancer.org.au/australiawiki/images/a/a1/20141015_Overall_cancer_pain_pathway.pdf. Accessed June 25, 2016; with permission.)

dimensions is paramount. See **Table 5** for examples of nonpharmacologic approaches that may be useful on their own or as adjuncts to pharmacologic management.

Communication, Continuity, and Coordination

When patients transition to palliative care, a variety of emotional responses reflecting fears and losses are experienced due to mixed messages, poor communication, and uncertainty.[25] Patients often report limited knowledge about the purpose and timing of transitions, limited involvement in decision making, and concern about the unrealistic information about the level of service available.[26,27] Effective communication is key to optimizing the integration of palliative care and symptom management. **Table 6** summarizes key elements of evidence-based guidelines for effective communication in palliative care.

Effective communication may also require discussion of preferences and wishes and development of advance care plans. **Box 4** summarizes key recommendations for establishing an advance care plan.

Achieving optimal outcomes also requires multiple service providers across many care settings over extended periods of time. Effective team work and interorganizational partnerships are integral to the new paradigm of palliative symptom management. Communication pathways and shared care models can be useful to achieve optimal symptom outcomes in palliative care as patients transition between service providers. **Fig. 2** provides an example of a pain management pathway developed to facilitate continuity and coordination of care.

SUMMARY

Modern cancer treatments have changed the landscape of cancer care. Cancer is now a chronic disease. For those diagnosed with more advanced disease, this can mean living many years with a range of physical and psychological symptoms associated with living with a life-limiting multisystem disease. There is strong evidence that early integration of palliative care can achieve improved quality of life as well as extended survival for those who receive such care. To optimize the outcomes from palliative care for this population, nurses need to have excellent skills in assessing and managing complex dynamic symptom profiles. Such practices include using etiology/evidence-based approaches to symptom management and tailoring management approaches to individual circumstances. Nurses also need to have specialized communication skills that elicit deep understanding of an individual's concerns, demonstrate support, and enable a person's preferences for care to be realized.

REFERENCES

1. Clark D. From margins to centre: a review of the history of palliative care in cancer. Lancet Oncol 2007;8(5):430–8.
2. Smith TJ, Temin S, Alesi ER, et al. American society of clinical oncology provisional clinical opinion: the integration of palliative care into standard oncology care. J Clin Oncol 2012;30:880–7.
3. Cherny NI, Catane R, Schrijvers D, et al. European society for medical oncology (ESMO) program for the integration of oncology and palliative care: a 5-year review of the designated centers' incentive program. Ann Oncol 2010;21:362–9.
4. Metastatic breast cancer network most common statistics cited for MBC. Available at: http://mbcn.org/education/category/most-commonly-used-statistics-for-mbc. Accessed June 26, 2016.

5. Lobb EA, Lacey J, Kearsley J, et al. Living with advanced cancer and an uncertain disease trajectory: an emerging patient population in palliative care? BMJ Support Palliat Care 2015. http://dx.doi.org/10.1136/bmjspcare-2012-000381.

6. William L, Jackson K, Bostanci A, et al. Diagnosis matters: the differing clinical trajectories for terminal prostate, lung and haematological cancers. Aust Fam Physician 2015;44(7):479–84.

7. Teunissen SC, Wesker W, Kruitwagen C, et al. Symptom prevalence in patients with incurable cancer: a systematic review. J Pain Symptom Manage 2007;34: 94–104.

8. Dong ST, Butow PN, Costa DS, et al. Symptom clusters in patients with advanced cancer: a systematic review of observational studies. J Pain Symptom Manage 2014 Sep;48(3):411–50.

9. Meyers FJ, Linder J, Beckett L, et al. Simultaneous care: a model approach to the perceived conflict between investigational therapy and palliative care. J Pain Symptom Manage 2004;28:548–56.

10. Ahmedzai SH, Walsh D. Palliative medicine and modern cancer care. Semin Oncol 2000;27:1–6.

11. Bakitas M, Byock IR, Ahle TA, et al. Effects of a palliative care intervention on clinical outcomes in patients with advanced cancer: the project ENABLE II randomized controlled trial. JAMA 2009;302:741–9.

12. Temel JS, Greer JA, Muzikansky A, et al. Early palliative care for patients with metastatic non–small-cell lung cancer. N Engl J Med 2010;363:733–42.

13. May P, Garrido M, Cassel J, et al. Prospective cohort study of hospital palliative care teams for inpatients with advanced cancer: earlier consultation is associated with larger cost-saving effect. J Clin Oncol 2015;33(25):2745–52.

14. Dodd M, Janson S, Facione N, et al. Advancing the science of symptom management. J Appl Nutr 2001;33:668–76.

15. Brant JM, Beck S, Miaskowski C. Building dynamic models and theories to advance the science of symptom management research. J Appl Nutr 2010;66: 228–40.

16. Lenz ER, Pugh LC, Milligan RA, et al. The middle-range theory of unpleasant symptoms: an update. Adv Nurs Sci 1997;19(3):14–27.

17. Watanabe SM, Nekolaichuk C, Beaumont C, et al. A multicenter study comparing two numerical versions of the edmonton symptom assessment system in palliative care patients. J Pain Symptom Manage 2012;41(2):456–68.

18. Portenoy RK, Thaler HT, Kornblith AB, et al. The memorial symptom assessment scale: an instrument for the evaluation of symptom prevalence, characteristics and distress. Eur J Cancer 1994;30A(9):1326–36.

19. Patient reported outcome version of the common terminology for criteria for adverse events. Available at: http://healthcaredelivery.cancer.gov/pro-ctcae/. Accessed June 26, 2016.

20. Brief pain inventory. Available at: https://www.mdanderson.org/education-and-research/departments-programs-and-labs/departments-and-divisions/symptom-research/symptom-assessment-tools/brief-pain-inventory.html. Accessed June 26, 2016.

21. Hardy J, Glare P, Yates P, et al. Palliation of nausea and vomiting. In: Cherny N, Fallon N, Kaasa S, et al, editors. Oxford textbook of palliative medicine. 5th Edition. Oxford: Oxford University Press; 2015. p. 1661–74.

22. Swarm, Paice J, Anghelescu, et al. NCCN Clinical Practice Guidelines in Oncology (NCCN Guidelines®) Adult Cancer Pain Version 2.2016. © 2016 National

Comprehensive Cancer Network, Inc. Available at: NCCN.org. Accessed December 18, 2016.

23. Yates P, Miaskowski C, Cataldo JK, et al. Differences in composition of symptom clusters between older and younger oncology patients. J Pain Symptom Manage 2015;49(6):1025–34.

24. Chou S, Gaysynsky A, Persoskie A. Health literacy and communication in palliative care. In: Wittenberg E, Ferrell B, Goldsmith J, et al, editors. Textbook of palliative care communication. Oxford: Oxford University Press; 2016. p. 90–101.

25. Larkin PJ, Dierckx de Casterlé B, Schotsmans P. Transition towards end of life in palliative care: an exploration of its meaning for advanced cancer patients in Europe. J Palliat Care 2007;23:69–79.

26. Larkin PJ, Dierckx de Casterlé B, Schotsmans P. Towards a conceptual evaluation of transience in relation to palliative care. J Adv Nurs 2007;59:86–96.

27. Australian cancer pain management pathway. Available at: http://www.cancer.org.au/news/news-articles/cancer-pain-management-in-adults.html.   Accessed June 26, 2016.

Cancer Survivorship, Models, and Care Plans
A Status Update

Lorrie L. Powel, PhD, RN[a],*, Stephen M. Seibert, BS[b]

KEYWORDS

- Cancer • Survivorship • Survivorship care plans • Adult cancer survivors

KEY POINTS

- Multifactorial challenges cancer survivors face after completion of active treatment necessitates an inspection of current models of survivorship care in order to refine and optimize ongoing surveillance and care.
- Formal survivorship care plans have the potential to bridge communication barriers between oncologists and primary care physicians in order to ensure continuity of care for cancer survivors.

INTRODUCTION

The advancements in cancer treatment realized since the National Cancer Act was signed in 1971 resulted in increased numbers of cancer survivors from 3 million in 1971 to 14 million in 2015—an increase of 11 million in 44 years.[1,2] Recent estimates show a continuation of this trend, as the 2016 data suggest that the number of survivors has now surpassed 16 million.[2] Earlier diagnosis and better treatment have resulted in more people living through and beyond cancer. The continual increase in cancer survivors has put a strain on already limited medical resources. If the number of long-term survivors increases at the current pace, the influx of cancer survivors will have a profound impact on health care and health care delivery for decades to come.

This health care burden has been shouldered largely by physicians whose practice focuses on chronic illness and cancer, namely primary care physicians (PCPs) and oncologists, respectively. PCPs and oncologists alike have not been able to keep pace with the growing number of patients with cancer who have completed active treatment.[3–5] Current research has elucidated a need to reorganize posttreatment cancer care in order

Disclosure Statement: The authors have nothing to disclose.
[a] Department of Nursing Research, Scholarship & Science, Louisiana State University Health Science Center School of Nursing, 1900 Gravier Street, New Orleans, LA 70112, USA; [b] Albert Einstein College of Medicine, Bronx, NY, USA
* Corresponding author. 4204 Ferran Drive, Metairie, LA 70002.
E-mail address: lpowe5@lsuhsc.edu

Nurs Clin N Am 52 (2017) 193–209
http://dx.doi.org/10.1016/j.cnur.2016.11.002

to more efficiently manage the growing population of cancer survivors while maintaining a high standard of care.[6,7] This refinement will necessitate an assumption of new roles for oncologists, PCPs, and nurses as well as increased institutional support.[8]

Ironically, the increasing number of cancer survivors has had the greatest effect on survivors themselves.[4] A growing body of cancer survivors faces continued late effects of active treatment, including both physical and psychological sequelae. These late effects compound other more immediate repercussions (ie, changes in function) and secondary effects of cancer treatment, such as adjustment to altered interpersonal, social, and economic circumstances. Managing late effects and comorbidities often falls under the purview of PCPs, yet some oncologists express concerns that PCPs lack the cancer-related expertise to adequately fulfill this role.[9]

Readjusting to day-to-day life after active cancer treatment not only necessitates management of physical and mental obstacles but also requires diligent self-monitoring for signs of recurrence and an assumption of a proactive healthy lifestyle. In order to navigate the complex issues characteristic of cancer survivorship, patients must become informed about the symptoms of recurrence, the presentation of late effects, and the nonphysiologic secondary effects of cancer treatment in order to be an active participant in their follow-up care. The assistance and oversight of a health care provider are pivotal to educating the patient and facilitating the transition from active treatment into survivorship. However, the aforementioned strain that the growing numbers of survivors place on health care resources often prevents patients from receiving adequate guidance.[6]

Considering the substantial advances in active cancer treatment, relatively modest progress has been made in the realm of survivorship care. Few survivors receive the attention and degree of ombudsmanship needed to manage this stage of their cancer trajectory.[7] However, this posttreatment care is not due to a lack of transparency of the needs of patients. In a qualitative study aimed at identifying the barriers to meeting health care needs of survivors, Chubak and colleagues[10] found that 97.5% of clinical leaders in primary and oncology care were able to identify unmet needs of cancer survivors and that most seemed to understand the difficulties patients face while transitioning from active cancer treatment into follow-up care.[10] Nevertheless, unmet need for information pertaining to late effects of cancer treatment, general health promotion, and better management of interpersonal and emotional problems remain endemic among cancer survivors.[11] Many attribute the shortcomings of survivorship care to multifactorial systemic issues that have allowed patients to simply fall through the cracks of an overburdened system.

In 1986, the National Coalition for Cancer Survivors (NCCS) was created to address survivorship issues. This organization was instrumental in redefining the individual's role in facing cancer by changing the label of cancer victim to cancer survivor. The NCCS published its first report concerning quality cancer care from the patient/survivor perspective in 1995. The report opened a dialogue regarding survivorship issues and ultimately led to the 1996 establishment of the Office of Cancer Survivorship (OCS) at the National Cancer Institute (NCI).[12,13]

It has been 2 decades since that initial report. Grassroots efforts of NCCS, coupled with the work of the OCS, the American Cancer Society (ACS), the National Comprehensive Cancer Network (NCCN), the Oncology Nursing Society, the American Society of Clinical Oncology, as well as other professional, nonprofit, and charitable organizations in the United States, Europe, and Canada have come together to address the ongoing needs of cancer survivors[14] (Table 1). The survivorship movement started to gain significant traction after the Institute of Medicine's (IOM) landmark report, *From Cancer Patient to Cancer Survivor: Lost in Transition*[15] (Table 2). It recommends every patient

Table 1 Survivorship organizations	
Survivorship Organization	**Web Address**
National Coalition for Cancer Survivorship (NCCS)	http://www.canceradvocacy.org/
The Office of Cancer Survivorship (OCS)	http://cancercontrol.cancer.gov/ocs/
American Cancer Society (ACS)	http://www.cancer.org/treatment/ survivorshipduringandaftertreatment/
Centers for Disease Control and Prevention (CDC)	https://www.cdc.gov/cancer/survivorship/
Institute of Medicine (IOM)	https://www.nationalacademies.org/ hmd/

receive a survivorship care plan (SCP) that includes a treatment summary, surveillance plan, and care after cancer treatment. The IOM report emphasizes 4 key elements: (1) Prevention of recurrent and new cancers as well as late effects; (2) Surveillance for spread of disease, recurrence, second cancers, and assessment of medical and psychosocial late effects; (3) Interventions for consequences of cancer and its treatments; and (4) Coordination between specialists and primary care providers (**Fig. 1**).[15] Hence, these organizations have initiated changes in the paradigm of cancer survivorship care with an additional focus that transcends the treatment phase.

This introduction provides the backdrop for this article. The purpose of this article is to provide an overview of survivorship; to describe the introduction to and implementation of various models of survivorship care and SCPs; and to identify barriers and facilitators influencing implementation of SCPs. The contradictory research regarding

Table 2 Health care educational programs should	
Physicians	• Add more survivorship-related continuing medical education opportunities. • Improve online survivorship information aimed at health care providers. • Expand training opportunities to promote interdisciplinary, shared care.
Nurses	• Increase survivorship content in undergraduate and graduate nursing programs. • Expand continuing education opportunities on survivorship for practicing nurses. • Increase the number of nursing schools that provide graduate training in oncology. • Increase the number of nurses who seek certification in oncology. • Endorse activities of those working to ease the nursing shortage.
Social workers and other providers of psychosocial services	• Support efforts of American Psychosocial Oncology Society to standardize and promote continuing education. • Endorse activities of those working to maintain social services in cancer programs.

From Hewitt M, Greenfield S, Stovall E. From cancer patient to cancer survivor: lost in transition. Washington, DC: The National Academies Press; 2006; with permission.

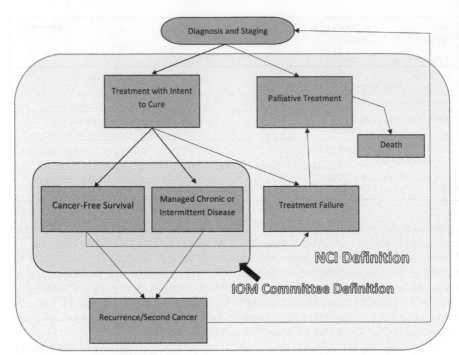

Fig. 1. Definitions of survivorship care. (*From* Hewitt ME, Ganz P. Implementing cancer survivorship care planning: workshop summary. Washington, DC: National Academies Press; 2007.)

the evidence-based benefits of SCPs will also be addressed as well as implications for practice and future research.

CANCER SURVIVORSHIP

The word survivor is derived from Middle French, *survivre*, to outlive, and from the Latin, *supervivere*, to live more. In a sentinel work on cancer survivorship, Fitzhugh Mullan described 3 phases of survivorship: acute survivorship (diagnosis and treatment), extended survivorship (posttreatment), and permanent survivorship (long-term survivorship).[16] In 2009, Miller[17] extended Mullan's survivorship phases to include transitional survivorship: the period of time when the survivor leaves the treatment team with mixed feelings of celebration and worry.

Today, the term survivorship can refer to different aspects of the cancer experience and is defined differently by different groups and organizations. The NCCS, the OCS, the ACS, and the Centers for Disease Control and Prevention (CDC), and others, define survivorship as the period of cancer trajectory from diagnosis until death. Meanwhile, the IOM acknowledges cancer itself as a chronic disease, but interprets survivorship as the distinct phase following completion of active treatment until the end of life.[3,15] Even less concordance regarding the definition of survivorship is observed among health care professionals both interinstitutionally and intrainstitutionally. In a sample of physicians, midlevel providers, nurses, and support service clinicians, 38.7% endorsed the definition of survivorship as "from initial cancer diagnosis on," 34.5% as "upon completion of active therapy and in remission," and 8.5% as "5 years from initial diagnosis."[18] This article uses the IOM definition of survivorship as "a distinct phase following completion of active treatment until the end of life" in order to focus on specific issues related to the juncture between active treatment and follow-up care.

THE IMPORTANCE OF COMMUNICATION IN SURVIVORSHIP CARE

Typically, PCPs hand off patients to oncologists once a patient has been diagnosed with cancer, sometimes before.[19] Afterward, the PCP may not reacquaint with that patient for several years. Over the course of active cancer treatment, oncologists often manage comorbidities (eg, hypertension) survivors may have because they assume several roles that would customarily be managed by the patient's PCP. This exchange introduces confusion on several levels on the completion of primary treatment. Although PCPs in some settings resume care of oncology patients in their practice following active treatment, they are invariably left out of the communication loop once active treatment has been completed and consequently are limited in their capacity to make informed clinical decisions.[5,20] Shortcoming is compounded by the PCP's scope of practice, that is, they are not trained as oncologists and therefore may not recognize clinical indicators of recurrence or other problems and/or may not order surveillance tests at the recommended intervals, and so forth.

Gilbert and colleagues,[21] among others, have acknowledged the imperative role that communication plays in interactions between oncology team members, other providers outside of the oncology team, and the survivors themselves. Without explicit communication and delineation of the roles of health care providers during the transition from primary to secondary care, the ongoing posttreatment needs of survivors have the potential to go unmet. This problem has been well documented in the substandard coordination of care between oncologists and PCPs. In the current system, up to 90% of patients with cancer transition from oncology to primary care without any formalized plan for ongoing treatment and surveillance.[10] The lack of formal communication between oncologists and PCPs has led to a great deal of confusion regarding the roles of each respective physician: 70% of oncologists perceive that they directly manage follow-up care of patients without input from other providers, whereas 50% of PCPs report having an active role in follow-up care.[22] This confusion has the potential to produce either a lack of needed surveillance, under the assumption that the other physician performs necessary screening, or the redundant duplication of surveillance.

The implementation of a formalized posttreatment care plan has the potential to ensure quality follow-up care by strengthening communication between providers and from provider to patient, while also equipping PCPs with the necessary knowledge and tools to efficiently and safely conduct follow-up care of patients.

MODELS OF SURVIVORSHIP CARE PLANS AND SURVIVORSHIP CARE

After the IOM report made the ongoing needs of cancer survivors more salient, a multitude of survivorship care models arose to fulfill the unmet needs of patients with hopes of improving clinical outcomes. Many studies have established that "one size does not fit all"[3] when it comes to survivorship care; each model must flexibly meet the specific needs of its patient population. Nevertheless, shared adherence to the IOM recommendations allows the various models to accomplish similar goals with respect to posttreatment care. The intermodel variation seen in survivorship care models and SCPs typically arises due to differences in health care setting (ie, academic hospital, community-based care center, ambulatory service), a patient's specific cancer diagnosis and/or treatment, and resources available at individual practices and institutions.[23] The 3 models that are discussed here include the longitudinal, consultative, and risk-stratified survivorship care models. **Table 3** highlights the central features of several care models.

Table 3
Survivorship models

Model	Main Features	Who Manages Care	SCP Use	Other Considerations
Consultative[23]	• One-time comprehensive visit • Visit covers treatment summary, follow-up plan, surveillance, late effects, and discusses health promotion	PCP, oncologist, or NP	Yes	• Explicit communication and strong patient involvement[26] • Lack of research-supported benefits[41] • Patients self-report satisfaction with program
Longitudinal[23]	• 1–5-y postactive treatment monitoring • Transfer to PCP once oncologist believes risk of recurrence is adequately low	Oncologist	Sometimes (<50%)	• Cost-intensive[23] • Survivorship care detracts oncologists' time from active treatment[23]
Risk-stratified[24,28]	Intensity of care is proportional to the patient's risk of long-term effects, recurrence, and secondary primaries	PCP, oncologist, or NP	Sometimes (<50%)	Only screening patients when clinically reasonable is more cost-effective[29]
Cancer-specific survivorship[24]	Each clinic focuses on a single cancer site, that is, breast, colorectal, and so forth	PCP, oncologist, or NP	Yes	Specialization to a specific cancer type may allow staff to deliver more focused and individualized information about specific cancer-related health problems[24]
Comprehensive/institutional[24]	Each clinic develops multidisciplinary programs with foci in multiple cancer groups	PCP, oncologist, or NP	Sometimes (<50%)	• Impacts a broader number of survivors than the Cancer-Specific Survivorship model[24] • Generally use various combinations of the other models[24]
Shared care[24]	A patient's oncologist and PCP closely collaborate to organize and execute both primary cancer treatment and survivorship care	PCP and oncologist	Yes	• Clear delineation of roles[24] • Formal points of communication[24]

The longitudinal model is the most frequently used and least formalized model of follow-up care. In this approach, the oncologist monitors the survivor for 1 to 5 years following acute treatment with a focus on surveillance for cancer recurrence and assessment for persistent toxicity of therapy.[24] Once the oncologist thinks that the aftereffects and the risk of recurrence are sufficiently small, ongoing care of the survivor is transferred to the PCP. An oncologist-led long-term follow-up may not be a practical allocation of limited medical resources. One of the corollaries of the longitudinal model is that oncologists' practices are overflowing with long-term survivors, which detracts from oncologists' available time to devote to new and active treatment planning.[23] The reluctance of oncologists to transfer patients to PCPs for follow-up care may be in part due to a pervasive belief among oncologists that PCPs do not possess adequate levels of cancer expertise.[25] However, recent research suggests that no significant statistical difference exists between oncologist-led, PCP-led, or nurse-led follow-up care for most clinical outcomes, including recurrence rate, time to detection of recurrence, death rate, and median time to death.[6,7] Moreover, a cost-effective analysis of the same providers demonstrated that nurse-led follow-ups are significantly more cost-effective than PCP- and oncologist-led follow-ups.[7] **Table 4** compares the different facets of oncologist-led, PCP-led, and nurse-led follow-up care.

The consultative model provides patients with a one-time comprehensive visit at a specialized survivorship clinic as a distinct supplement from ongoing oncology care. During this consultation, a patient will typically meet with an oncologist, PCP, or nurse practitioner (NP) in order to review his/her treatment summary and obtain a newly prescribed SCP. The SCP is a central tenet to the consultative care model; this document provides patients with a detailed and individualized treatment summary, personal recommendations for a healthier lifestyle, information on signs and symptoms of cancer recurrence, and guidelines for follow-up care. The administration of an SCP explicitly delineates the expectations and responsibilities of patients and physicians in an effort to encourage patients to play a more active role in their follow-up care and preclude lapses in patient-provider communication.[23] Some preliminary research has shown that patients demonstrate improved knowledge of relevant follow-up care information and report a higher quality of life after attending a consultative care appointment.[26] Adversaries of SCP use often cite a lack of reimbursement for the extensive time

Table 4
Provider led survivorship models

Who Manages Care	Cost-Effective	Recurrence and Death Rates	Limitations
PCP-led[6]	Less than NP[7]	No difference[6]	Poor communication with oncologist,[9] insufficient knowledge of cancer survivor issues[9]
Oncologist-led[6]	Less than NP[7]	No difference[6]	Survivorship care detracts oncologists' time from active treatment[23]
Nurse-led[7]	Yes[7]	No difference[7]	Poor communication with oncologist,[9] insufficient knowledge of cancer survivor issues,[9] physicians report lack of trust in SCPs created by NPs[38]

required to extract the necessary information to construct the SCP. Tevaarwek and colleagues[27] have demonstrated that using the electronic medical record in order to develop an automated, programmable application that extracts information for SCPs may circumvent this problem by reducing the amount of time required to fill out an SCP to less than 10 minutes. However, the lack of standardization of the EMR and its inconsistent use have delayed any widespread use of the extraction tool. **Table 5** displays the IOM content recommendation for SCPs.

At the core of the risk-stratified survivorship care model is the idea that the intensity of follow-up care should be proportional to the level of risk of long-term effects, recurrence, and secondary primaries.[24,28] Research has demonstrated that among patients without metastatic disease, providing routine cancer screening every 3 months compared with 6 months did not yield any benefit in detection of cancer recurrence.[29] Therefore, providing this low-risk group with a lower intensity of follow-up care is more cost-conscious without being a detriment to the patients' health. By providing a tiered approach, oncologists can reallocate care to those survivors who require closer observation and dedicate more time to addressing the care of both new patients and those undergoing active treatment.[23]

The consultative, longitudinal, and risk-stratified survivorship care models demonstrate an evolution of thought, resultant of both trial-and-error and clinical research,

Table 5 Elements of a survivorship care plan	
Record of care	• Diagnostic tests performed and results • Tumor characteristics • Dates of treatment initiation and completion • Surgery, chemotherapy, radiotherapy, transplant, hormonal therapy, gene or other therapy • Psychosocial, nutritional, and other supportive services provided • Full contact information on treating institutions and key individual providers • Identification of a key point of contact and coordinator of continuing care
Standards of care	• The likely course of recovery from treatment toxicities as well as need for ongoing health maintenance/adjuvant therapy • A description of recommended cancer screening and other periodic testing and examinations and the schedule on which they should be performed • Information on possible late and long-term effects of treatment and symptoms of such effects • Information on possible signs of recurrence and second tumors • Information on possible effects of cancer on marital/partner relationship, sexual functioning, work, and parenting, and the potential future need for psychosocial support • Information on the potential insurance, employment, and financial consequences of cancer and, as necessary, referral to counseling, legal aid, and financial assistance • As appropriate, information on counseling and testing to identify high-risk individuals who could benefit from more comprehensive cancer surveillance, chemoprevention, or risk-reduction surgery • As appropriate, information on known effective chemoprevention strategies for secondary prevention • Referrals to specific follow-up care providers, support groups, and/or the patient's primary care provider • A listing of cancer-related resources and information

From Refs.[15,47,48]

pertaining to the manner in which survivorship care ought to be managed. Traditional follow-up care somewhat mirrored the longitudinal survivorship model, in which a patient's oncologist continues to provide post–active treatment survivorship care; however, as oncologists' practices became saturated with survivors, a need to reorganize the standard of survivorship care emerged. This realignment necessitated an elicitation of increased PCP and NP involvement in survivorship care administration. As such, alternative approaches began to materialize that delegated survivorship care responsibility to members of the health care team aside from oncologists, particularly to PCPs. Although this new standard of follow-up care allowed oncologists to dedicate more time to active treatment planning, it often came at the consequence of continuity of care as patients transitioned from primary oncology to a PCP-led follow-up. In order to meet the transitional needs of patients, the consultative model arose in an effort to explicitly delineate survivorship responsibilities of both the patient and the physician. The enlistment of NPs and PCPs allows the consultative model to be more cost-effective than the longitudinal follow-up, and the generation of an SCP encourages increased patient involvement, which has been linked to improved clinical outcomes.[30] The risk-stratified model is not necessarily mutually exclusive from the consultative or longitudinal models; instead, it can be used in concert with the other survivorship care models in order to further improve cost-effectiveness. For example, at a patient's consultative model appointment, a PCP or NP may deem the patient to be "low risk" in terms of possibility of recurrence. The patient may then subsequently be assigned to a less rigorous follow-up, which has proven to be more cost-effective without detracting from positive health outcomes.

Examples of other models include the Institutional/comprehensive care model and the shared-care model.[21,31] Although the intent of all of the models is to provide tailored care centering on quality, comprehensive, and coordinated care,[31] each approach enlists different medical resources, and the cost-effectiveness of each model must be considered in order to most efficiently direct follow-up care.

BARRIERS AND FACILITATORS TO SURVIVORSHIP CARE PLAN IMPLEMENTATION

Providers and institutions alike struggled to implement SCPs in the years following the IOM report. A study of 53 NCI-designated cancer centers revealed that only 44% reported SCP use after 8 years. Even among the centers that reported SCP use, 69% reported using SCPs for less than half of all patients.[32] Moreover, the content of currently used SCPs shows an inadequate level of concordance with several IOM recommendations, especially pertaining to information regarding psychosocial services, physical therapy and nutritional services, recommendations for ongoing care, where to receive future testing, and the possibility of late effects.[8] Although many thought that the introduction of the IOM recommendations would bolster the prevalence of SCP use and better address the needs of patients transitioning from active treatment to survivorship, a myriad of inherent deficiencies and institutional obstacles has stymied the implementation of SCPs[33] (Table 6).

The ineffectual guidelines for SCP implementation have likely produced a formidable barrier to ubiquitous application. A study by Birken and colleagues[32] reviewed 16 SCP implementation guidelines and maintained that nearly all of the guidelines lacked practical applicability; namely, most of the guidelines neglected to discuss barriers to SCP implementation and only half recommended a specific SCP template. Furthermore, the study highlighted a disagreement concerning when SCPs should be implemented. Although some guidelines suggested an SCP should be provided upon the completion of active treatment, others thought it should be provided upon

Table 6	
Facilitators and barriers to survivorship care plan use	
Facilitators	**Barriers**
• CoC standards	• Time required to extract relevant
• NCCN guidelines	information
• Grant funding	• Obtaining medical records from other
• Institutional commitment	clinics
• Flexibility, team meetings, appointment	• Poor reimbursement
of a team leader	• Poor institutional support
• Strong communication between PCP	• Insufficient training of staff
and oncologist	• Inadequate oncologist recommendations
• Regular and complete IT documentation	• Poor information technology

Data from Refs.[8,9,32]

initial diagnosis.[34] This discrepancy is likely embedded in the aforementioned absence of an agreed upon definition of a "cancer survivor." The IOM established a high standard for the quality of SCPs; however, without a practical means of application, the objectives of the IOM cannot come to fruition.

Another commonly cited barrier to implementation of SCPs is that it is a resource-intensive process; recent studies have reported the development of SCPs takes from 1 to 4 hours to complete.[9,35] As previously mentioned, preliminary evidence may suggest that the enlistment of the EMR in conjunction with an automated programmable application may streamline the process of developing SCPs. Nonetheless, the fragmentary, incomplete status of the EMR and the fact that some information needs human interpretation have perhaps slowed widespread implementation of such an automated program.[9,36,37] A common source of contention has been determining whom among the professional and support staff should extrapolate and interpret the necessary information from the medical record to develop the treatment summary and the plan of care. There has also been debate about which provider, that is, physician, NP, or physician's assistant, should discuss the plan with the patient and coordinate care with the PCP.[31] Although recent research has established that no difference in recurrence rates exists between nurse-led and physician-led survivorship follow-ups,[7] physicians report being skeptical about the quality of SCPs developed by NPs.[38]

Other institutionally engrained obstacles likely further contribute to low levels of SCP use. The LIVESTRONG Foundation assessed the barriers and facilitators to implementing SCPs across 8 NCI-designated Comprehensive Cancer Centers and LIVE-STRONG Centers of Excellence (COE) from 2004 to 2008[33] (**Box 1**). They conducted both qualitative and quantitative methods of inquiry using the Chronic Care Model as the overarching framework. Methodologies used included document reviews, semistructured telephone interviews with 39 key informants, an online survey (N = 40), and 3 site visits. Models of care across the COE sites included survivorship, integrative, and consultative models. The study found that numerous health system factors contributed as barriers as well as facilitators to SCP implementation. Having strong leadership support with program champions at various levels of the organization played a key role in facilitating SCP implementation. Predictably, the lack of these components served as a barrier. Other impediments included reimbursement issues (ie, no specific financial mechanism to support care specific to cancer survivors), lack of space, and lack of leadership commitment to changes in clinical programs. Common to all programs was a lack of information systems infrastructure and a lack of focus on survivor self-management.[33]

Box 1
Goals of the LIVESTRONG Survivorship Centers of Excellence Network

- Transform how survivors are perceived, treated, and served
- Help create a body of knowledge, evidence, and understanding of survivorship care
- Develop and deliver evidence-based treatment and care interventions
- Improve the quality and integration of survivorship services
- Strengthen the link between primary care treatment and survivorship care
- Increase accessibility to services among ethnically diverse and underserved survivors
- Help find sources of support to sustain survivorship centers over the long term
- Create insurance or reimbursement mechanisms to cover survivor care and services

From LIVESTRONG Survivorship Centers of Excellence. Available at: https://www.livestrong.org/what-we-do/program/centers-of-excellence-network. Accessed May 19, 2016.

One strong driving force behind SCP implementation has been the requirement of the American College of Physicians Commission on Cancer (CoC) that centers accredited by the CoC must have SCPs in place by 2019. Implementation has been repeatedly stymied because institutions including university teaching hospitals, community institutions, private practices, and many cancer centers—even NCI-designated comprehensive cancers—have not been prepared to overcome the various impediments to SCP implementation. Consequently, the "deadline" for implementation has been repeatedly extended as further measures have been put in place to facilitate the integration of SCPs into routine care.[39,40] **Box 2** details the current CoC accreditation requirements.

IMPACT OF SURVIVORSHIP CARE PLAN ON PATIENT OUTCOMES

A decade following the IOM report, evidence of improved patient outcomes from SCP usage has been limited. For example, in a 2014 systematic review of SCPs that included 10 prospective studies of 2286 survivors (5 randomized controlled trials), the use of SCPs showed no significant effect on survivor distress, satisfaction with care, cancer care coordination, or oncologic outcomes.[35] This result been corroborated by other studies. In a 2011 randomized trial of 408 breast cancer survivors, the use of SCPs produced no advantage in cancer-specific distress, general psychological distress, or

---

Box 2
Commission on cancer accreditation requirements

- January 1, 2015: Implement a pilot survivorship care plan process involving 10% of eligible patients.
- January 1, 2016: Provide survivorship care plans to 25% of eligible patients.
- January 1, 2017: Provide survivorship care plans to 50% of eligible patients.
- January 1, 2018: Provide survivorship care plans to 75% of eligible patients.
- January 1, 2019: Provide survivorship care plans to all eligible patients.

From Accreditation Committee Clarifications for Standard 3.3 Survivorship Care Plan. Available at: https://www.facs.org/publications/newsletters/coc-source/special-source/standard33. Accessed May 18, 2016.

physical- and mental-related quality of life.[41] Similarly, in a 2015 randomized trial of breast cancer survivors, the use of SCPs did not influence a patient's adherence to treatment, the patient's ability to correctly identify the physician primarily responsible for their follow-up care, or the frequency of postdischarge visits.[42]

There are likely many contributory factors preventing a demonstrable benefit of SCPs, many of which have already been acknowledged. As previously mentioned, although stakeholders seem clear on the elements of the IOM report, its implementation is less clear—there are so many variations on the theme. The various configurations of health care settings require flexibility in order to meet the needs of patients they treat; however, the resultant lack of a standardized approach makes it difficult to assess outcomes empirically.[25,28] Moreover, as previously addressed, current SCPs do not incorporate many of the IOM recommendations that may be paramount to improving patient outcomes. Attempts to develop a plan that addresses the care of patients transitioning from active treatment to survivorship have accentuated problems revolving around coordination of care at that juncture and on into survivorship. The handoff between the oncology team and the PCPs remains a major concern. Even with the introduction of nascent SCPs, communication—the common bond between the patient and the providers—continues to be inadequate. These weaknesses, namely the lack of SCP standardization, only partial fulfillment of IOM recommendations, and poor communication between the survivor and providers, are likely key barriers to studying and demonstrating improved patient outcomes.[43]

One area that has received less attention than the mechanics of implementation and outcomes of SCPs is the degree to which survivors understand information communicated to them by their health care providers.[44] Another explanation for the lack of significant evidence supporting the benefits of SCPs is patients may not always understand the information in the SCP. They may be embarrassed to admit that they do not clearly understand what the provider told them, do not know the correct questions to ask, or are afraid to challenge their provider. Some may not know they have the right and responsibility to understand medical information given to them.

This explanation is particularly reasonable for survivors with low health literacy (LHL). Indeed, these are the survivors who would likely benefit most from an SCP. Simply providing individuals of low income and low literacy with information at discharge is insufficient to affect understanding of communicated cancer information or incorporation of risk reduction behaviors. Only 12% of US adults are proficient enough in health literacy to understand and use health information effectively.[44] It should be noted that LHL is not specific to survivors of low general literacy or those representative of minority and underserved populations, although it is more of a problem in these groups. Kent and colleagues[11] demonstrated that nonwhite cancer survivors report a higher number of unmet needs and a lower physical and mental quality of life. Recent studies have examined interventions specific to minority and non-English speaking survivors. However, overall, the impact on minority groups and those of LHL has not been well studied. **Fig. 1** provides evidence-based guidelines from the Agency for Healthcare Research and Quality for health care professionals to promote universal understanding of health care information for all patients, irrespective yet inclusive of all levels of health literacy (**Table 7**).[45]

CLINICAL PRACTICE AND RESEARCH IMPLICATIONS

Despite the progress made in cancer treatment, prevention, and detection, assisting patients to transition to survivorship has not been addressed in a comprehensive manner. As survivors complete the treatment phase of their cancer trajectory—a

Table 7
Agency for health research and quality low health literacy recommendations

Spoken Communication	Written Communication	Self-Management and Empowerment	Supportive Systems
• Use clear, direct communication	• Ensure all written documents provided to patients have a patient-appropriate level of readability and understandability	• Invite questions, use strategies to elicit questions, that is, asking what can we review again?	• Link patients with available community resources that provide assistance with transportation, food, employment, budgeting, and housing
• Ask patients to repeat in their own words what they need to know or do about their health (teach-back method)	• Ask patients to evaluate forms and other written materials	• Remind patients to bring questions to appointments and help patients prioritize questions	• Review patients' insurance coverage and connect them with medicine assistance programs
• Use follow-ups to check in on a patient's progress	• Do not assume patients will read all health-related pamphlets and materials given them. Guide patient through written material using the teach-back method	• Create an action plan that outlines one or more easy steps for patients to take in order to achieve goals	• Refer patients to an adult learning center for literacy and math enhancement
• Ensure the health care facility has patient-friendly telephone access	• Ensure a welcoming practice	• Help patients remember how and when to take their medications	• Do not rely on patients to relay information from other health care team members
• Have patients bring all of their medications and supplements to review them	• Offer help with the forms patients are asked to fill out or sign	• Provide patients with a list of medications, provide pill boxes, synchronize refills, and enlist help from family members	• Offer help with referrals, make sure patients understand reasons for referrals, provide clear instructions, and follow up on referrals
• Ask patients for their preferred language and use an interpreter or other language assistance if necessary	• Create a brochure that highlights key elements of your practice		
• Remain sensitive to religious, cultural, ethnic, or any other beliefs that may influence health care decision making and the way advice is received	• Use the waiting room to display important information		

From AHRQ Health Literacy Universal Precautions Toolkit. 2016. Rockville (MD): Agency for Healthcare Research and Quality. Available at: http://www.ahrq.gov/professionals/quality-patient-safety/quality-resources/tools/literacy-toolkit/index.html; and Health Literacy. 2014. Rockville (MD). Agency for Healthcare Research and Quality. Available at: http://www.ahrq./gov/research/findings/factsheets/literacy/healthlit/index.html. Accessed April 15, 2016.

phase that has become their norm over the last 6 months or year, depending on their treatment—they face a pivotal point in their care, the transition from the active phase of treatment to cancer survivorship. As such, they are faced with new norms and adjustments to their interpersonal, social, and economic circumstances.

As survivors take a more active role in their own care, they need to have an understanding of the treatment they have undergone and what to expect going forward, be it adjusting to changes in physical function, recognizing and managing late-term effects of treatment, or making a plan for surveillance follow-up. It is not uncommon for patients to find themselves feeling as though they are in a whole new world, unaware of how to manage their new reality. Nurses play an important role in easing the angst survivors often feel as they transition to a survivorship phase. They can be instrumental in closing the gaps in the development and coordination of SCPs through collaborative efforts with oncologists and PCPs.[46,47]

The literature is replete with articles on the various facets of survivorship and SCPs, be it models, implementation, timing, communication, types of providers, and if and how these do or do not have an impact on addressing the myriad of issues survivorship entails. One issue that has not been well studied is the degree to which survivors adopt and sustain behaviors articulated in their SCPs. That is, it is not clear if survivors assume behaviors that promote a healthy lifestyle or other aspects of their SCP. Nurse researchers could examine if SCP booster sessions are necessary to support survivorship, for example, sessions following the initial SCP discussion. Within that context, it would be important to determine the content of the booster session, the intervention dosage, and the degree to which the booster session or sessions influence self-management of components of the SCP, for example, actively participate in healthy behaviors, such as diet and exercise.

Survivorship research will benefit from more clinical trials on the influence of SCPs on specific clinical outcomes, including both short- and long-term effects. Although preliminary trials that fail to establish any appreciable benefit of SCPs on patient outcomes may be disconcerting, a lack of SCP standardization and failure to customarily adhere with certain IOM standards may undermine the potential benefits of SCPs. Meanwhile, although there have been a few studies on the development and use of SCPs for survivors who are members of minority populations, the authors are unaware of studies that specifically assess health literacy or examine the degree to which survivors understand the SCP, education, and/or counseling received. Studies like these will contribute to evidence needed to provide comprehensive survivorship care.

SUMMARY

The number of cancer survivors is increasing and will continue to grow exponentially as prevention and detection, imaging, and cancer treatment modalities advance. The sheer number of survivors creates challenges in providing comprehensive care to cancer survivors. The 2006 IOM report underscored the prevalence of substandard care recommending every patient receive a treatment summary and plan for future care (SCP) at the conclusion of active cancer treatment. Regrettably, there have been obstacles to the broad adoption and implementation of SCPs and ultimately comprehensive survivorship care. An appropriate balance between individualization and standardization of SCPs needs to be established. Little conclusive information is known regarding the impact of the SCPs on patient outcomes and how, when, or by whom they should be implemented. It is also not clear how SCPs should be administered in specific populations, for example, those with LHL, minority groups, and non-English speakers.[31] These issues challenge us to conduct more research to evaluate the effectiveness of current strategies and determine the next steps in the development of methods that enable providers to offer comprehensive care for cancer survivors.

REFERENCES

1. Valdivieso M, Kujawa AM, Jones T, et al. Cancer survivors in the United States: a review of the literature and a call to action. Int J Med Sci 2012;9(2):163–73.
2. American Cancer Society. Cancer Facts & Figures 2016. Atlanta (GA): American Cancer Society; 2016.
3. Ganz PA. Quality of care and cancer survivorship: the challenge of implementing the Institute of Medicine recommendations. J Oncol Pract 2009;5(3):101–5.
4. Potosky AL, Han PKJ, Rowland J, et al. Differences between primary care physicians' and oncologists' knowledge, attitudes and practices regarding the care of cancer survivors. J Gene Med 2011;26(12):1403–10.
5. Shulman LS, Jacobs LA, Greenfield S, et al. Cancer care and cancer survivorship care in the United States: will we be able to care for these patients in the future? J Oncol Pract 2009;5(3):119–23.
6. Wattchow DA, Weller DP, Esterman A, et al. General practice vs surgical-based follow-up for patients with colon cancer: randomised controlled trial. Br J Cancer 2006;94(8):1116–21.
7. Knowles GH, Jodrell DI. Recent developments in adjuvant chemotherapy for colorectal cancer. Eur J Cancer Care 1997;6(1):18–22.
8. Salz T, Oeffinger KC, McCabe MS, et al. Survivorship care plans in research and practice. CA Cancer J Clin 2012;62(2):101–17.
9. Dulko D, Pace CM, Dittur KL, et al. Barriers and facilitators to implementing cancer survivorship care plans. Oncol Nurs Forum 2013;40(6):575–80.
10. Chubak J, Tuzzio L, Hsu C, et al. Providing care for cancer survivors in integrated health care delivery systems: practices, challenges, and research opportunities. J Oncol Pract 2012;8(3):184–9.
11. Kent EE, Arora NK, Rowland JH, et al. Health information needs and health-related quality of life in a diverse population of long-term cancer survivors. Patient Educ Couns 2012;89(2):345–52.
12. Clark EJ, Stovall EL, Leigh S, et al. Imperatives for quality cancer care. Silver Springs (MD): National Coalition for Cancer Survivorship; 1995.
13. Office of cancer survivorship. 2016. Available at: http://www.canceradvocacy.org/about-us/our-history. Accessed May 27, 2016.
14. Rowland JH, Kent EE, Forsythe LP, et al. Cancer Survivorship Research in Europe and the United States: where have we been, where are we going, and what can we learn from each other? Cancer 2014;119(11):2094–108.
15. Hewitt M, Greenfield S, Stovall E. From cancer patient to cancer survivor: lost in transition. Washington, DC: The National Academies Press; 2006.
16. Mullan F. Seasons of survival: reflections of a physician with cancer. N Engl J Med 1985;313:270–3.
17. Miller K. Revisiting the seasons of survival. Available at: http://www.curetoday.com/publications/cure/2009/summer2009/revisiting-the-seasons-of-survival?p=2. Accessed May 1, 2016.
18. Gage EA, Pailler M, Zevon MA, et al. Structuring survivorship care: discipline-specific clinician perspectives. J Cancer Surviv 2011;5(3):217–25.

19. Sussman J, Balwin L. The interface of primary and oncology specialty care: treatment through survivorship. J Natl Cancer Inst Monogr 2010;40:18–24.
20. Blanch-Hartigan D, Forsythe LP, Alfano CM, et al. Provision and discussion of survivorship care plans among cancer survivors: results of a nationally representative survey of oncologists and primary care physicians. J Clin Oncol 2014;32:1–8.
21. Gilbert SM, Miller DC, Hollenbeck BK, et al. Cancer survivorship—challenges and changing paradigms. J Urol 2008;179(2):431–8.
22. Klabunde CN, Han PKJ, Earle CC, et al. Physician roles in the cancer-related follow-up care of cancer survivors. Fam Med 2013;45(7):463–74.
23. McCabe MS, Jacobs LA. Clinical update: survivorship care–models and programs. Semin Oncol Nurs 2012;28(3):e1–8.
24. Oeffinger KC, McCabe MS. Models for delivering survivorship care. J Clin Oncol 2006;24(32):5117–24.
25. Kantsiper M, McDonald EL, Geller G, et al. Transitioning to breast cancer survivorship: perspectives of patients, cancer specialists, and primary care providers. J Gen Intern Med 2009;24(Suppl 2):459–66.
26. Curcio KR, Lambe C, Schneider S, et al. Evaluation of a cancer survivorship protocol. Clin J Oncol Nurs 2012;16(4):400–6.
27. Tevaarwek AJ, Wisinski KB, Buhr KA, et al. Leveraging electronic health record systems to create and provide electronic cancer survivorship care plans: a pilot study. J Oncol Pract 2014;10(3):e150–9.
28. McCabe MS, Partridge AH, Grunfeld E, et al. Risk-based health care, the cancer survivor, the oncologist, and the primary care physician. Semin Oncol 2013;40(6):804–12.
29. Kokko R, Hakama M, Holli K. Follow-up cost of breast cancer patients with localized disease after primary treatment: a randomized trial. Breast Cancer Res Treat 2005;93(3):255–60.
30. Mazor HM, Rubin DL, Roblin DW, et al. Health literacy-listening skill and patient questions following cancer prevention and screening discussions. Health Expect 2016;19(4):920–34.
31. Wolin KY, Colditz GA, Proctor EK. Maximizing benefits for effective cancer survivorship programming: Defining a dissemination and implementation plan. Oncologist 2011;16:1189–96.
32. Birken SA, Presseau J, Ellis SD, et al. Potential determinants of health-care professionals' use of survivorship care plans: a qualitative study using the theoretical domains framework. Implement Sci 2014;9:167.
33. Campbell MK, Tessaro I, Gellin M, et al. Adult cancer survivorship care: experiences from the LIVESTRONG centers of excellence network. J Cancer Surviv 2011;5(3):271–82.
34. Birken SA, Ellis SD, Walker JS, et al. Guidelines for the use of survivorship care plans: a systematic quality appraisal using the AGREE II instrument. Implement Sci 2015;10:63.
35. Brennan ME, Gormally JF, Butow P, et al. Survivorship care plans in cancer: a systematic review of care plan outcomes. Br J Cancer 2014;111(10):1899–908.
36. De Moor JS, Mariotto AB, Parry C, et al. Cancer survivors in the United States: prevalence across the survivorship trajectory and implications for care. Cancer Epidemiol Biomarkers Prev 2013;22(4):561–70.
37. Available at: https://www.livestrong.org/what-we-do/program/centers-of-excellence-network. Accessed May 19, 2016.
38. Shalom MM, Hahn EE, Casillas J, et al. Do survivorship care plans make a difference? A primary care provider perspective. J Oncol Pract 2011;7(5):314–8.

39. Cancer program standards: ensuring patient-centered care. American College of Surgeons, 2016 edition. Chicago, IL.
40. Hershman DL, Ganz PA. Quality of care, including survivorship care plans. Adv Exp Med Biol 2015;862:255–69.
41. Grunfield E, Julian JA, Pond G, et al. Evaluating survivorship care plans: results of a randomized, clinical trial of patients with breast cancer. J Clin Oncol 2011; 29(36):4755–62.
42. Boekhout AH, Maunsell E, Pond GP, et al. A survivorship care plan for breast cancer survivors: extended results of a randomized clinical trial. J Cancer Surviv 2015;9(4):683–91.
43. Mayer DK, Birken SA, Check DK, et al. Summing it up: an integrative review of studies of cancer survivorship care plans (2006-2013. Cancer 2015;121(7): 978–96.
44. Department of Health & Human Services. Americans health literacy: why we need accessible health information. Washington, DC: US Department of Health and Human Services; 2008.
45. Health Literacy. 2014. Agency for healthcare research and quality. Rockville (MD). Available at: http://www.ahrq.gov/research/findings/factsheets/literacy/healthlit/index.html. Accessed March 3, 2016.
46. Cooper JM, Loeb SJ, Smith CA. The primary care nurse practitioner and cancer survivorship care. J Am Acad Nurse Pract 2010;22(8):394–402.
47. Institute of Medicine of the National Academies, Cancer Survivorship Care Planning Fact Sheet, November 2005. In: Hewitt M, Greenfield S, Stovall E, editors. From Cancer Patient to Cancer Survivor: Lost in transition. National Cancer Policy Board. Institute of Medicine and National Research Council of the National Academies. Washington, DC: The National Academies Press; 2005. p. 24.
48. Hewitt M, Greenfield S, Stovall E. From cancer patient to cancer survivor: Lost in transition. National Cancer Policy Board. Institute of Medicine and National Research Council of the National Academies. Washington, DC: The National Academies Press; 2005. p. 24.

Equity in Cancer Care
Strategies for Oncology Nurses

Tracy Truant, RN, MSN, PhD(c)

KEYWORDS

• Oncology • Cancer • Nursing • Inequities • Advocacy • Leadership

KEY POINTS

• Despite improvements in cancer treatment and outcomes, inequities have been increasingly documented in the cancer population, particularly among those experiencing marginalizing conditions within society.

• Oncology nurses have a social justice imperative to address inequities in cancer care, although this aspect of their role is underdeveloped.

• Equity-oriented strategies that draw on a social justice imperative consider the social determinants of health, as well as those factors, contexts, and structures that influence individuals' ability to optimize their health.

• To effectively address inequities, oncology nurses may take a two-pronged approach, including equity-oriented strategies focusing on the direct care of individuals and communities, as well as addressing the root causes of inequity through leadership, policy influence, advocacy, education, and research.

INTRODUCTION

A central tenet of high quality cancer care includes equitable care for all.[1–4] However, even within high-resource countries, such as Canada and the United States, achieving equitable and quality cancer care largely remains unrealized. Increasingly, health inequities (sometimes called health disparities) are documented among people living with cancer, particularly individuals living in rural and remote settings, of lower socioeconomic status, who are older with advanced disease at diagnosis, indigenous groups, ethnic minorities, and immigrants.[1,5–9] Most efforts to address cancer care inequities are aimed at improving access to care (eg, through the introduction of nurse navigator roles), or by attempting to change behaviors (eg, smoking cessation, healthy eating, exercise programs). Despite these efforts, cancer care inequities persist and are increasing in many areas.[5] These narrowly focused efforts may never fully address inequities and may unintentionally marginalize vulnerable people. A broader view is needed that incorporates the social determinants of health (SDH), including factors

School of Nursing, University of British Columbia, T201-2211 Wesbrook Mall, Vancouver, British Columbia V6S1R6, Canada
E-mail address: Tracy.truant@nursing.ubc.ca

Nurs Clin N Am 52 (2017) 211–225
http://dx.doi.org/10.1016/j.cnur.2016.11.003
0029-6465/17/© 2016 Elsevier Inc. All rights reserved.

nursing.theclinics.com

such as contexts and structures that shape and influence abilities to optimize health and ensure equity during the cancer experience.[10–15]

Oncology nurses have an important yet underdeveloped role to play in addressing cancer care inequities. Nurses have an ethical and social justice imperative to support and advocate for optimal health for individuals and groups. Addressing inequities is a core philosophic tenet and code of ethics standard.[10–12,16] It is vital that oncology nurses understand and embrace their role in promoting equity and reducing cancer care inequities.

This article provides a backdrop for understanding and explaining oncology nurses' role and action imperative in addressing cancer care inequities. Although the discussion focuses on the Canadian and North American context, there are opportunities for application to oncology nurses and cancer care settings around the world. This article begins by unpacking concepts central to inequities, such as equity, inequality, and justice (**Fig. 1**). With equity as a goal in cancer care, it is important to incorporate the SDH in oncology nursing care, including key factors, contexts, ideologies, and structures shaping inequities (**Fig. 2**). Recommendations promoting equity-oriented care are presented, informing oncology nurses' participation in addressing inequities in the cancer care context. A two-pronged approach to address cancer care inequities offers oncology nurses strategies to use in their practice with individuals, families, and communities, and addresses root causes of inequities through policy, leadership, advocacy, education, and research perspectives (**Box 1**).

ALL CANCERS ARE NOT EQUAL

A complex array of factors interact to determine the disease trajectory for individuals diagnosed with any of over 200 types of cancer. Certain cancers, such as pancreatic, liver, lung, and head and neck cancer, are associated with greater morbidity and shorter survival time.[17,18] Risk factors for these cancers may include lower socioeconomic status, male sex, alcohol use, smoking, and viral infections such as hepatitis B and C.[6] Conversely, breast and prostate cancer, although diagnosed more frequently, are associated with longer survival times and less morbidity when compared with pancreatic, liver, lung, and head and neck cancer.[18] The biology of the cancer itself

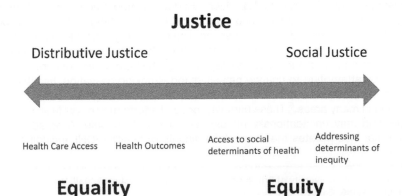

Fig. 1. Equity, equality, and justice in health care. (*From* Varcoe C. Health disparities in cancer care: foundational concepts. In: Varcoe C, Habib S, Sinding C, et al. Health disparities in cancer care: exploring Canadian, American and international perspectives. Can Oncol Nurs J 2015;25:73–4; with permission.)

Box 1
Two-pronged mandate for oncology nurses to promote equity in cancer care

1. Practice (individual and/or community level)
   - Emancipatory knowing
   - Assessment, interventions, and evaluations that include the SDH
   - Understand intersectional effects of the SDH; avoid essentializing individuals
   - Support self-care strategies; attention to structures influencing agency to adopt self-care
   - Culturally sensitive care
   - Sensitivity to issues of power, trust, and respect

2. Address root causes (structural determinants)
   - Leadership, policy, and advocacy
     - Nursing conceptual frameworks include the SDH, contexts, and structures, and focus at collective level.
     - Build cancer care models
       - Focus on patient needs (vs system needs)
       - Embed oncology nursing expertise where it is most needed and/or accessible to patients across health systems (vs adding navigator role)
       - Build relationships between patients and health care professionals
     - Strengthen nurses' political competence (policy analysis and advocacy)
     - Workplace policy commitment to address the SDH
     - Advocate for health in all policies
     - Include vulnerable groups to inform advocacy and policy agendas
     - Collaborative action among oncology professional organizations regarding social justice and the SDH
   - Education
     - Undergraduate nursing education to include the SDH and social justice concepts
     - Graduate nursing programs to include policy courses (skills in policy analysis and advocacy)
   - Research
     - Generate contextual knowledge (ie, qualitative methods) to better understand inequities in cancer care
     - Research policy analysis to better understand links between evidence and policy uptake and/or utilization
     - Determine policy advocacy best practices

Adapted from Reutter L, Kushner KE. 'Health equity through action on the social determinants of health': taking up the challenge in nursing. Nurs Inq 2010;17:269; with permission.

---

accounts for some of the morbidity and mortality but some of the differences also can be explained by the social, political, historical, and economic context in which individuals with these types of cancer live. Race, sex, gender, minority status, poverty, low socioeconomic status, and rural and remote geography, for example, all have been demonstrated to affect the stage of diagnosis and access to high-quality treatment, which, in turn, affects quality of life and survival.[7,19–27]

The complex social, economic, and environmental circumstances in which people live also influences options for health behaviors and health care access and utilization.[23,25,27–30] "The receipt of health care is the outcome of many different complex processes, of which all need to be recognized if access is to be properly understood."[31]

UNPACKING INEQUITIES: EQUITY, EQUALITY, AND SOCIAL JUSTICE

It is important for oncology nurses to understand the concepts of equity, equality, and justice (see **Fig. 1**) to more fully inform their role and strategies to address inequities and to move the equity agenda forward. Dialogues about equity must first be framed

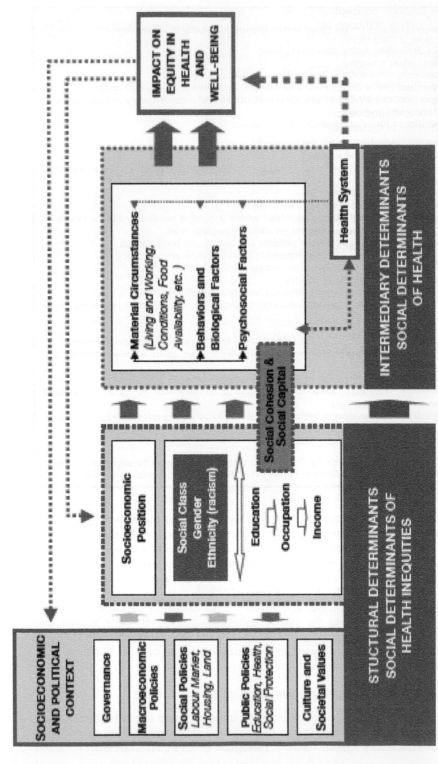

Fig. 2. Commission on the Social Determinants of Health framework. (*From* Solar O, Irwin A. A conceptual framework for action on the social determinants of health. Social determinants of health discussion paper 2 (policy and practice). Geneva (Switzerland): World Health Organization; 2010. Available at: http://www.who.int/sdhconference/resources/ConceptualframeworkforactiononSDH_eng.pdf; with permission of the publisher.)

within the broader concept of justice (fairness), differentiating social justice from distributive justice. Although social justice begins with understanding differences between groups, it also highlights the conditions that shape inequities.[32,33]

According to the World Health Organization, health equity is "the absence of unfair and avoidable or remediable differences in health among population groups defined socially, economically, demographically or geographically."[34] Health, as a social phenomenon, is shaped by the interplay of structural (eg, socioeconomic, political, and historical context; socioeconomic position) and intermediary (eg, material circumstances, biological factors, behaviors, psychosocial factors, health system) factors[34] (**Fig. 2**). Health inequities, then, are health differences that are socially produced, systematically distributed across a population, unfair, and potentially remediable.[35] **Box 2** highlights definitions of social justice versus distributive justice.

An example of distributive justice includes promoting patient access to oncology nursing care and treatment expertise through navigator roles. Improved access for individuals fortunate enough to have a nurse navigator will have positive benefits for that individual. This distributive justice approach does not consider factors, conditions, or contexts that shape the lack of access for individuals nor does it consider other individuals who lack access to a nurse navigator. This type of justice alone may unwittingly set up further health inequities between groups. It is essential that oncology nurses also take a social justice perspective addressing upstream factors. Structural determinants (eg, race, class, gender) are referred to as upstream factors because they sustain hierarchies, ultimately shape individuals' health outcomes, and may reinforce inequities.[34,35,38] Effective strategies to address health inequities must include attention to upstream factors, disrupting power hierarchies, creating healthy policies, and shifting social and cultural values. Without a social justice perspective, adding a nurse navigator becomes a bandage for a broken system that lacks capacity to optimize health equity for all individuals at risk for and/or living with cancer.

ONCOLOGY NURSING AND THE SOCIAL DETERMINANTS OF HEALTH

A social justice approach to promoting equity requires oncology nurses to understand the SDH and their role in promoting high quality cancer care for individuals, groups, and populations. **Fig. 2** illustrates how structural determinants affect intermediary SDH (ie, material circumstances, biological factors, behaviors, psychosocial factors, health system). Structural determinants influence the distribution of money, power, and resources, and are shaped by governmental and social policies, as well as societal and cultural values.

Box 2
Definitions: social justice versus distributive justice

According to Kirkham and Browne, "social justice draws attention to the application of justice to social groups; brings into focus how justice and injustices are sustained through social institutions and social relationships; and highlights the embeddedness of individual experience in a larger realm of political, economic, cultural, and social complexities".[36]

Distributive justice, although also about fairness, deals with the allocation of resources, commonly based on neoliberal, economic, and biomedical reductionist foundations for redistributing and improving access to resources. Attention to distributive justice alone ignores the social interconnectedness of individuals and the influence of structures (eg, health care institutions, policies) that may subtly oppress.[36,37]

In oncology nursing, a focus on the SDH demonstrates the interplay of social, environmental, political, and economic factors shaping cancer risk, experiences, and outcomes, instead of looking for a single biological factor or health behavior accounting for cancer risk and/or outcomes. For example, **Box 3** offers an exemplar of this interplay of factors related to smoking cessation as an important health promoting nursing intervention.

CONTEXTS AND STRUCTURES SHAPING INEQUITIES

If high-quality cancer care that includes equity is a goal, Canada and other developed nations have a long road ahead to achieve this goal. Inequities in access to care and cancer outcomes continue to rise, particularly in socially disadvantaged groups.[5,8,9] A variety of structures and contexts play a role in shaping these inequities, including social, economic, and political factors. It is important to examine how structures and contexts play a role in shaping cancer care inequities and how oncology nurses may address and reduce inequities.

Specialization and the Biomedical Model

The biomedical and cancer treatment-focused system creates tensions to enact person-centered care that focuses on the whole person and the context in which they live.[41] The lack of attention to context minimizes opportunities to achieve optimal health during the cancer experience, especially for individuals who are vulnerable due to marginalizing conditions (eg, poverty, unstable housing, racism).[34] The complexity of the cancer care system with its various silos has been identified as a significant barrier to equitable care.[42,43] In addition to the effects of fragmenting care, specialization compartmentalizes health professionals, limiting collaborative opportunities for addressing structural constraints that perpetuate health inequities.[44]

The concept of navigation, embraced by many cancer care organizations, as a solution to the disjointed cancer care system, may also unwittingly further fragment

---

Box 3
Exemplar: smoking cessation with an social determinants of health lens

There is causal evidence linking smoking to lung and other cancers. Data supports quitting after a cancer diagnosis because it improves prognosis and treatment outcomes while decreasing risk of a secondary cancer and death.[39] Nursing interventions lacking a SDH perspective include providing access to smoking cessation programs and/or self-care management strategies to support smoking cessation behaviors.[40] Such evidence-informed interventions draw on distributive justice (ie, improving access to care by placing the responsibility for health solely with the individual). In this scenario, one might be inclined to assign responsibility for failure to the individual if the individual is not successful in reducing or quitting smoking. This action may thwart future attempts to quit smoking.

Conversely, using a social justice perspective, the scenario might look different. In addition to interventions aimed at the individual, nursing interventions would be broader, addressing political, economic, social, and other structures and contexts shaping smoking behavior. Nurses could address the lack of health-promoting policies in the workplace. Enacting policies for a smoke-free working environment, having easy access to a work-site smoking cessation program, and including extended health benefit coverage of nicotine replacement patches is likely to boost and sustain smoking cessation efforts. The SDH barriers of income, transportation, and access to smoking cessation services may be minimized by changing health behavior policies. For many, smoking is a social inclusion strategy and social isolation should be included in smoking cessation programs. Strategies that shift group social norm from smoking to health promoting activities is another example of addressing the SDH to improve smoking cessation rates.

care.[45–47] Since the introduction of patient navigator roles in the United States to address inequities in breast cancer outcomes between minority African American and other vulnerable population groups, there has been a plethora of navigator roles and strategies implemented worldwide.[48–50] Founded on a distributive justice model to improve access to cancer care, navigation conceptualizes health as a commodity that is something to be handed out by nurses and passively received by patients.[51] The focus on health care access without consideration of the SDH may undermine health professionals' ability to promote optimal, equitable health outcomes for people experiencing cancer.[36] Strategies are required to embed navigation within the health care system, without the need for another layer of health professionals that further divides practices and system fragmentation.

Corporatization of Cancer Care

Corporatization of the cancer care environment is underpinned by ideologies of scarcity and views of health care as a commodity. While attempting to improve efficiency, corporatization inadvertently also may objectify individuals and health care providers, reducing quality and access to care and health resources.[52–54] Corporatization can have negative impacts on people who experience marginalizing conditions within society (eg, due to race, gender inequality, poverty, unemployment, disability, low health literacy, inadequate social supports, and other barriers).[55] The impact of corporatization on clinical systems encourage efficient movement of individuals through the cancer care system, possibly at the expense of other needs, such as addressing psychosocial issues or support for health promotion behaviors.[54] Development of therapeutic relationships and relational practice is limited, while those with complex needs may be referred to another health professional, further fragmenting care. The growing evidence of inequities specific to unmet psychosocial, informational, and supportive care, as well as health promotion needs, in the cancer survivor population[1,56,57] attest to the negative effects of an efficiency driven system.[41,58]

Individualism and Self-care

A neoliberal ideology purports individual free choice and equal opportunity in which individual benefit is valued over collective and societal benefit.[59,60] Self-care strategies are an example of neoliberal ideologies operating within cancer care, in which responsibility rests with individual choices and actions to restore and preserve health, while social, political, and cultural norms and contexts are negated.[61,62] In cancer care, individual responsibility for health is observed frequently regarding lifestyle interventions related to cancer prevention and recurrence.[63] Interventions focusing on mediating individuals' behaviors, without attention to the social, political, economic and other forces shaping health behavior, can lead to victim-blaming, oppression and inequities. This is particularly apparent in those who experience marginalizing conditions within society (eg. discrimination due to gender, ethnicity, socioeconomic status).[64–67]

STRATEGIES FOR ACTION: LESSONS LEARNED FROM OTHER HEALTH CARE SYSTEMS

A brief review of research, systematic reviews, and expert roundtables on enacted and recommended health equity strategies from a variety of settings and systems at local, national, and international levels revealed a common set of themes. **Box 4** lists the themes from the literature.

These themes reflect the importance of addressing inequities at the individual and community level, as well as working to effect change in policies and structural factors that are the root cause of inequities. In particular, oncology nurses can draw from the

---

Box 4
Common themes in recommended health equity strategies

1. The quality of care at the individual or community level is shaped by policies at the local, regional, and national level. Influencing policy is an essential aspect of equitably high-quality care. Policy advocacy requires an intersectoral approach (beyond the health sector).[1,13,68–70]

2. Interventions to address the SDH should be a routine aspect of health care, often as a main priority.[13,70,71]

3. Culturally and linguistically competent care is essential to deliver patient-centered care that takes into consideration cultural meanings of health and illness, as well as effects of racialization, discrimination, and marginalization.[1,71,72]

4. Provider communication can influence inequities in terms of content and time to develop relationships.[1,71–73]

5. Reinforce the centrality of patient-centered care, tailoring care, programs, and services to the context of people's lives.[1,71]

6. Community-based, collaborative, and participatory engagement approaches are essential.[1,71,74]

7. Navigation can be an effective strategy to improve coordination of care if the SDH and other structural factors are considered.[1,71,75,76]

8. The primary care setting is more effective than specialty care (as it is currently configured) in addressing the SDH and promoting health.[1,71,77]

---

themes and data to inform strategies tailored to address inequities within specialized oncology environments.

PROMOTING EQUITY: A TWO-PRONGED MANDATE FOR ONCOLOGY NURSES

A growing body of nursing scholars, researchers, and nursing professional associations, such as Canadian Nurses Association,[10–12] Community Health Nurses of Canada,[78] and International Council of Nurses,[79] have begun to highlight important strategies for nurses to adopt to promote equity across practice, education, research, and leadership roles. Building on this collective work, Reutter and Kushner[13] articulated a two-pronged mandate for nurses to address health inequities: (1) providing culturally sensitive empowering care at the individual and/or community level to those at risk for or who are experiencing inequities and (2) addressing social, environmental, and other structural conditions that are the root causes of inequities. This approach is a useful template to guide the development of a social justice approach for action by oncology nurses to address inequities in cancer care.

Addressing Inequities in the Care of Individuals and Communities

Addressing inequities at the practice level begins by taking a perspective of emancipatory knowing. Chinn and Kramer[80] recommend reconceptualizing Carper's[81] work on nurses' ways of knowing to include emancipatory knowing, which emphasizes attention to the social, historical, economic, and political factors leading to inequity.[13,82] This perspective encourages oncology nurses to assess health status not only in terms of what is, but also in terms of why.[13] Emancipatory knowing necessitates the use of nursing conceptual frameworks that include considerations of the SDH in nursing assessment, planning, intervention, and evaluation, including social and political factors that shaped an individual's health or disease status, such as poverty.

Recommendations for equitably high quality care point to the importance of culturally sensitive care.[1,71,72] An individual's culture is influenced to varying degrees by factors such as race, gender, religion, ethnicity, socioeconomic status, sexual orientation, and life experiences. Culturally sensitive care also necessitates understanding an individual's beliefs, values, and goals in relation to cancer. Culture is not the same as identifying with a particular cultural or ethnic group; although some individuals self-identify with ethnic groups that form part of their cultural identity. Culturally sensitive care goes hand in hand with relational nursing practice that encourages respectful, compassionate, and authentic inquiry into individual experiences, along with an awareness of one's own values and biases that may affect culturally sensitive care.[83,84]

Considering an individual's culture highlights inherent challenges to developing group interventions. Such interventions are used to enhance access to care for vulnerable populations, such as, for example, Indigenous groups who are disproportionately marginalized in society which is compounded when diagnosed with cancer.[83,85] Each individual is complex and has their own unique culture; oncology nurses should avoid essentializing individuals to a specific ethnic group. Inequities unintentionally created through group interventions or programs should be considered so as not to set up "have" and "have-not" groups that create the "Other".[64,65] Development of programs must include the end users, patients and families with cancer, to ensure their individuals and collective priorities and needs are met.

Addressing the Root Causes of Inequities

In addition to directly caring for individuals, families, or communities to address inequities, a broader approach by the oncology nurse is needed that also targets the root causes of inequities (ie, the social, political, historical, and environmental contexts and structures within society). These broader approaches can be considered in terms of (1) leadership, policy influence, and advocacy; (2) education; and (3) research strategies.

Leadership, policy influence, and advocacy
Influencing policy targeting the SDH has been identified as the key strategy to reduce inequities.[10–13,86,87] Although political advocacy is considered an important part of nursing's role, most nurses confess to having little knowledge or competency to engage in political advocacy strategies. However, political advocacy can take many forms, from increasing public and stakeholder awareness of the impact of inequities on everyday care, to participating in advocacy that tackles national health and social policies to promote equity in cancer care.

Nurses are situated "at the intersection of public policy and personal lives; they are, therefore, ideally situated and morally obligated to include sociopolitical advocacy in their practice."[88] Nurses must critically question why and how inequities are occurring across individuals or groups within their practice. Storytelling regarding the impact of policy on peoples' lives can be an effective awareness-raising strategy to engage the pubic, stakeholders, and policymakers regarding inequities.[13] Policy also can encompass and give direction to nursing frameworks, models of care, standards, competencies, and other structures that shape the nursing care environment for patients with cancer. National oncology nursing professional organizations (eg, Canadian Association of Nurses in Oncology) must articulate practice standards that include promoting equity and reducing inequities as an expectation of high-quality nursing care.

Oncology nurses must advocate for nursing frameworks and models of care that include the SDH and address the structural factors influencing inequities. Oncology nurses, as patient advocates, must proactively take a leadership role to promote the added value of the shift to equity-oriented cancer care. Examples include leveraging advocacy by patient, family, or community groups; learning from the equity-focused initiatives within primary care that are transferrable across settings; and bringing together oncology health professional organizations to develop joint position statements and other policies that direct cancer care organizations to consider equity strategies as core to their business.

Another political advocacy focus for oncology nurses is at the government level (local, provincial, national, international) to advocate for "health in all policies".[12,15,79] With the aim to break down silos across social, health, and other sectors, this advocacy effort targets policies in development, such as those addressing income, employment, education, housing, and transportation, regarding their impact on health. A diagnosis of cancer affects all of these areas, so that having healthy social policies ensures individuals are not marginalized in terms of income, employment, transportation, and other social determinants, due to the effects of cancer and its treatment. Including individuals who are experiencing marginalizing conditions with society (eg, racism, stigma, poverty, low socioeconomic status) also is an important strategy to inform advocacy and policy agendas.

Education

Undergraduate nursing programs are beginning to include social justice concepts and the SDH in their core curriculum.[89] Clinical placements should reinforce and apply these concepts across a variety of clinical oncology and primary care settings. Graduate nursing education should include policy and advocacy courses in which students gain competencies in creating, critiquing, positioning, and advocating for policies that shape health. Specialized oncology nursing certification blueprints (eg, Canadian Nurses Association[90]) and study programs must also include concepts of equity and social justice that lift nurses' gaze beyond the individual nurse-patient-environment relationship.

Research

Most published research on inequities in cancer care is derived from epidemiologic and other quantitative studies. Contextual knowledge is needed, generated using qualitative research and/or critical perspectives. Research that critically explores and explains how social, political, economic, and other factors layer and intersect to influence inequity in cancer care have been not yet been examined in detail. This area of research is in its nascent stages and ripe for development by oncology nursing researchers, particularly those with qualitative expertise. Another area for research is policy analysis to better understand the links between evidence and policy uptake and utilization. Investigations into policy best practices will support nurses and other health professionals' efforts in moving the equity agenda forward.[13]

SUMMARY

Oncology nurses have an opportunity to take a leadership role to affect inequities in cancer care. Aligned with their ethical imperative for social justice, oncology nurses are optimally situated to take a social justice approach to addressing inequities that considers the SDH, as well as those factors, contexts, and structures that shape and influence inequities. Enhanced understanding of how various contexts and structures, such as the biomedical model, specialization, corporatization, and neoliberalism, may promote inequities in the cancer care environment offers oncology nurses insights into areas for intervention to promote equity. A two-pronged approach to addressing inequities offers oncology nurses strategies to use in practice with individuals and communities, as well as in addressing the root causes of inequity through leadership, policy influence, advocacy, education, and research. Through these sustained strategies, it is anticipated that oncology nurses may disrupt the power hierarchies that sustain inequities within the cancer care system, ultimately promoting equitably high-quality care for all.

REFERENCES

1. Palaty C, BC Cancer Agency, Canadian Partnership Against Cancer. Cancer care for all Canadians: improving access and minimizing disparities for vulnerable populations in Canada. Vancouver (Canada): BC Cancer Agency; 2008.
2. Canadian Partnership Against Cancer. Sustaining action toward a shared vision. 2012. Available at: http://www.partnershipagainstcancer.ca/wp-content/uploads/Sustaining-Action-Toward-a-Shared-Vision-Full-Document.pdf. Accessed March 30, 2016.
3. Canadian Partnership Against Cancer. Examining disparities in cancer control: a system performance special focus report. 2014. Available at: www.cancerview.ca/systemperformancereport. Accessed March 30, 2016.
4. Levit LA, Balogh E, Nass SJ, et al, National Academies Press Free eBooks, Institute of Medicine (U.S.), Committee on Improving the Quality of Cancer Care: Addressing the Challenges of an Aging Population. Delivering high-quality cancer care: charting a new course for a system in crisis. Washington, DC: National Academies Press; 2013.
5. Ahmed S, Shahid RK. Disparity in cancer care: a Canadian perspective. Curr Oncol 2012;19:e376.
6. Blinder VS, Griggs JJ. Health disparities and the cancer survivor. Semin Oncol 2013;40:796.
7. Casillas J, editor. Disparities in care for cancer survivors. New York: Springer New York; 2011. p. 153–68.
8. Maddison AR, Asada Y, Urquhart R. Inequity in access to cancer care: a review of the Canadian literature. Cancer Causes Control 2011;22:359–66.
9. Sheppard AJ, Chiarelli AM, Marrett LD, et al. Detection of later stage breast cancer in First Nations women in Ontario, Canada. Can J Public Health 2010;101: 101–5.
10. Canadian Nurses Association. Ethics in practice for Registered Nurses: Social justice in practice. 2009. Available at: http://www.cna-aiic.ca/~/media/cna/page%20content/pdf%20en/2013/07/26/10/38/ethics_in_practice_april_2009_e.pdf. Accessed March 11, 2016.
11. Canadian Nurses Association. Social Justice. 2nd edition. 2010. Available at: http://www.cna-aiic.ca/~/media/cna/page%20content/pdf%20en/2013/07/26/10/38/social_justice_2010_e.pdf. Accessed March 11, 2016.
12. Canadian Nurses Association. Social determinants of health: Position statement. 2013. Available at: http://www.cna-aiic.ca/~/media/cna/files/en/ps124_social_determinants_of_health_e.pdf. Accessed March 11, 2016.
13. Reutter L, Kushner KE. 'Health equity through action on the social determinants of health': taking up the challenge in nursing. Nurs Inq 2010;17:269.
14. Varcoe C, Habib S, Sinding C, et al. Health disparities in cancer care: Exploring Canadian, American and international perspectives. Can Oncol Nurs J 2015;25:73.
15. World Health Organization, WHO Commission on Social Determinants of Health. Closing the gap in a generation: health equity through action on the social

determinants of health: final report of the Commission on Social Determinants of Health. Geneva (Switzerland): World Health Organization; 2008.

16. Canadian Association of Nurses in Oncology. Standards and Competencies for the Specialized Oncology Nurse. 2006. Available at: http://www.cano-acio.ca/practice-standards. Accessed March 11, 2016.

17. American Cancer Society. Cancer facts and figures. Atlanta (GA): American Cancer Society; 2015.

18. Canadian Cancer Society's Steering Committee on Cancer Statistics. Canadian Cancer statistics 2015. Toronto: Canadian Cancer Society; 2015.

19. Dunn BK, Agurs-Collins T, Browne D, et al. Health disparities in breast cancer: biology meets socioeconomic status. Breast Cancer Res Treat 2010;121:281–92.

20. Niu X, Roche LM, Pawlish KS, et al. Cancer survival disparities by health insurance status. Cancer Med 2013;2:403–11.

21. Ayanian JZ. Racial disparities in outcomes of colorectal cancer screening: biology or barriers to optimal care? J Natl Cancer Inst 2010;102:511–3.

22. Kagawa-Singer M, Valdez Dadia A, Yu MC, et al. Cancer, culture, and health disparities: time to chart a new course? CA Cancer J Clin 2010;60:12–39.

23. Laiyemo AO, Doubeni C, Pinsky PF, et al. Race and colorectal cancer disparities: health-care utilization vs different cancer susceptibilities. J Natl Cancer Inst 2010; 102:538–46.

24. Lantz PM, Mujahid M, Schwartz K, et al. The influence of race, ethnicity, and individual socioeconomic factors on breast cancer stage at diagnosis. Am J Public Health 2006;96:2173–8.

25. Miller AM, Ashing KT, Modeste NN, et al. Contextual factors influencing health-related quality of life in African American and Latina breast cancer survivors. J Cancer Surviv 2015;9:441–9.

26. Skinner D. The gendering of cancer survivorship. Health 2012;3:63–76.

27. Weaver KE, Palmer N, Lu L, et al. Rural–urban differences in health behaviors and implications for health status among US cancer survivors. Cancer Causes Control 2013;24:1481–90.

28. Boehmer U, Miao X, Ozonoff A. Health behaviors of cancer survivors of different sexual orientations. Cancer Causes Control 2012;23:1489–96.

29. Guy GP Jr, Ekwueme DU, Yabroff KR, et al. The economic burden of cancer survivorship among adults in the United States. Value Health 2013;16:A136–7.

30. McNulty JA, Nail L. Cancer survivorship in rural and urban adults: a Descriptive and Mixed Methods Study: cancer survivorship, rural and urban. J Rural Health 2015;31:282–91.

31. Dixon-Woods M, Cavers D, Agarwal S, et al. Conducting a critical interpretive synthesis of the literature on access to healthcare by vulnerable groups. BMC Med Res Methodol 2006;6:35.

32. Buettner-Schmidt K, Lobo ML. Social justice: a concept analysis: Social justice. J Adv Nurs 2012;68:948–58.

33. Young IM. Justice and the politics of difference. Princeton (NJ): Princeton University Press; 1990.

34. Solar O, Irwin A. A conceptual framework for action on the social determinants of health. Social determinants of health discussion paper 2 (policy and practice). Geneva (Switzerland): World Health Organization; 2010. Available at: http://www.who.int/sdhconference/resources/ConceptualframeworkforactiononSDH_eng.pdf. Accessed March 30, 2016.

35. Whitehead M, Dahlgren G. Levelling up (part 1): a discussion paper on concepts and principles for tackling social inequities in health. Studies on social and

economic determinants of population health, No. 2. Copenhagen (Denmark): WHO Collaborating Centre for Policy Research on Social Determinants of Health, University of Liverpool; 2006.

36. Kirkham SR, Browne AJ. Toward a critical theoretical interpretation of social justice discourses in nursing. ANS Adv Nurs Sci 2006;29:324.

37. Pauly BM. Challenging health inequities: enacting social justice in nursing practice. In: Storch JL, Rodney PA, Starzomski RC, editors. Toward a moral horizon: nursing ethics for leadership and practice. 2nd edition. Toronto: Pearson; 2013. p. 430–47.

38. Braveman P, Gottlieb L. The social determinants of health: it's time to consider the causes of the causes. Public Health Rep 2014;129(Suppl 2):19–31.

39. U.S. Department of Health and Human Services. The health consequences of smoking—50 years of progress: a report of the surgeon general. Atlanta (GA): U.S. Department of Health and Human Services, Centers for Disease Control and Prevention, National Center for Chronic Disease Prevention and Health Promotion, Office on Smoking and Health; 2014. Available at: http://www.surgeongeneral.gv/library/reports/50-years-of-progress/index.html. Accessed March 20, 2016.

40. Rice VH, Hartmann-Boyce J, Stead LF. Nursing interventions for smoking cessation. Cochrane Database of Systematic Reviews 2013;(8):CD001188.

41. McMurtry R, Bultz BD. Public policy, human consequences: the gap between biomedicine and psychosocial reality. Psychooncology 2005;14:697–703.

42. Canadian Strategy for Cancer Control. A cancer plan for Canada: discussion paper. Toronto: Canadian Strategy for Cancer Control; 2016.

43. Hewitt ME, Greenfield S, Stovall E, National Cancer Policy Board (U.S.). Committee on Cancer survivorship: improving care and quality of life. From Cancer patient to Cancer survivor: lost in transition. Washington, DC: National Academies Press; 2006.

44. Dzurec LC. Poststructuralist musings on the mind/body question in health care. ANS Adv Nurs Sci 2003;26(1):63–76.

45. Pedersen A, Hack TF. Pilots of oncology health care: a concept analysis of the patient navigator role. Oncol Nurs Forum 2010;37:55–60.

46. Pedersen AE, Hack TF. The British Columbia Patient Navigation Model: a critical analysis. Oncol Nurs Forum 2011;38:200–6.

47. Thorne S, Truant T. Will designated patient navigators fix the problem? Oncology nursing in transition. Can Oncol Nurs J 2010;20:116–21.

48. Fillion L, Cook S, Veillette A, et al. Professional navigation framework: elaboration and validation in a Canadian context. Oncol Nurs Forum 2012;39:E58–69.

49. Freeman HP, Chu KC. Determinants of cancer disparities: barriers to cancer screening, diagnosis, and treatment. Surg Oncol Clin N Am 2005;14:655.

50. Shockney LD. The Evolution of Breast Cancer Navigation and Survivorship Care. Breast J 2015;21:104–10.

51. Jennings B. Beyond distributive justice in health reform. Hastings Cent Rep 1996; 26:14–5.

52. Austin WJ. The incommensurability of nursing as a practice and the customer service model: an evolutionary threat to the discipline. Nurs Philos 2011;12:158–66.

53. Ritzer G. The McDonaldization of society. 20th anniversary. 7th edition. Thousand Oaks (CA): Sage; 2013.

54. Varcoe C, Rodney P. Constrained agency: The social structure of nurses' work. In: Bolaria BS, Dickinson HD, editors. Health, illness and health care in Canada. 4th edition. Toronto: Nelson; 2009. p. 122–51.

55. Henderson A, Semeniuk P, Anderson J, et al. Healthcare restructuring with a view to equity and efficiency: reflections on unintended consequences. Nurs Leadersh 2003;16:112–40.
56. Campbell HS, Sanson-Fisher R, Turner D, et al. Psychometric properties of cancer survivors' unmet needs survey. Support Care Cancer 2011;19:221–30.
57. Hodgkinson K, Butow P, Hobbs KM, et al. After cancer: the unmet supportive care needs of survivors and their partners. J Psychosoc Oncol 2007;25:89–104.
58. Sofaer S. Navigating poorly charted territory: patient dilemmas in health care "non-systems". Med Care Res Rev 2009;66:75S–93S.
59. Browne AJ. The influence of liberal political ideology on nursing science. Nurs Inq 2001;8:118–29.
60. Coburn D. Beyond the income inequality hypothesis: class, neo-liberalism, and health inequalities. Soc Sci Med 2004;58:41–56.
61. Dean K, Kickbusch I. Health related behavior in health promotion: utilizing the concept of self care. Health Promot Int 1995;10:35–40.
62. Foster C, Fenlon D. Recovery and self-management support following primary cancer treatment. Br J Cancer 2011;105(Suppl 1):S21–8.
63. Pekmezi DW, Demark-Wahnefried W. Updated evidence in support of diet and exercise interventions in cancer survivors. Acta Oncol 2011;50:167–78.
64. Anderson JM. Empowering patients: issues and strategies. Soc Sci Med 1996;43: 697–705.
65. Anderson JM, Rodney P, Reimer-Kirkham S, et al. Inequities in health and healthcare viewed through the ethical lens of critical social justice: contextual knowledge for the global priorities ahead. ANS Adv Nurs Sci 2009;32:282.
66. Bell K. Cancer survivorship, mor(t)ality and lifestyle discourses on cancer prevention. Sociol Health Illn 2010;32:349–64.
67. Sinding C, Miller P, Hudak P, et al. Of time and troubles: patient involvement and the production of health care disparities. Health (London) 2012;2011(16):400–17.
68. Kelly UA. Integrating intersectionality and biomedicine in health disparities research. ANS Adv Nurs Sci 2009;32:E42.
69. Moy B, Polite BN, Halpern MT, et al. American Society of Clinical Oncology Policy Statement: opportunities in the patient protection and affordable care act to reduce cancer care disparities. J Clin Oncol 2011;29:3816–24.
70. Raphael D. Health equity in Canada. In Bryant, Toba and Raphael, Dennis (eds). Social Alternatives 2010;29:41–9.
71. Browne AJ, Varcoe CM, Wong ST, et al. Closing the health equity gap: evidence-based strategies for primary health care organizations. Int J Equity Health 2012; 11:59.
72. Printz C. Addressing survivorship in diverse populations. Cancer 2010;116:4894.
73. Mack JW, Paulk ME, Viswanath K, et al. Racial disparities in the outcomes of communication on medical care received near death. Arch Intern Med 2010; 170:1533–40.
74. Ramanadhan S, Salhi C, Achille E, et al. Addressing cancer disparities via community network mobilization and intersectoral partnerships: a social network analysis. PLoS One 2012;7:e32130.
75. Campbell C, Craig J, Eggert J, et al. Implementing and measuring the impact of patient navigation at a comprehensive community cancer center. Oncol Nurs Forum 2010;37:61–8.
76. Esparza A, Calhoun E. Measuring the impact and potential of patient navigation: proposed common metrics and beyond. Cancer 2011;117:3537–8.

77. Starfield B, Shi L, Macinko J. Contribution of primary care to health systems and health. Milbank Q 2005;83:457–502.
78. Community Health Nurses of Canada. Canadian community health nursing professional practice model and standards of practice. 2011. Available at: https://chnc.ca/documents/chnc-standards-eng-book.pdf. Accessed March 30, 2016.
79. International Council of Nurses. The ICN code of ethics for nurses. 2014. Available at: http://www.icn.ch/images/stories/documents/about/icncode_english.pdf. Accessed March 31, 2016.
80. Chinn PL, Kramer MK. Integrated theory and knowledge development in nursing. 8th edition. St Louis (MO): Mosby/Elsevier; 2011.
81. Carper B. Fundamental patterns of knowing in nursing. Advances in nursing science 1978;1:13.
82. Bryant T. An introduction to health policy. Toronto: Canadian Scholars' Press; 2009.
83. College of Nurses of Ontario. Culturally sensitive care. 2009. Available at: http://www.cno.org/globalassets/docs/prac/41040_culturallysens.pdf. Accessed March 30, 2016.
84. Hartrick Doane G, Varcoe C. How to nurse? Relational inquiry with individuals and families in changing health and healthcare contexts. Philadelphia: Lippincott, Williams & Wilkins; 2015.
85. Olson RA, Howard F, Turnbull K, et al. Prospective evaluation of unmet needs of rural and aboriginal cancer survivors in Northern British Columbia. Curr Oncol 2014;21:e179.
86. Mahony D, Jones EJ. Social determinants of health in nursing education, research, and health policy. Nurs Sci Q 2013;26:280–4.
87. Yanicki SM, Kushner KE, Reutter L. Social inclusion/exclusion as matters of social (in)justice: a call for nursing action. Nurs Inq 2015;22:121–33.
88. Falk-Rafael A. Speaking truth to power: nursing's legacy and moral imperative. ANS Adv Nurs Sci 2005;28:212.
89. Cohen BE, Gregory D. Community health clinical education in Canada: part 2-developing competencies to address social justice, equity, and the social determinants of health. Int J Nurs Educ Scholarsh 2009;6:2–15.
90. Canadian Nurses Association. Exam blueprint and specialty competencies: Blueprint for the oncology nursing certification exam. 2013. Available at: https://www.nurseone.ca/~/media/nurseone/files/en/cert_oncology_2013_e.pdf. Accessed April 8, 2016.

Index

Note: Page numbers of article titles are in **boldface** type.

Moving?

Make sure your subscription moves with you!

To notify us of your new address, find your **Clinics Account Number** (located on your mailing label above your name), and contact customer service at:

Email: journalscustomerservice-usa@elsevier.com

800-654-2452 (subscribers in the U.S. & Canada)
314-447-8871 (subscribers outside of the U.S. & Canada)

Fax number: 314-447-8029

**Elsevier Health Sciences Division
Subscription Customer Service
3251 Riverport Lane
Maryland Heights, MO 63043**

*To ensure uninterrupted delivery of your subscription, please notify us at least 4 weeks in advance of move.

Printed and bound by CPI Group (UK) Ltd, Croydon, CR0 4YY

03/10/2024

01040390-0005